FESTIVALS U.S.A.

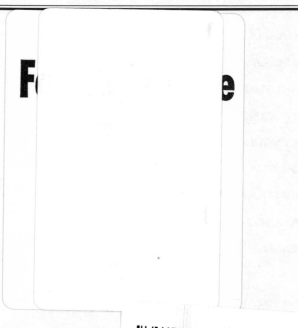

TRAVEL AND LANGUAGE BOOKS FROM WILEY

DO'S AND TABOOS AROUND THE WORLD: A GUIDE TO INTERNATIONAL BEHAVIOR, Roger E. Axtell

THE PINYIN CHINESE-ENGLISH DICTIONARY, Compiled by the Beijing Foreign Languages Institute under the supervision of Professor Wu Jingrong

PASSPORT TO EUROPE'S SMALL HOTELS AND INNS, 26TH EDITION, Beverly Beyer

STREET FRENCH: HOW TO SPEAK AND UNDERSTAND FRENCH SLANG, A SELF-TEACHING GUIDE, David Burke

EXPERIENCING AMERICA'S PAST: A TRAVEL GUIDE TO MUSEUM VILLAGES, Gerald & Patricia Gutek

FRENCH: A SELF-TEACHING GUIDE, Suzanne A. Hershfield

FESTIVALS U.S.A., Kathleen Thompson Hill

ENGLISH-RUSSIAN/RUSSIAN-ENGLISH DICTIONARY, Kenneth Katzner

ITALIAN: A SELF-TEACHING GUIDE, Edoardo Lebano

CHINESE/ENGLISH PHRASE BOOK FOR TRAVELLERS, John S. Montanaro

PRACTICAL SPANISH GRAMMAR, Marcial Prado

MORE PRACTICAL SPANISH GRAMMAR, Marcial Prado

GERMAN: A SELF-TEACHING GUIDE, Heimy Taylor & Werner Haas

A NEW ENGLISH-CHINESE DICTIONARY (Second Revised Edition), Zheng Yi Li, Dhang Fend De, Xu Shi Gu, Hu Xue Yuan, Liu Bang Shen & Shen Feng Wei

Available at your local bookstore or direct from John Wiley & Sons, 605 Third Avenue, New York, New York, 10158 (212) 850-6000

FESTIVALS
U.S.A.

Kathleen Thompson Hill

JOHN WILEY & SONS, INC.
New York · Chichester · Brisbane · Toronto · Singapore

PUBLISHER: Stephen Kippur
EDITOR: Katherine Schowalter
MANAGING EDITOR: Andrew B. Hoffer
PRODUCTION SERVICES: Folio Graphics Company, Inc.

This publication is designed to provide accurate and authoritative information in regard to the subject matter covered. It is sold with the understanding that the publisher is not engaged in rendering professional services in the subject matter discussed. Due to the ever changing marketplace, we suggest that you contact the addresses given to verify information.

Library of Congress Cataloging-in-Publication Data
Hill, Kathleen.
  Festivals U.S.A.
  1. Festivals—United States. I. Title.
II. Title: Festivals USA.
GT4803.H54   1987   394.2'6973   87-3479
ISBN 0-471-62636-8

Printed in the United States of America

88 89 10 9 8 7 6 5 4 3 2 1

To Gerald, Erin, and Mack
for their patience
and love.

festival *n* (1589) 1 a: a time of celebration marked by special observances b: FEAST *2* 2: a periodic season or program of cultural events or entertainment 3: GAIETY, CONVIVIALITY *

FOREWORD

Festivals—I love 'em.

Every year more than eighty million people prove their love of festivals by packing up their car, camper, or RV and heading out to enjoy the music, art, pageantry, history, and foods of our great fifty states. Ah, yes, the foods of all the nations whose people make up this wonderful country as well as hundreds of local and regional specialties from crab, quahog, and salmon bakes to shoofly pie, enchiladas and kolache.

Festivals are fun—fun for children and centenarians, yuppies and truckers, gourmands and gourmets, Mozart and Bach lovers, country and bluegrass fans, artists and craftspeople, lovers of Appalachian life and native American artifacts, as well as sportslovers who enjoy fishing derbies, rattlesnake hunts, golf and tennis tournaments, fun runs and triathlons. At festivals there is something for everyone.

Now we have FESTIVALS U.S.A., a guide for all seasons. Use it to discover where the fun is when you're planning a trip anywhere in the U.S. or wondering where you can find the festivals with your special interests.

FESTIVALS U.S.A. is written by Kathleen Thompson Hill, the country's foremost authority on festivals. She is known from the Country Music Association in Nashville to the BBC in London as "The Festival Lady." She has been researching festivals for years and out of the 9,000 in her files, Hill has chosen over 1000 of the best to share with you!

FESTIVALS U.S.A. is a handy book which can be used over and over again to find yourself healthy entertainment, either nearby for a weekend getaway or for an extended vacation. It is chock-full of helpful information such as telephone numbers, admission costs, accommodations and restaurants available in the area, along with clear and realistic descriptions of events. FESTIVALS U.S.A. is charmingly written and a necessity for any travel bookshelf. You will certainly find it on mine!

So whether you're planning a trip or just want to sit at home and reap vicarious pleasure from a travel guide, this is the one for you!

WILLARD SCOTT

Contents

INTRODUCTION   XXV

Northeast   1

CONNECTICUT   3

Dogwood Festival / 3 ■ A Taste of Hartford / 3 ■ Lobster Weekend / 3 ■ Sea Music Festival / 3 ■ Barnum Festival / 3 ■ New Haven Jazz Festival / 4 ■ Sail Festival Weekend / 4 ■ Santa Maria Magdelana Feast / 4 ■ Pillar Polkabration / 4 ■ Sharon Audubon Festival / 4 ■ Festival Italiano / 4 ■ Mystic Outdoor Arts Festival / 5 ■ Oyster Festival / 5 Long Island Sound America Festival / 5 ■ Norwalk Seaport Oyster Festival / 5 ■ New Haven Greek Festival / 5 ■ Bristol Chrysanthemum Festival and International Festival / 5 ■ Apple Harvest Festival / 6

MAINE   6

Winter Wonderland Week / 6 ■ Kennebec Whatever Week and Race / 6 ■ Festival De La Bastille / 6 ■ Molly Ockett Day / 6 ■ Maine Potato Blossom Festival /70 ■ Yarmouth Clam Festival / 7 ■ Maine Lobster Festival / 7 ■ International Festival / 7 ■ Winter Harbor Lobster Festival / 8 ■ Maine Festival of the Arts / 8 ■ Fall Foliage Country Fair / 8 ■ New Year's/Portland / 8

MASSACHUSETTS   9

Daffodil Festival / 9 ■ Rockport Music Festival / 9 ■ St. Peter's Fiesta and Blessing of the Fleet / 9 ■ Whaling City Festival / 9 ■ National Folk Festival / 9 ■ Feast of the Blessed Sacrament / 9 ■ Center Street Festival / 10 ■ Waterfront Festival / 10 ■ Festival By The Sea / 10 ■ Dennis Festival Days / 10 ■ Lower Cape Arts Festival / 10 ■ World Kielbasa Festival / 10 ■ Cranberry Harvest Festival / 11 ■ Bourne Scallop Festival / 11 ■ Greek Food Festival / 11 ■ Northern Berkshire Fall Foliage Festival / 11 ■ First Night New Bedford / 11

NEW HAMPSHIRE   12

Lakes Region Fine Arts and Crafts Festival / 12

NEW JERSEY   12

Thompson Park Day / 12 ■ Fishawack / 12 ■ Victorian Plainfield Festival of Art / 12 ■ Frogtown Frolic / 12 ■ Festival on the Green / 12 ■ Turkey Swamp Park Day / 13

NEW YORK   13

Winter Carnival / 13 ■ International Festival / 13 ■ Tulip Festival / 13 ■ Catskills Irish Festival / 13 ■ Woodstock Festival of the Arts / 14 ■ Allentown Art Festival and Juneteenth Festival / 14 ■ Strawberry Festival / 14 ■ Bach Aria Festival / 14 ■ Summerscape Arts Festival / 14 ■ Wednesdays and Sundays at the Plaza / 14 ■ Italian Festival / 14 ■ Harbor Festival / 15 ■ Corn Hill Art Festival / 15 ■ Taste of Buffalo / 15 ■ Christmas in July / 15 ■ Potsdam Summer Festival / 15 ■ Lake George Opera Festival / 15 ■ German Alps Festival / 16 ■ Julyfest / 16 ■ International Seaway Festival / 16 ■ Country Music Festival Parts I and II / 16 ■ Interarts Festival / 16 ■ Coxsackie Riverside Festival / 16 ■ National Polka Festival / 17 ■ Sauerkraut Festival / 17 ■ Harlem Week / 17 ■ Festival of North Country Folklife / 17 ■ Athens Street Festival / 17 ■ Italian American Festival / 17 ■ New York State Woodsmen's Field Days / 18 ■ International Celtic Festival / 18 ■ Golden Oldies Festival / 18 ■ Iroquois Indian Festival / 18 ■ Native American Festival / 18 ■ Irish Festival / 19 ■ Polka Holidays of the Finger Lakes / 19 ■ Golden Harvest Festival / 19 ■ Finger Lakes Dixieland Jazz Festival / 19 □ Old Time Gas and Steam Show / 19 ■ Festival of Grapes / 19 ■ Autumn Harvest Festival / 20 ■ Adirondack Balloon Festival / 20 ■ Fall Festival / 20 ■ Salamanca Falling Leaves Festival / 20 ■ Oyster Festival / 20 ■ Fall Foliage Festival / 21 ■ Festival of Lights / 21 ■ Sparkle of Christmas / 21

PENNSYLVANIA   22

Pennsylvania Maple Festival / 22 ■ Pulaski Festival / 22 ■ Shad Festival / 22 ■ Apple Blossom Festival / 22 ■ Bach Festival / 22 ■ National Pike Festival / 23 ■ Pittsburgh Folk Festival / 23 ■ Greater Uniontown All Ethnic Festival / 23 ■ Italian Festival / 23 ■ Mayfair / 23 ■ Three Rivers Arts Festival / 24 ■ Portuguese Heritage Days / 24 ■ Western Pennsylvania Laurel Festival / 24 ■ Monessen's Cultural Heritage Festival / 24 ■ Susquehanna Boom Festival / 24 ■ Ellwood City Arts, Crafts, and Food Festival / 25 ■ Lehigh River Canal Festival / 25 ■ Central Pennsylvania Festival of the Arts / 25 ■ Christmas City Fair / 25 ■ Marlboro Music Festival / 25 ■ Lehigh Valley Balloon Festival / 26 ■ Fort Armstrong Folk Festival / 26 ■ The Pittsburgh Three Rivers Regatta / 26 ■ Daw Awkscht Fescht (The August Festival) / 26 ■ Musikfest / 26 ■ Dankfest / 27 ■ Springs Folk Festival / 27 ■ The Great Allentown Fair / 27 ■ Philadelphia Ceili Group's Irish Music and Dance Festival / 27 ■ Keystone Country Festival / 27 ■ Fort Ligonier Days / 28 ■ Autumn Leaf Festival / 28

RHODE ISLAND   28

Providence Festival of Historic Homes / 28 ■ Newport Jazz Festival / 28 ■ Fall
Harvest Festival / 29 ■ Autumn Fest / 28

VERMONT   29

Maple Sugar Festival / 29 ■ Festival of the Arts / 29 ■ Discover Jazz Festival / 30 ■
Vermont Mozart Festival / 30 ■ Stratton Arts Festival / 30 ■ Festival of Vermont
Crafts / 31

MID-ATLANTIC   33

DELAWARE   35

Spring Fest / 35 ■ Delmarva Chicken Festival / 35 ■ River and Harvest Festival / 35

DISTRICT OF COLUMBIA   35

Smithsonian Kite Festival / 35 ■ Cherry Blossom Festival / 35 ■ Potomac Riverfest
/ 36 ■ Mostly Mozart Festival / 36 ■ Festival of American Folklife / 36 ■ Latin
American Festival / 36 ■ National Frisbee Festival / 36 ■ Washington Reggae
Festival / 36

MARYLAND   37

Winterfest / 37 ■ Southern Maryland Celtic Festival and Highland Gathering / 37 ■
Salisbury Festival / 37 ■ Preakness Stakes and Festival Week / 37 ■ Chestertown
Tea Party / 37 ■ Halfway Park Days / 38 ■ Cumberland Heritage Days / 38 ■ Polish
Festival / 38 ■ Pocomoke City Cypress Festival / 38 ■ Frostburg Italian Festival /
38 ■ Grantsville Days / 38 ■ Old Fashioned Weekend in the Park / 39 ■ Tidewater
Music Festival / 39 ■ Park Arts Festival / 39 ■ Tuckahoe Steam and Gas Engine
Show / 39 ■ Italian Festival / 39 ■ Lotus Blossom Festival / 39 ■ American Indian
Pow Wow / 40 ■ University of Maryland International Piano Festival and William
Kapell Competition / 40 ■ J. Millard Tawes Crab and Clam Bake / 40 ■ Old
Fashioned Corn Roast Festival / 40 ■ Frontier Craft Days / 40 ■German Festival /
41 ■ C&O Canal Boat Festival / 41 ■ National Hard Crab Derby / 41 ■
Boonesborough Days / 41 ■ Hancock Lions Apple Canal Festival / 41 ■ Baltimore
City Fair / 41 ■ Seafood Festival / 42 ■ Maryland Wine Festival / 42 ■ Sunfest / 42 ■
Westminster Fallfest / 42 ■ Furnace Town Fall Festival / 42 ■ Autumn Glory
Festival / 43 ■ Catoctin Colorfest / 43

VIRGINIA   43

Kite Festival / 43 ■ Spring Seaport Festival / 43 ■ Heart of Virginia Festival / 43 ■
RiverFair / 43 ■ Virginia Poultry Festival / 44 ■ Viva! Vienna! / 44 ■ Celebrate

Summer At Wolf Trap / 44 ■ Fredericksburg Art Festival / 44 ■ Beach Music Festival / 44 ■ Heritage Festival / 45 ■ Bluegrass Music Festival / 45 ■ Lakefest / 45 ■ Hungry Mother Park Arts and Crafts Festival / 45 ■ Old Fiddlers Convention / 45 ■ Wine Festival / 45 ■ Hampton Bay Days / 45 ■ Chilhowie Apple Festival / 45 ■ Virginia Beach Neptune Festival / 45 ■ Poquoson Seafood Festival / 45 ■ Medley of the Arts / 46 ■ Newport News Fall Festival / 47 ■ Fall Foliage Festival / 47 ■ Oyster Festival / 47 ■ Historic Appomattox Railroad Festival / 47 ■ Suffolk Peanut Fest / 47 ■ Yorktown Day / 48 ■ Fall Foliage Festival / 48

MID-SOUTH
49

KENTUCKY
51

Tater Day / 51 ■ Mountain Folk Festival / 51 ■ International Bar-B-Q Festival / 51 ■ Maifest / 51 ■ The Great Inland Seafood Festival / 51 ■ Owensboro Summer Festival / 51 ■ Berea Crafts Festival / 52 ■ Corbin Nibroc Festival / 52 ■ Pioneer Days Festival / 52 ■ Oktoberfest / 52 ■ Louisville Bluegrass Festival / 52 ■ Black Gold Festival / 52 ■ Golden Armor Festival / 53 ■ International Bluegrass Music Festival / 53 ■ Festival of the Horse / 53 ■ Country Ham Days / 53 ■ Big Rivers Arts and Crafts Festival / 53 ■ Washington County Sorghum Festival / 53 ■ Lincoln Days Celebration / 54 ■ Poage Landing Days Celebration / 54 ■ Aurora Country Festival / 54 ■ Bloomfield Tobacco Festival / 54 ■ Traditional Music Festival / 54 ■ Corn Island Storytelling Festival / 54

NORTH CAROLINA
55

Grifton Shad Festival / 55 ■ Carolina Dogwood Festival / 55 ■ Dogwood Festival / 55 ■ National Whistlers Convention / 55 ■ Apple Chill / 56 ■ ArtsPlosure Spring Festival / 56 ■ Watauga County Spring Festival / 56 ■ Pleasure Island Spring Festival / 56 ■ White Lake Water Festival / 56 ■ Mayfest International Festival / 56 ■ Old Time Fiddlers' and Bluegrass Festival / 56 ■ Charlotte Folk Music Festival / 57 ■ North Carolina Blue Crab Derby and Festival / 57 ■ American Dance Festival / 57 ■ Cullowhee Music Festival / 57 ■ Rhododendron Festival / 57 ■ Festival of Festivals / 57 ■ Blue Ridge Mountain Fair Week / 58 ■ Grandfather Mountain Highland Games and Gathering of Scottish Clans / 58 ■ Eastern Music Festival / 58 ■ Sourwood Festival / 58 ■ Mountain Dance and Folk Festival / 58 ■ North Carolina Apple Festival / 58 ■ Piney Woods Festival / 59 ■ North Carolina Pickle Festival / 59 ■ Centerfest / 59 ■ National Balloon Rally / 59 ■ Mountain Heritage Day / 59 ■ Brushy Mountain Apple Festival / 60 ■ Fall Festival / 60 ■ Cherokee Indian Fall Festival / 60 ■ Mountain Glory Festival / 60 ■ North Carolina Oyster Festival / 60 ■ Autumn Leaves Festival / 61 ■ John Blue Cotton Festival / 61 ■ Chrysanthemum Festival / 61 ■ Woolly Worm Festival / 61 ■ Old Salem Christmas / 61

TENNESSEE 62

State of Tennessee Old-Time Fiddler's Championships / 62 ■ Mule Day Country Living / 62 ■ Dogwood Arts Festival / 62 ■ Blount County Dogwood Arts Festival / 63 ■ World's Biggest Fish Fry / 63 ■ Mid-South Jazz Festival / 63 ■ Lake Chickamauga Spring Festival / 63 ■ Memphis in May International Festival / 63 ■ Downtown Arts Festival / 64 ■ Fair on the Square / 64 ■ Tennessee Crafts Fair / 64 ■ Azalea Festival / 64 ■ East Main Street Festival / 64 ■ East Tennessee Strawberry Festival / 65 ■ Andrew Jackson Days / 65 ■ Great Smokey Mountain-Gatlinburg Highland Games / 65 ■ Summer Lights Festival / 65 ■ Tullahoma Fine Arts and Crafts Festival / 65 ■ Great River Carnival / 66 ■ International Country Music Fan Fair / 66 ■ Covered Bridge Celebration / 66 ■ The Martha White-Lester Flatt Hometown Memorial Festival / 66 ■ Defeated/Cordell Hull Bluegrass Music Festival / 66 ■ High Forest Jamboree / 66 ■ Roan Mountain Rhododendron Festival / 67 ■ Folk Medicine Festival / 67 ■ Winfield Appalachian Dumplin' Festival / 67 ■ Old Time Fiddlers' Jamboree and Crafts Festival / 67 ■ Horseshoe Bend Festival / 67 ■ Dollywood National Mountain Music Festival / 68 ■ Cedar City Summer Celebration / 68 ■ Fun Fest / 68 ■ Arts and Crafts Fair / 68 ■ Italian Street Fair / 68 ■ The Memphis Music Festival / 68 ■ Old Time Music Day / 69 ■ Old Timer's Day / 69 ■ Tennessee Apple Festival / 69 ■ Folklife Festival / 69 ■ Artfest / 69 ■ Tennessee Grass Roots Days / 70 ■ Dollywood National Crafts Festival / 70 ■ Pigeon Forge Rotary Craft Festival / 70 ■ Madison Hillbilly Days / 70 ■ Festival / 71 ■ Nillie Bipper Art and Craft Festival / 71 ■ Fayette County Egg Festival / 71 ■ Black Folklife Festival / 71 ■ Octoberfest / 71 ■ Unicoi County Apple Festival / 72 ■ Octoberfest and Carroll County Pork Festival / 72 ■ Autumn Gold Festival / 72 ■ National Storytelling Festival / 72 ■ Michelob Traditional Jazz Festival / 72 ■ Heritage Days / 73 ■ Oktoberfest / 73 ■ Mountain Makins Festival / 73 ■ Monroe County Tobacco and Harvest Festival / 73 ■ Gatlinburg's Christmas Festival / 73 ■ Nashville's Country Holidays / 74 ■ Festival of Lessons and Carols / 74

WEST VIRGINIA 74

Dogwood Arts and Crafts Festival / 74 ■ Webster County Woodchopping Festival / 74 ■ Three Rivers Coal Festival / 74 ■ West Virginia Dandelion Festival / 75 ■ Mountain Festival / 75 ■ Vandalia Gathering / 75 ■ West Virginia Strawberry Festival / 75 ■ Mountain Heritage Arts and Crafts Festival / 75 ■ Tri-State Fair and Regatta / 75 ■ West Virginia State Folk Festival / 76 ■ Mountain State Art and Craft Fair / 76 ■ Jamboree-In-The-Hills / 76 ■ Upper Ohio Valley Italian Festival / 76 ■ West Virginia Water Festival / 76 ■ Appalachian Arts and Crafts Festival / 76 ■ Charleston Sternwheel Regatta Festival / 77 ■ West Virginia Italian Heritage Festival / 77 ■ Stonewall Jackson Arts and Crafts Jubilee / 77 ■ West Virginia Railroad Heritage Festival / 77 ■ King Coal Festival / 77 ■ Preston County Buckwheat Festival / 78 ■ Fall Mountain Heritage Arts and Crafts Festival / 78 ■ West Virginia Honey Festival / 78 ■ Mountain State Forest Festival / 78 ■ West Virginia Black Walnut Festival / 78 ■ Bridge Walk Festival / 79 ■ Mountain State Apple Harvest Festival / 79

DEEP SOUTH   81

ALABAMA   83

Mardi Gras / 83 ■ Historic Selma Pilgrimage and Antique Show / 83 ■ Mobile International Festival / 83 ■ Birmingham Festival of Arts / 83 ■ Greek Food Festival / 83 ■ Cahawba Festival / 84 ■ Alabama Jubilee Hot Air Balloon Classic / 84 ■ Alabama June Jam / 84 ■ Alabama Blueberry Festival / 84 ■ Blessing of the Fleet / 84 ■ Summer Music Festival / 84 ■ Mentone Crafts Festival / 85 ■ Alabama Shakespeare Festival / 85 ■ W. C. Handy Music Festival / 85 ■ Octoberfest / 85 ■ Outdoor Arts and Crafts Show / 85 ■ Harvest Festival / 86 ■ Kentuck Festival / 86 ■ Riverfront Market / 86 ■ Alabama Tale Tellin' Festival / 86 ■ National Shrimp Festival / 86 ■ National Peanut Festival / 87

ARKANSAS   87

Arkansas Folk Festival / 87 ■ Dogwood Festival / 87 ■ Festival of Two Rivers / 87 ■ Toad Suck Daze / 87 ■ Arkansas Fun Festival / 88 ■ Wynne Funfest / 88 ■ Pink Tomato Festival / 88 ■ Hope Watermelon Festival / 88 ■ Beaver Lake Water Festival / 88 ■ Texarkana Quadrangle Arts and Crafts Festival / 89 ■ Bella Vista Arts and Crafts Festival / 89 ■ Oktoberfest / 89 ■ Ozarks Arts and Crafts Fair / 89 ■ Original Ozark Festival / 89 ■ World's Championship Duck Calling Contest and Wings Over the Prairie Festival / 90

FLORIDA   90

Old Island Days / 90 ■ Florida Keys Renaissance Faire / 90 ■ Orlando Scottish Highland Games / 90 ■ Pirate Fest and Gasparilla Invasion / 91 ■ Fiesta Day / 91 ■ Miami Beach Outdoor Festival of the Arts / 91 ■ Florida Citrus Festival / 91 ■ Grant Seafood Festival / 91 ■ Swamp Cabbage Festival / 92 ■ Coconut Grove Arts Festival / 92 ■ Hatsume Fair / 92 ■ Gasparilla Sidewalk Arts Festival / 92 ■ Chalo Nitka / 92 ■ River Festival / 93 ■ Florida Strawberry Festival and Hillsborough County Fair / 93 ■ Bach Festival at Winter Park / 93 ■ Strawberry Festival / 93 ■ Delius Festival / 93 ■ Kissimmee Bluegrass Festival / 94 ■ Pioneer Park Days / 94 ■ Carnaval Miami / 94 ■ Down Home Days / 94 ■ Orange Blossom Festival / 95 ■ Speckled Perch Festival / 95 ■ Winter Park Sidewalk Art Festival / 95 ■ St. Petersburg Festival of States / 95 ■ Country Music Festival / 95 ■ Catfish Festival / 95 ■ Spring Arts Festival / 96 ■ De Soto Celebration / 96 ■ Cocoa Beach Easter Surfing Festival / 96 ■ Apopka Art and Foliage Festival / 96 ■ Week of the Ocean Festival / 96 ■ Chautauqua Festival / 97 ■ International Festival / 97 ■ Spring Music Festival / 97 ■ Palm Harbor Day Arts Crafts and Music Festival / 97 ■ Isle of Eight Flags Shrimp Festival / 97 ■ Florida Folk Festival / 97 ■ Zellwood Sweet Corn Festival / 98 ■ Music Festival of Florida / 98 ■ Billy Bowlegs Festival / 98 ■ Florida Pro / 98 ■ Destin Seafood Festival / 98 ■ Fall Festival / 99 ■ Jacksonville Jazz Festival / 99 ■ Indian Summer Seafood Festival / 99 ■ Winter Park Autumn Art Festival / 99 ■ Boggy Bayou Mullet Festival / 99 ■ Brandon Balloon Festival / 100 ■

John's Pass Seafood Festival / 100 ■ Pioneer Days Folk Festival / 100 ■ Florida Forest Festival / 100 ■ Guava-Ween Halloween Extravaganza / 100 ■ Florida Seafood Festival / 101 ■ Festival of the Arts / 101 ■ Highlands Art League Sidewalk Art Festival / 101 ■ Ybor City Folk Festival / 101 ■ Collard Festival / 101 ■ St. Cloud Art Festival / 101 ■ Palm Harbor Arts, Crafts, and Music Festival / 102

GEORGIA 102

St. Patrick's Festival / 102 ■ Old South Celebration / 102 ■ Lindbergh Days: A Festival of Light / 102 ■ Springfest and BBQ Pork Cook-off / 103 ■ Prater's Mill Country Fair / 103 ■ Vidalia Onion Festival / 103 ■ Georgia Folk Festival / 103 ■ Putnam Co. Dairy Festival / 103 ■ Winterville Marigold Festival / 104 ■ Powers' Crossroads Country Fair & Art Festival / 104 ■ Yellow Daisy Festival / 104 ■ Barnesville Buggy Days / 104 ■ Heritage Holidays / 105 ■ Georgia Sweet Potato Festival / 105

LOUISIANA 105

River City Blues Festival / 105 ■ FestForAll / 105 ■ Louisiana Balloon Festival and Airshow / 105 ■ Mudbug Madness / 105 ■ Jambalaya Festival and Art Show / 106 ■ Black Arts Festival / 106 ■ Gospel Music Festival / 106 ■ Cajun Bastille Day / 106 ■ Natchitoches-Northwestern Folk Festival / 106 ■ Louisiana Shrimp and Petroleum Festival / 106 ■ Festivals Acadiens / 107 ■ Rayne Frog Festival / 107 ■ Red River Revel / 107 ■ International Alligator Festival / 107 ■ Natchitoches Christmas Festival of Lights / 108

MISSISSIPPI 108

World Catfish Festival / 108 ■ Amory Railroad Festival / 108 ■ Gum Tree Festival / 108 ■ Great River Days / 109 ■ Greenwood Arts Festival / 109 ■ Jimmie Rodgers Memorial Festival / 109 ■ Red Hills Festival / 109 ■ Mississippi Deep Sea Fishing Rodeo / 109 ■ Choctaw Indian Fair / 110 ■ C.R.O.P. Day (Cotton Row on Parade Day) / 110

SOUTH CAROLINA 110

Lowcountry Oyster Festival / 110 ■ Flowertown Festival / 110 ■ Bethune Chicken Strut / 111 ■ Palmetto Balloon Classic / 111 ■ Come-See-Me / 111 ■ Abbeville Spring Festival / 111 ■ South Carolina Festival of Roses / 111 ■ Spoleto Festival U.S.A. / 112 ■ Apple Festival / 112 ■ Atalaya Arts and Crafts Festival / 112 ■ Catfish Festival / 112 ■ The Taste of Charleston / 112 ■ Carolina Golden Leaf Festival / 113 ■ Jubilee: Festival of Heritage / 113 ■ Moja Arts Festival / 113 ■ International Arts Festival / 113 ■ Autumnfest / 113 ■ South Carolina Sweet Potato Festival / 113 ■ Fall Fiesta of the Arts / 114 ■ Oktoberfest / 114 ■ Christmas in Charleston / 114 ■ Elgin Catfish Stomp / 114

MIDWEST 115

ILLINOIS 117

Celebration: A Festival of the Arts / 117 ■ Heritage Days Festival / 117 ■ A Taste of the Illinois Valley / 117 ■ Harvard Milk Day Festival / 117 ■ Dance of the Nations / 117 ■ Old Canal Days / 118 ■ Steamboat Days / 118 ■ Swedish Days / 118 ■ Oglesby Celebration Days / 118 ■ Dixon Petunia Festival / 118 ■ Lincolnfest / 118 ■ Taste Chicago / 119 ■ West Chicago Railroad Days / 119 ■ Fiesta Days / 119 ■ Rediscover Cahokia / 119 ■ National Sweet Corn Festival / 119 ■ Frankfort Fall Festival / 119 ■ National Sweetcorn Festival / 120 ■ Jubilee Days / 120 ■ Pekin Marigold Festival / 120 ■ Cedarhurst Craft Fair / 120 ■ Festival of the Vine / 120 ■ Oktoberfest / 121 ■ Bureau County Homestead Festival and Pork BBQ / 121 ■ Sweetcorn and Watermelon Festival / 121 ■ Little Vermillion Fall Festival / 121 ■ Morton Pumpkin Festival / 121 ■ Honey Bee Festival / 121 ■ Ethnic Fest for All / 122

INDIANA 122

Renaissance Faire / 122 ■ Wabash Valley Festival / 122 ■ Heritage Days Festival / 122 ■ Riverfront Festival / 123 ■ Three Rivers Festival / 123 ■ Iron Horse Festival / 123 ■ Swiss Days / 123 ■ Banks of the Wabash Dixieland Jazz Festival / 123 ■ Van Buren Popcorn Festival / 124 ■ Village Art Festival / 124 ■ Turkey Trot Festival / 124 ■ Cumberland Covered Bridge Festival and Antique Engine Show / 124 ■ Lafayesta: Family Festival of the Arts / 124 ■ Little Italy Festival / 125 ■ Steamboat Days / 125 ■ Oktoberfest / 125 ■ Hoosier Heritage Days / 125 ■ Fairmount Museum Days / 125 ■ Harvest Homecoming / 125 ■ Covered Bridge Festival / 126

IOWA 126

St. Pat's Celebration / 126 ■ Pella Tulip Time / 126 ■ DubuqueFest / 126 ■ Two Rivers Festival / 127 ■ Frontier Days / 127 ■ North Iowa Band Festival / 127 ■ Grant Wood Art Festival / 127 ■ Glenn Miller Birthplace Society Festival / 127 ■ Sturgis Falls Celebration / 128 ■ Clinton Riverboat Days / 128 ■ Mississippi Valley Blues Festival / 128 ■ Czech Folk Festival / 128 ■ Nordic Fest / 129 ■ Bix Arts, Crafts and Food Fest / 129 ■ National Hobo Convention / 129 ■ Art in the Park / 129 ■ National Hot Air Balloon Championships / 129 ■ Great River Days / 130 ■ Family Fest / 130 ■ Old Time Country Music Festival and Pioneer Exposition of Arts and Crafts / 130

KANSAS 130

Pancake Day / 130 ■ St. Patrick's Road Race and Parade / 131 ■ Wichita River Festival / 131 ■ Downtown Manhattan Fun Festival / 131 ■ Good Ol' Days / 131 ■ Beef Empire Days / 131 ■ Smoky Hill River Festival / 132 ■ Festival International / 132 ■ Wheat Festival / 132 ■ Dodge City Days and Ford County Fair / 132 ■ Renaissance Festival / 132 ■ Walnut Valley Festival / 133 ■ Maple Leaf Festival / 133 ■ Neewollah / 133

MICHIGAN
133

Winterfest / 133 ■ National Trout Festival / 134 ■ Alma Highland Festival and Games / 134 ■ Garden City Community Flower and Garden Festival / 134 ■ National Asparagus Festival / 134 ■ Frankenmuth Bavarian Festival / 134 ■ Detroit/Windsor International Freedom Festival / 135 ■ Three Rivers Water Carnival / 135 ■ Belleville Area Strawberry Festival / 135 ■ Chesaning Showboat / 135 ■ National Cherry Festival / 136 ■ Alpenfest / 136 ■ National Blueberry Festival / 136 ■ Kalamazoo County Flowerfest / 136 ■ Hiawatha Music Co-op Festival / 136 ■ Plainwell Island City Festival / 137 ■ Harbor Days / 137 ■ Danish Festival / 137 ■ Montreux Detroit Jazz Festival / 137 ■ Michigan Wine and Harvest Festival / 137 ■ Festival of the Pines / 137 ■ Festival of the Forks / 138 ■ Tuscola County Pumpkin Festival / 138 ■ Oktoberfest / 138

MINNESOTA
138

Saint Paul Winter Carnival / 138 ■ Festival of Nations / 139 ■ Hagar's Lutefisk Festival / 139 ■ Western Fest / 139 ■ White Bear Lake Area Manitou Days / 139 ■ Kaffe Fest / 139 ■ Lake City Water Ski Days / 139 ■ Scandinavian Hjemkomst Festival / 140 ■ Taste of Minnesota / 140 ■ Wheels, Wings, and Water Festival / 140 ■ Riverfront Music Festival / 140 ■ Viennese Sommerfest / 140 ■ Sinclair Lewis Days / 141 ■ Minneapolis Aquatennial / 141 ■ Art in the Park / 141 ■ Heritagefest / 141 ■ Rivertown Days / 141 ■ Glenwood Waterama / 142 ■ "We" Minnesota Country Music Fest / 142 ■ Songs of the Lumberjack / 142 ■ Defeat of Jesse James Days / 142 ■ Big Island Rendezvous and Festival / 142 ■ Oktoberfest / 143

MISSOURI
143

Storytelling Festival / 143 ■ Richmond Mushroom Festival / 143 ■ International Festival / 143 ■ Scott Joplin Ragtime Festival / 143 ■ National Ragtime and Traditional Jazz Festival / 144 ■ National Tom Sawyer Days / 144 ■ Veiled Prophet Fair / 144 ■ St. Louis Strassenfest / 144 ■ Japanese Festival / 144 ■ Santa-Call-Gon Days / 145 ■ Shoe-Me Sho-Off Selebration / 145 ■ Bevo Day / 145 ■ Mexico Jaycees Soybean Festival / 145 ■ Prairie View Festival / 145 ■ Autumn Historic Folklife Festival / 145

NEBRASKA
146

St. Patrick's Day Celebration / 146 ■ Arbor Day Celebration / 146 ■ German Heritage Days / 146 ■ Nebraskaland Days / 146 ■ Stromsburg Swedish Festival / 147 ■ Fur Trade Days / 147 ■ Summerfest Celebration / 147 ■ Wayne Chicken Show / 147 ■ Nebraska Czech Festival / 147 ■ Applejack Festival / 148 ■ Oktoberfest / 148

NORTH DAKOTA
148

Winter Festival / 148 ■ Arts and Humanities Festival / 148 ■ Pioneer Days / 148 ■ United Tribes Days / 149 ■ Oktoberfest / 149

OHIO 149

Winterfest / 149 ■ International Festival / 149 ■ Moonshine Festival / 149 ■ Holy Toledo! It's Spring / 150 ■ Troy Strawberry Festival / 150 ■ Jonathan Bye Days / 150 ■ Festival of the Fish / 150 ■ International Week / 150 ■ Ohio Scottish Games / 150 ■ Downtown Euclid Community Festival / 151 ■ Crosby Gardens Festival of the Arts / 151 ■ Midwest Tobacco Spittin' Championship / 151 ■ Columbia Homecoming and Blueberry Festival / 151 ■ Westerville Music and Arts Festival / 151 ■ Celina Lake Festival / 151 ■ Pro Football Hall of Fame Festival / 152 ■ North Ridgeville Corn Festival / 152 ■ The Potato Festival / 152 ■ Salt Fork Arts and Crafts Festival / 152 ■ Bratwurst Festival / 152 ■ Toledo Festival: A Celebration of the Arts / 152 ■ Clinton County Corn Festival / 153 ■ Pioneer Days Festival / 153 ■ Ohio Honey Festival / 153 ■ Elyria Apple Festival / 153 ■ Ravenna Balloon A-Fair / 153 ■ Tipp City Mum Festival / 153 ■ Jackson County Apple Festival / 154 ■ Ohio Pumpkin Festival / 154 ■ Middfest International / 154 ■ Ohio Swiss Festival / 154 ■ Ohio Gourd Show / 154 ■ Apple Festival / 154 ■ Ohio Sauerkraut Festival / 155 ■ New Music Festival / 155

OKLAHOMA 155

Azalea Festival / 155 ■ Waynoka Rattlesnake Hunt / 155 ■ Kolache Festival / 155 ■ Stilwell Strawberry Festival / 156 ■ Tulsa International Mayfest / 156 ■ World Championship Cow Chip Throwing Contest / 156 ■ Italian Festival / 156 ■ Festival Del Paseo / 156 ■ Sante Fe Trail Daze / 157 ■ Kiamichi Owa-Chito / 157 ■ Blue Grass Show / 157 ■ Grant's Bluegrass and Old Time Music Festival / 157 ■ Frontier Days Celebration / 157 ■ Chili Bluegrass Festival / 158 ■ Calf Fry Festival and Cook-Off / 158 ■ Fall Festival of the Arts / 158 ■ Czech Festival / 158 ■ Sorghum Day / 158 ■ Cheese-Sausage Festival / 158 ■ Watonga Cheese Festival / 159

SOUTH DAKOTA 159

Arts and Crafts Festival / 159 ■ Black Hills Heritage Festival / 159 ■ Gold Discovery Days Pageant of Paha Sapa (Sacred Land of the Sioux Indians) / 159 ■ Yankton Riverboat Days / 159 ■ Fall Festival / 160 ■ Corn Palace Week / 160

WISCONSIN 160

Winter Festival / 160 ■ Wisconsin State Sled Dog Championships / 160 ■ Great River Festival of the Arts / 161 ■ Great Wisconsin Dells Balloon Rally / 161 ■ Walleye Weekend Festival and National Walleye Tournament / 161 ■ Lakefront Festival of the Arts / 161 ■ Musky Festival / 161 ■ Summerfest / 161 ■ Hodag Country Festival / 162 ■ Bastille Days / 162 ■ Port Washington Fish Day / 162 ■ Festa Italiana / 162 ■ Holland Festival / 162 ■ German Fest / 162 ■ Afro Fest / 163 ■ Irish Fest / 163 ■ North Hudson Pepper Festival / 163 ■ Sweet Corn Festival / 163 ■ Fiesta Mexicana / 163 ■ Rutabaga Festival / 163 ■ Polish Fest / 164 ■ Wo-Zha-Wa Days Fall Festival / 164 ■ Wine and Harvest Festival / 164 ■ Polka Fest Celebration / 164 ■ Fall-O-Rama / 164

WEST   165

ALASKA   167

Tent-City Festival / 167 ■ Cordova Iceworm Festival / 167 ■ Fur Rendezvous ("Rondy") / 167 ■ Great Sitka Herring Festival / 167 ■ Fairbanks Ice Festival / 167 ■ Little Norway Festival / 168 ■ Kodiak Crab Festival / 168 ■ Sitka Summer Music Festival / 168 ■ Golden Days / 168 ■ Alaska Day Festival / 168

CALIFORNIA   169

National Date Festival / 169 ■ Holtville Carrot Festival / 169 ■ World Champion Crab Races / 169 ■ Santa Barbara International Film Festival / 169 ■ Snowfest! / 170 ■ Whale Festival / 170 ■ Slug Fest / 170 ■ Desert Cavalcade Parade / 170 ■ San Francisco Film Festival / 170 ■ Apple Blossom Festival / 171 ■ Pacific Coast Collegiate Jazz Festival / 171 ■ Cherry Blossom Festival / 171 ■ Calico Pitchin', Cookin', and Spittin' Hullabaloo / 171 ■ Santa Barbara Arts Festival / 171 ■ Bodega Bay Fishermen's Festival / 172 ■ San Dimas Festival of Western Arts / 172 ■ Westwood Art Show / 172 ■ Calico Spring Festival / 172 ■ Fair Oaks Fiesta / 172 ■ Celebrate the Arts / 172 ■ Campbell Wine and Arts Music Festival / 173 ■ Fiesta La Ballona / 173 ■ Strawberry Festival / 173 ■ Calaveras County Fair and Jumping Frog Jubilee / 173 ■ Russian River Winefest / 173 ■ Mule Days Celebration / 173 ■ Grubstake Days / 174 ■ Fiesta De Las Artes / 174 ■ Sacramento Dixieland Jubilee / 174 ■ Union Street Spring Festival / 174 ■ Apricot Fiesta / 174 ■ Festival / 175 ■ Sunnyvale Art and Wine Festival / 175 ■ Scandinavian Midsummer Festival / 175 ■ Music in the Mountains Summer Festival / 175 ■ New North Beach Fair / 175 ■ Celtic Festival / 175 ■ Huck Finn's Jubilee / 176 ■ Lake Tahoe Summer Music Festival / 176 ■ Easter in July Lily Festival / 176 ■ Twain Harte Summer Craft Festival / 176 ■ Carmel Bach Festival / 176 ■ Gilroy Garlic Festival / 176 ■ San Anselmo Art and Wine Festival / 177 ■ Shakespeare at Sand Harbor / 177 ■ Old Spanish Days Fiesta / 177 ■ Klamath Salmon Festival and Boat Races / 177 ■ Palo Alto Celebrates the Arts / 178 ■ Mountain Festival / 178 ■ Russian River Jazz Festival / 178 ■ Bishop Homecoming Rodeo and Wild West Weekend / 178 ■ Concord Fall Fest / 178 ■ Oakland Festival of the Arts: Arts Explosion / 178 ■ Wasco Festival of Roses / 179 ■ Powwow Days / 179 ■ Castro Valley Fall Festival / 179 ■ Mountain View Art and Wine Festival / 179 ■ 16th of September Fiesta / 179 ■ Art and Wine Festival / 179 ■ Monterey Jazz Festival / 180 ■ Pan Pacific Exposition Art and Wine Festival / 180 ■ Danish Days / 180 ■ Pacific Coast Fog Fest / 180 ■ Santa Clara Arts and Wine Festival / 180 ■ Valley of the Moon Vintage Festival / 181 ■ Columbus Day Celebration / 181 ■ Autumn Jubilee / 181 ■ Italian American Culture Festival / 181 ■ Festa Italiana / 181 ■ Jazz and All That Art on Fillmore / 182 ■ Calico Days / 182 ■ Brussels Sprout Festival / 182 ■ Goleta Valley Days / 182 ■ Riverbank Cheese and Wine Exposition / 182 ■ Half Moon Bay Pumpkin Festival / 182 ■ Hangtown Jazz Jubilee / 183 ■ Borrego Days Desert Festival / 183 ■ Fine Arts Festival / 183 ■ Auburn Craft Festival and Christmas Marketplace / 183 ■ Brawley Cattle Call / 183 ■ Sonora Christmas Craft Festival / 183

HAWAII 184

Narcissus Festival / 184 ■ Cherry Blossom Festival / 184 ■ Captain Cook Festival / 184 ■ Merrie Monarch Festival and Concert at Ka'auea / 184 ■ Festival of the Pacific / 184 ■ Gotcha Pro Surf Championships / 184 ■ King Kamehameha Celebration / 185 ■ Establishment Day Cultural Festival / 185 ■ Prince Lot Hula Festival / 185 ■ Macadamia Nut Harvest Festival / 185 ■ Okinawan Festival / 185 ■ Aloha Week Festivals / 185 ■ Kanikapila (Let's Play Music) / 186 ■ Kamehameha Schools Festival / 186 ■ Kona Coffee Festival / 186 ■ Na Mele O'Maui Festival / 186 ■ Hawaii International Film Festival / 186

IDAHO 187

Winter Festival / 187 ■ McCall Winter Carnival / 187 ■ Dogwood Festival / 187 ■ Payette Apple Blossom Festival / 187 ■ National Oldtime Fiddlers' Contest / 187 ■ Art on the Green / 188 ■ Pend Oreille Arts Council's Arts and Crafts Festival / 188 ■ Idaho Huckleberry Festival / 188 ■ McCall Summer Arts and Crafts Fair "Love in the Arts" / 188

MONTANA 188

Whitefish Winter Carnival / 188 ■ Flathead Cherry Blossom Festival / 189 ■ Red Lodge Music Festival / 189 ■ Art in Washoe Park / 189 ■ Libby Logger Days / 189 ■ Lewis and Clark Expedition Festival / 189 ■ Festival of Nations / 190 ■ Crow Fair / 190 ■ Heritage of the Yellowstone Folklife Festival / 190 ■ Nordicfest / 190 ■ Herbstfest / 190

NEVADA 191

Elks Helldorado Days / 191 ■ Basque Festival / 191 ■ Festival Reno / 191 ■ Dixieland Jazz Festival / 191 ■ Tombola / 191 ■ Ely Basque Club Festival / 192 ■ Reno Basque Festival / 192 ■ World's International Whistle-Off / 192

OREGON 192

Oregon Shakespearean Festival / 192 ■ Newport Seafood and Wine Festival / 193 ■ Tillamook County Mid-Winter Festival / 193 ■ Pear Blossom Festival / 193 ■ Rhododendron Festival / 193 ■ Boatnik Festival / 193 ■ Portland Rose Festival / 194 ■ Lebanon Strawberry Festival / 194 ■ Phil Sheridan Days / 194 ■ Rooster Crow Festival / 194 ■ Oregon Bach Festival / 194 ■ Western Days / 194 ■ Festival Corvallis—Midsummer Music / 195 ■ Obon Odori (Obon Festival) / 195 ■ Salem Art Fair and Festival / 195 ■ Renaissance Arts Festival / 195 ■ Mt. Hood Festival of Jazz / 195 ■ Wild Blackberry Festival / 196 ■ Junction City Scandinavian Festival / 196 ■ Depoe Bay Salmon Bake / 196 ■ Pendleton Round-Up and Happy Canyon / 196 ■ Corvallis Fall Festival / 196

WASHINGTON 197

Rain Or Shine Jazz Festival / 197 ■ Rhododendron Festival / 197 ■ Viking Fest / 197 ■ Walla Walla Hot Air Balloon Stampede / 197 ■ Ski To Sea Festival / 198 ■ Moses Lake Spring Festival / 198 ■ Northwest Folklife Festival / 198 ■ Greek Festival / 198 ■ Skandia Midsommar Fest / 198 ■ Berry-Dairy Days / 199 ■ Sedro Woolley Loggerodeo / 199 ■ Capital Lakefair / 199 ■ Walla Walla Sweet Onion Festival / 199 ■ Loggers Jubilee / 199 ■ Omak Stampede and World Famous Suicide Race / 200 ■ Chief Seattle Days / 200 ■ Wooden Boat Festival / 200

WYOMING 200

Cultural Festival / 200 ■ Encampment Woodchoppers Jamboree / 200 ■ Flaming Gorge Days / 201 ■ Lander Pioneer Days / 201 ■ Grand Teton Music Festival / 201 ■ World Open Atlatl Championships, Crafts Fair and Community Trout Fry / 201 ■ Cheyenne Frontier Days / 201 ■ Lander Valley Apple Festival / 201

SOUTHWEST 203

ARIZONA 205

Gold Rush Days / 205 ■ Lost Dutchman Days / 205 ■ Coolidge Cotton Festival / 205 ■ Tombstone Territorial Days / 205 ■ Tucson Festival / 205 ■ Bill Williams Rendezvous Days / 206 ■ Arizona Summer Arts Festival / 206 ■ Oldtime Country Music & Bluegrass Festival / 206 ■ Loggers Sawdust Festival / 206 ■ Old Time Fiddlers Contest & Festival / 207 ■ Call of the Canyon Festival of the Arts / 207 ■ Fall Festival / 207 ■ London Bridge Days / 207 ■ Rex Allen Days / 207 ■ Billy Moore Days / 207 ■ Four Corner States Bluegrass Festival / 207

COLORADO 208

Ullr Fest / 208 ■ Winterskol / 208 ■ White River Winter Rendezvous / 208 ■ Winter Fest / 208 ■ Snowmass/Aspen Banana Season / 208 ■ Sunshine Festival / 209 ■ Central City Arts Festival / 209 ■ Telluride Bluegrass and Country Music Festival / 209 ■ Strawberry Days / 209 ■ Aspen Music Festival and School / 209 ■ Oro City Rebirth of a Miner's Camp / 210 ■ Bach, Beethoven or Breckenridge: Festival of Music at the Summit / 210 ■ Range Call Celebration / 210 ■ Telluride Jazz Festival / 210 ■ Ski Hi Stampede / 211 ■ Top of the Rockies Leadville Music Festival / 211 ■ AMC Summitfest / 211 ■ Boom Days Celebration/International Pack Burro Races / 211 ■ Central City Jazz Festival / 211 ■ Telluride Film Festival / 212 ■ Oktoberfest / 212 ■ Breckenridge Festival of Film / 212

NEW MEXICO 212

Gathering of Nations Powwow / 212 ■ Mayfair / 212 ■ Taos Spring Arts Celebration / 213 ■ Taos School of Music Summer Chamber Music Festival / 213 ■ Piñata / 213

■ Southeastern New Mexico Fourth of July Celebration / 213 ■ Ruidoso Art Festival / 213 ■ Inter-Tribal Indian Ceremonial / 213 ■ Music From Angel Fire Festival / 214 ■ Fiesta De Santa Fe / 214 ■ Taos Arts Festival / 214 ■ The Whole Enchilada Fiesta / 214 ■ Albuquerque International Balloon Fiesta / 215 ■ Southeastern New Mexico Arts and Crafts Festival / 215

TEXAS   215

Lovelady Love Fest / 215 ■ Sweetwater "World's Largest Rattlesnake Roundup" / 215 ■ Derrick Days / 215 ■ Tyler County Dogwood Festival / 216 ■ Prairie Dog Chili Cook-Off and World Championship of Pickled Quail Egg Eating / 216 ■ RioFest / 216 ■ Humble Good Oil Days / 216 ■ Lubbock Arts Festival / 216 ■ Strawberry Festival / 217 ■ Neches River Festival / 217 ■ Texas State Festival of Ethnic Cultures and Arts and Crafts Show / 217 ■ Wildflower Trails of Texas / 217 ■ Scarborough Faire / 218 ■ Cinco De Mayo Festival / 218 ■ Ennis Polka Festival / 218 ■ Fort Bend County Czech Fest / 218 ■ Kaleidoscope / 218 ■ Kerrville Folk Festival / 219 ■ Texas State Arts and Crafts Fair / 219 ■ Strange Family Bluegrass Festival / 219 ■ Luling Watermelon Thump / 219 ■ Saints Roost Celebration / 220 ■ Black-Eyed Pea Jamboree / 220 ■ Austin Aqua Festival / 220 ■ Texas Folklife Festival / 220 ■ Schulenburg Festival / 221 ■ XIT Rodeo and Reunion / 221 ■ St. Louis Day / 221 ■ Westfest / 221 ■ National Championship Indian Powwow / 222 ■ Kolache Festival / 222 ■ Oak Cliff Urban Pioneer Festival and Homes Tour / 222 ■ City Fest-Highland Games / 222 ■ Texas International Wine Classic / 223 ■ Texas Rice Festival / 223 ■ Shrimporee / 223 ■ Seafair / 223 ■ East Texas Yamboree / 223 ■ Western Days Celebration / 224 ■ Old Fiddler's Festival / 224 ■ Czhilispiel / 224 ■ Peanut Festival / 224 ■ Symphony of Trees / 224

UTAH   225

United States Film Festival / 225 ■ Utah Shakespearean Festival / 225 ■ Days of '47 Pioneer Celebration / 225 ■ Festival of the American West / 225 ■ Main Street U.S.A. Summerfest / 226 ■ Park City Art Festival / 226 ■ Springville World Folkfest / 226 ■ Swiss Days / 226 ■ Peach Days / 226

GLOSSARY   229

INDEX   233

INTRODUCTION

America's festivals have escalated rapidly in popularity as sources of entertainment, artistic display, and cultural enlightenment. Attending a festival can be an integral part of a vacation or an inexpensive way to spend an afternoon or evening full of fun and recreation close to home.

We view more arts and crafts at American festivals than in all the museums across the country. More people hear live music at festivals than at gigantic rock or classical concerts.

Festivals are the backbones of the cultural life of any country: unifying communities that prepare and execute the events, while at the same time showing the world their most cherished traditions. Renewed interest in one's national origins is replacing the old American trend toward "blending in" with American society. We now feel free to take pride in celebrating and discovering our heritage.

Festivals are not new. The earliest historical reference to a festival is the Jewish Passover in celebration of the escape to freedom from Egypt more than 3,000 years ago. The "Dragon Boat Festival" in China dates back more than 2,000 years, as does the Jewish harvest festival, Sukkot.

As early as 776 B.C., annual sports festivals were held, including the Olympic games. By 500 B.C., the Greeks were presenting dramatic festivals and enjoying the winter festival of Dionysus in honor of both wine and song.

Julius Caesar was warned of the plot to kill him during the Festival of Lupercalia in 44 B.C. when half-naked young men chased women through the streets, lashing them with thongs.

The word "carnival" is derived from the Latin *carne vale* (farewell to flesh), a three-day holiday preceding Lent in early Christian times and today known as Mardi Gras ("Fat Tuesday").

May Day festivals called "Florida" were held in Roman times, while selecting and crowning a May Day Queen dates back to medieval England. The first winter carnival in the United States was in 1886, and by 1900 there were many festivals celebrating the harvest, historical events, and national origins.

Today's festivals vary tremendously and one can easily enjoy or study American culture at festivals through their entertainment, arts, and foods.

Music plays a role in most festivals and is the main attraction at many, including Bach, Mozart, W. C. Handy, country/western, Beethoven, bluegrass, whistling, mariachis, folk, jazz, beach music, along with Celtic, Italian,

Czechoslovakian, German, Polish, Dutch, reggae, Japanese, big band and high school band sounds, Hawaiian, mountain, traditional, blues, and just about every variation of the above imaginable.

Arts and crafts ranging from fine arts by renowned artists to cottage crafts are displayed and sold at 95 of American festivals, representing local products and national origins of residents.

Festivals celebrating the harvest feature a wide variety of products typifying the vast resources of America, such as quahog, mullet, carrots, brussels sprouts, sorghum, wheat, all sorts of fruits, garlic, wines, rhododendrons and azaleas, petunias, tree blossoms, musky, mushrooms, peanuts, oysters and crabs, rice, and potatoes.

Dramatic productions range from lavish Shakespearean festivals to puppet shows, while some festivals honor local and nationally known historical personages.

Americans' vast range of national origins and ethnic backgrounds is reflected in the costuming, pageantry, and the foods served at festivals. You will find enchiladas and tacos at a Mexican fiesta, bratwurst and sauerkraut at a German Oktoberfest, kolache at Czech festivals, seafoods where they abound, Cuban sandwiches in Ybor City, macadamia nuts in Hawaii, onions in Georgia, mountain specialties in Appalachia, Indian fry bread on reservations, and Cajun and Creole delicacies in Louisiana. I challenge you to find ghost bread!

Promotion of festivals evokes the use of superlatives and a rash of world "capitals" such as those of agate, artichokes, garlic, uranium, Indian, fiddling, and even a "festival capital," and two claims of the "World's Largest Fish Fry." Throughout FESTIVALS U.S.A. one will find more than one festival claiming to be the "capital" source of the same product.

Many festivals have intriguing names such as the Boggy Bayou Mullet Festival, Swamp Cabbage Festival, Narcissus Festival, Na Mele O'Maui Festival, Mudbug Madness, Cajun Bastille Day, Lotus Blossom Festival, Woolly Worm Festival, the World Championship Cow Chip Throwing Contest, the Bethune Chicken Strut, and The Whole Enchilada Fiesta.

America's festivals are truly "the whole enchilada" of our national character and culture. Now it's time to pack up the car, the van, RV, or motor home, get on your bike or buy a bus, train, or plane ticket and go.

And don't forget, most festivals benefit local charities, so they welcome and seek outsiders to visit and participate. Many offer road or foot races, golf and tennis tournaments, chess tournaments, and many other activities in which one can take part for free or a small fee.

TIPS ON USING FESTIVALS U.S.A.

For easy referencing, all festivals in the book are organized by geographic region and then by state. The festivals within each state are listed by month. You'll note that many states don't have any festivals until the spring, so the spring months are the first to be listed.

Be sure to phone or write each festival to confirm dates and costs. While food costs are rarely mentioned herein, there are almost always charges for food and beverages, except in the instances indicated. Often there are charges to play games and for admittance to special areas or events, so be sure to bring cash or traveler's checks, although smaller festivals will not be accustomed to the traveler's checks.

Comments in quotation marks are direct quotes from local festival organizers and are included for their special charm of phrasing, and sometimes for humor. You'll note a figure at the end of some festival descriptions. This figure represents estimated annual attendance for the festival. Unfortunately, this figure was not available for all the festivals, since many festival organizers find it difficult to assess attendance. If a festival does not serve food, or if there are no accommodations or restaurants in the locale of a festival, then these categories are omitted from the festival's listing. Neither the author nor the publisher is responsible for those opinions quoted, or for inaccurate information provided to the author by festival organizers.

Assessments of restaurants' qualities are always subjective, and while fast foods and family style are fairly constant, "elegant" may vary widely in the eyes of the beholders. B&B's refer to Bed and Breakfasts, and RV parks refer to specific camping parks that specialize in gradations of electrical and water hook-ups for recreational vehicles.

Should any reader find a festival or festivals to be in any way different from the descriptions in FESTIVALS U.S.A., please write and let me know of your views. If you should discover or know of a festival you think should be included in our next edition, please send the information to Kathleen Thompson Hill, P.O. Box 654, Sonoma, CA 95476.

And finally, sit back or pack up and enjoy the fun of FESTIVALS U.S.A.

KATHLEEN THOMPSON HILL
January 1988

Northeast

Connecticut / 3

Maine / 6

Massachusetts / 9

New Hampshire / 12

New Jersey / 12

New York / 13

Pennsylvania / 22

Rhode Island / 28

Vermont / 29

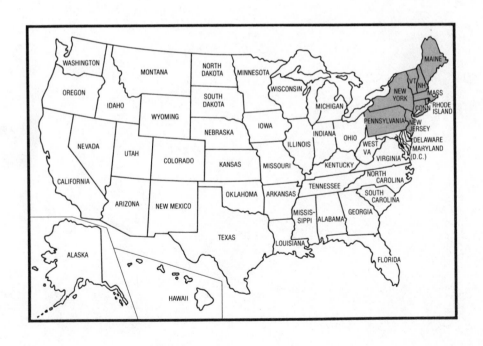

CONNECTICUT

DOGWOOD FESTIVAL *second week in May*, Fairfield, Fairfield Co., to celebrate the blooming of the dogwood trees. Guided garden tours, musical programs, professional art show and crafts, children's crafts, slide show, shops and shows featuring gifts, plants, flowers, and "attic treasures." FOODS SERVED: seated luncheon and picnic lunches. ADMISSION: free. ACCOMMODATIONS: motels and hotels. RESTAURANTS: fast foods, elegant. CONTACT: Women's Guild, The Greenfield Hill Congregational Church, 1045 Old Academy Rd., Fairfield, CT 06430, (203) 259-5596. 5,000

A TASTE OF HARTFORD *third weekend in May*, Hartford, Hartford Co., in Constitution Plaza. More than fifty restaurants prepare and sell their specialties "under colorful tents," cooking demonstrations, wine tasting, "and other spontaneous entertainment," continuous entertainment on two stages including local music, dance, magic, and comedy. FOODS SERVED: wide range of gourmet delectables. ADMISSION: free. ACCOMMODATIONS: motels and hotels, B&B's, campgrounds. RESTAURANTS: fast foods, family, elegant. CONTACT: Greater Hartford Convention and Visitors Bureau, One Civic Center Plaza, Hartford, CT 06103, (203) 728-6789. 120,000

LOBSTER WEEKEND *fourth weekend in May*, Mystic Seaport, New London Co., to celebrate the abundance of local lobster. Fresh native lobster and other seafoods served outdoors under tents along the river's edge, sea chanties, entertainment. FOODS SERVED: lobster and other local seafoods. ADMISSION: free, charge for food. ACCOMMODATIONS: motels and hotels, B&B's, campgrounds, RV parks. RESTAURANTS: fast foods, family, elegant, seafood. CONTACT: Public Affairs Office,

Mystic Seaport Museum, Rte. 27, Mystic, CT 06355, (203) 572-0711. 12,000

SEA MUSIC FESTIVAL *second weekend in June*, Mystic Seaport, New London Co., at the Mystic Seaport Museum, to celebrate traditional and contemporary music of the sea. Historic Mystic preserves musical history by offering the talents of folk musicians specializing in songs of the sea such as Louis Killen, Jeff Warner, The Boarding Party, and 80-year-old Stan Jugill from Wales, "a chanteyman on squarereiggers in his youth, and a great raconteur." Concerts, mini-concerts, symposia, featured artist concert, workshops, country music dance. FOODS SERVED: American, British, French. ADMISSION: $25.00 advance for weekend. ACCOMMODATIONS: motels and hotels, B&B's, campgrounds, RV parks. RESTAURANTS: fast foods, family, elegant, "the very best of seafood," Chinese, Italian, Mexican. CONTACT: Geoff Kaufman, Sea Music Festival at (203) 572-0711 ext. 337 or write Mystic Seaport Museum, Rte. 27, Mystic, CT 06355. 5,000

BARNUM FESTIVAL *last week in June through July 5th*, Bridgeport, New Haven Co., to honor Phineas Taylor Barnum's birthday, his service to Bridgeport as its "mayor and mentor," and the circus he created. Ringmaster's Ball, fashion show, Jai Alai Night, Cruise Night featuring classic cars, senior olympics, King and Queen Coronation, Women's Predicted Power Boat Log Race, Wing Ding children's parade including wheelchairs, Whip and Whistle Luncheon, Jenny Lind Contest, Tom Thumb and Lavinia Contest, air show including sailplanes, parachute teams, aerobatic teams, flying clown acts, and landing of the Emery 727; Black Rock Day, art and auto shows, parade, fireworks, carnival. Entertainers have included stars such as Julio Iglesias and the Beach Boys. FOODS SERVED: "all nationalities." ADMISSION: free to many events, charges for others. ACCOMMODATIONS: motels and hotels, campgrounds, RV parks. RESTAURANTS: fast foods, family, elegant. CONTACT: Barnum Festival, 303 State St., Bridgeport, CT 06604, (203) 367-8495. 250,000

NEW HAVEN JAZZ FESTIVAL *Saturdays throughout July*, New Haven, New Haven Co., on the Green. Twilight concerts feature nationally and internationally kown jazz artists such as Count Basie, Lionel Hampton, the Glenn Miller Orchestra, the Tommy Dorsey Orchestra, and the Duke Ellington Orchestra. FOODS SERVED: international. ADMISSION: free. ACCOMMODATIONS: motels and hotels, B&B's, campgrounds, RV parks. RESTAURANTS: fast foods, family, elegant, international. CONTACT: New Haven Convention and Visitors Bureau, 155 Church St., New Haven, CT 06510, (203) 787-8367. 300,000

SAIL FESTIVAL WEEKEND *early July*, New London, New London Co. Arts and crafts, cruises, waterfront fireworks, live entertainment, and games. FOODS SERVED: lots of seafood. ADMISSION: free. ACCOMMODATIONS: motels and hotels, B&B's, campgrounds, RV parks. RESTAURANTS: fast foods, family, elegant, international, seafood. CONTACT: Marine Commerce and Development, One Whale Oil Row, New London, CT 06320, (203) 443-8331.

SANTA MARIA MAGDELANA FEAST *third weekend in July*, New Haven, New Haven Co., on Wooster Street. "New Haven's largest and oldest ethnic festival" featuring rides, clowns, mimes, large processions down Wooster Street honoring Saint Mary Magdalen. FOODS SERVED: area restaurants serve their ethnic specialties at booths along the street. ADMISSION: free. ACCOMMODATIONS: motels and hotels, B&B's, campgrounds, RV parks.

RESTAURANTS: fast foods, family, elegant, international. CONTACT: Santa Maria Magdelana Society, New Haven, CT 06511, or the New Haven Convention and Visitors Bureau, 155 Church St., New Haven, CT 06510, (203) 787-8367. 120,000

PILLAR POLKABRATION *third and fourth weeks in July*, New London, New London Co., at Ocean Beach Park. More than forty bands from throughout the United States provide music for day and evening dancing, Polish dancers perform in costume. FOODS SERVED: Polish. ADMISSION: free. ACCOMMODATIONS: motels and hotels, B&B's, campgrounds, RV parks. RESTAURANTS: fast foods, family, elegant, international, seafood. CONTACT: Ocean Beach Park, New London, CT 06320, (203) 447-3031, or the Southeastern Connecticut Chamber of Commerce, One Whale Oil Row, New London, CT 06320, (203) 443-8332. 30,000

SHARON AUDUBON FESTIVAL *last weekend in July*, Sharon, Litchfield Co. Environmental exhibits and programs concerning New England weather, trees, wildflowers, wolves, whales and dolphins, wildlife landscaping, water studies, mosses and lichens, ponds and streams, exhibits of common knots and ropes, home-grown produce, native wildflowers, rocks and minerals, basket making, music by folksingers Bill Oliver and Glen Waldek. FOODS SERVED: beverages, salads, hot dogs, hamburgers, ice cream. ADMISSION: 12 and over $4.00, ages 5-11 $1.00, 5 and under free. ACCOMMODATIONS: motels and hotels, B&B's, campgrounds, RV parks. RESTAURANTS: fast foods, family, elegant. CONTACT: National Audubon Society and Housatonic Audubon Society, Northeast Audubon Center, R. R. 1. Box 171, Sharon, CT 06069, (203) 364-0520.

FESTIVAL ITALIANO *second week in August*, New London, New London Co., to celebrate residents' Italian heritage and culture. Opera, travelogue on Italy, "alta moda" fashions, Italian folk music and outdoor concerts, gallant ball, Miss Italia Pageant, wine tasting, religious processions, fireworks, professional bicycle racing, film festival, art exhibits. FOODS SERVED: Italian. ADMISSION: free, charges for some events. ACCOMMODATIONS: motels and hotels, B&B's, campgrounds. RESTAURANTS: fast foods, elegant, international. CONTACT: Festival Italiano, Inc., P.O. Box 870, New London, CT 06320, (203) 443-1884. 10,000

MYSTIC OUTDOOR ARTS FESTIVAL
second weekend in August, Mystic, New London Co. Festival is "one of New England's biggest and best outdoor art shows, spreading itself along the sidewalks of this picturesque shoreline village." More than 400 artists display and sell their works. FOODS SERVED: food booths and sit-down luncheons. ADMISSION: free. ACCOMMODATIONS: motels and hotels, B&B's, campgrounds, RV parks. RESTAURANTS: fast foods, family, elegant, "the very best of seafood," Chinese, Italian, Mexican. CONTACT: Mystic Chamber of Commerce, P.O. Box 143, Mystic, CT 06355, (203) 536-4730. 100,000

OYSTER FESTIVAL *third Saturday in August,* Milford, New Haven Co., on Long Island Sound. Arts and crafts, boat race, oyster shucking and oyster eating contests, live entertainment. FOODS SERVED: loads of food booths featuring oysters and other local seafoods. ADMISSION: free. ACCOMMODATIONS: motels and hotels, campgrounds. RESTAURANTS: fast foods, family, elegant, seafood. CONTACT: Peter Nagle, 28 Cardinal Dr., Milford, CT 06460, (203) 335-3111. 50,000

LONG ISLAND SOUND AMERICA
FESTIVAL *late August through Labor Day (early September),* headquartered at Milford, New Haven Co. Events all "over, under, on, and around Long Island Sound," including balloon races, fly-ins, boat races, theatrical performances, foot races, concerts, sky-diving, rafting and more. FOODS SERVED: concessions. AD-

MISSION: free. ACCOMMODATIONS: motels and hotels, campgrounds. RESTAURANTS: fast foods, family, elegant, seafood. CONTACT: LISA, Milford, CT 06460, (203) 877-3262.

NORWALK SEAPORT OYSTER FESTIVAL *second weekend in September,* Norwalk, Fairfield Co., as a celebration of Long Island Sound's "seafaring past." Arts and crafts show, boat parade, fireworks nightly, beer garden, display vessels, boat rides, fun park, contests, polka, jazz, and folk dancing. FOODS SERVED: seafood and ethnic foods. ADMISSION: $2.00, children under 6 free. ACCOMMODATIONS: motels and hotels, campgrounds. RESTAURANTS: fast foods, family, elegant, international, seafood. CONTACT: Norwalk Seaport's Association, 203 Liberty Sq., Norwalk, CT 06855, (203) 866-0184. 150,000

NEW HAVEN GREEK FESTIVAL *second weekend in September,* New Haven, New Haven Co., at Lighthouse Point Park. Live Greek music by "well-known Greek bands," belly dancing and ethnic dancers in traditional costumes, cultural and educational events, Greek marketplace, Greek coffee house by the seashore. FOODS SERVED: moussaka, shish-ke-bob, gyro, Greek demitasse and American coffee, baklava, honey puffs, sweet Greek breads, imported Greek gourmet foods. ADMISSION: free. ACCOMMODATIONS: motels and hotels, B&B's. RESTAURANTS: fast foods, family, elegant, international. CONTACT: Helen Proestakis at (203) 669-2122, or the New Haven Convention and Visitors Bureau, 900 Chapel St., Suite 520, New Haven, CT 06510, (203) 787-8367. 6,000

BRISTOL CHRYSANTHEMUM FESTIVAL AND INTERNATIONAL FESTIVAL *third weekend through the fourth weekend in September,* Bristol, Hartford Co. Art show, crafts fair, dog show, auction, fireworks, carnival, parade, food festival, lots of music. FOODS SERVED: Greek,

Lebanese, Spanish, Italian, Mexican, American. ADMISSION: free, charges for some events. ACCOMMODATIONS: B&B's. RESTAURANTS: fast foods, family, elegant. CONTACT: Chamber of Commerce, 55 N. Main St., Bristol, CT 06010, (203) 589-4111.

APPLE HARVEST FESTIVAL *first two weekends in October,* Southington, Hart-ford Co., to celebrate the harvest of apples from local orchards. Arts and crafts, bicycle races, parade, bed races, road races, apple products. FOODS SERVED: apple concoctions and apple products galore, other foods. ADMISSION: free. ACCOMMODATIONS: motels and hotels. RESTAURANTS: fast foods, family. CONTACT: Ann Hauver, 7 North Main St., Southington, CT 06489, (203) 628-8036. 350,000

MAINE

WINTER WONDERLAND WEEK *second week in February,* Bethel, Oxford Co., in the Bethel resort community of southwestern Maine. Hot air balloon flights, cross country race, scavenger hunt in the snow, cross country ski tours, skating party, ski movies, Moosehead Giant Slalom, sweetheart ski by lamplight, dog sled races, tours of historic Bed and Breakfast with hot refreshments, Morgan horse sleigh rides. FOODS SERVED: hors d'oeuvres, beverages, fish chowder, and other refreshments served at B&B's, inns. ADMISSION: free. ACCOMMODATIONS: motels and hotels, B&B's. RESTAURANTS: fast foods, family, elegant. CONTACT: Sunday River Ski Resort, Bethel, ME 04217, (207) 824-2187.

KENNEBEC WHATEVER WEEK AND RACE *ten days around July 4th,* Augusta, Kennebec Co., in the Kennebec Valley, to celebrate "the return of the Kennebec River to the people." Ten days of carnival, marathons, Mud Run, queen contest, softball, tennis, and volleyball tournaments, dances, climaxing in the Whatever Floats Raft Race featuring "homemade craft muscled by man or wind—no motors allowed," live entertainment which has included stars such as Charlie Pride. FOODS SERVED: chicken barbecues, concessions. ADMISSION: free, with $10.00 charge to register for a race.

ACCOMMODATIONS: motels and hotels, B&B's, campgrounds, RV parks. RESTAURANTS: fast foods, family, Italian, Chinese, Mexican. CONTACT: Kennebec Valley Chamber of Commerce, P. O. Box E, Augusta, ME 04330, (207) 623-4559. 40,000

FESTIVAL DE LA BASTILLE *second weekend in July (nearest the 14th),* Augusta, Kennebec Co., at the Calumet Club, to celebrate the French heritage of Augusta residents. Arts and crafts, eating and drinking, French Canadian entertainers. FOODS SERVED: French. ADMISSION: $1.00 per day. ACCOMMODATIONS: motels and hotels, B&B's, campgrounds, RV parks. RESTAURANTS: fast foods, family, Italian, Chinese, Mexican. CONTACT: Kennebec Valley Chamber of Commerce, P. O. Box E, Augusta, ME 04330, (207) 623-4559. 10,000

MOLLY OCKETT DAY *third Saturday in July,* Bethel, Oxford Co., on the Common. Molly Ockett was a Pequawket Indian who lived among the early settlers of western Maine, and was known as "the great Indian doctress," as a storyteller, and as an accomplished Indian craftswoman about whom legends abound. Molly Ockett Day Classic including 1 mi, 5k, and 10k foot races, Western Maine

Frog Jumping Contest, bed races, Professional Lumberjack Competition, Ronald McDonald Show, parade, golf tournament, arts and crafts, games on the Common, square dance exhibition, Old-Time Fiddlers Contest, fireworks display, music by the Last Straw Band. FOODS SERVED: barbecued chicken and fried clams, lobster rolls, concessions. ADMISSION: free. ACCOMMODATIONS: motels and hotels, B&B's, campgrounds, RV parks. RESTAURANTS: fast foods, family, elegant. CONTACT: Bethel Area Chamber of Commerce, Box 121, Bethel, ME 04217, (207) 824-2282. 5,000

MAINE POTATO BLOSSOM FESTIVAL third weekend in July, Fort Fairfield, Aroostook Co., to celebrate the blooming of Maine potatoes. Fishing derby, trapshoot, swim meet, bicycle rodeo, Queen's Tea, Potato Industry Dinner, horseshoe, archery, softball, and basketball tournaments, street dance in the municipal parking lot, Border City Classic 5k Road Race, Potato Blossom 5-Miler featuring the Aroostook Joggernauts, sidewalk arts and crafts sale, giant flea market, celebrity dunking booth, Mashed Potato Wrestling Contest, parade, Queen Scholarship Pageant, Roostook River Raft Race, Beautiful Baby Contest, golf tournament and horse show. FOODS SERVED: chicken barbecue and concessions. ADMISSION: free. ACCOMMODATIONS: B&B's. RESTAURANTS: fast foods, family. CONTACT: Fort Fairfield Chamber of Commerce, P.O. Box 607, Fort Fairfield, ME 04742, (207) 472-3381. 15,000

YARMOUTH CLAM FESTIVAL third weekend in July, Yarmouth, Cumberland Co., in the greater Portland area, to enjoy Maine seafood, especially clams. "Maine's biggest and best parade," Downeast Tennis Classic, art show featuring Littlejohn's Artists' Association, Great Royal River Canoe Race, aerobic and karate demonstrations, Fireman's Muster Ladder and Hose Contest, fireworks, bicycle race, ecumenical service, diaper derby, carnival,

balloon zoo, craft show, pink elephant sale, horse-drawn wagon rides, musical performances including Doc's Banjo Band, Devonsquare, Crazy Moonbeam, Bellamy Jazz Band, Oktoberfest Band, the Downeasters Barbershop Chorus and Quartets, Royal River Philharmonic Band, The Wicked Good Band, Joy Spring Jazz, Royal River Chapter of Sweet Adelines, Inc., and the Community Orchestra of The Portland Symphony. FOODS SERVED: blueberry pancake breakfast, breakfast bar, ham and turkey supper, loads of clam and seafood booths. ADMISSION: free. ACCOMMODATIONS: motels and hotels, nearby B&B's, and campgrounds. RESTAURANTS: family, seafood. CONTACT: Yarmouth Chamber of Commerce, Inc., P. O. Box 416, Yarmouth, ME 04096, (207) 846-3984. 60,000

MAINE LOBSTER FESTIVAL last weekend in July, Rockland, Knox Co., at the Public Landing. "The Original Lobster Festival" recognizes and serves Maine seafoods. Crafts, marine and commercial exhibits, lobster crate and trap hauling contests, crowning of Maine Sea Goddess, children's activities, art and photo exhibits, live entertainment including local and professional groups, talent show, and lobster eating contest. FOODS SERVED: lobster and seafoods, some other concessions. ADMISSION: $1.00 per person per day. ACCOMMODATIONS: (nearby) motels and hotels, B&B's, campgrounds, RV parks. RESTAURANTS: (nearby) fast foods, family, elegant, Maine seafood. CONTACT: Rockland Chamber of Commerce, Box 508, Rockland, ME 04841, (207) 596-0376. 25,000

INTERNATIONAL FESTIVAL first full week in August, Calais, Washington Co., and St. Stephen, New Brunswick, Canada, to celebrate and foster "international cooperation and friendship." Parade from one country to the other, 5 mi run through both countries; Miss International, Little Miss and Cutie Baby Pageants, street fair, craft fair, bingo, golf tournament, blue-

grass, country, Irish, and rock music performed outdoors and at dances; dinners, beerfest. FOODS SERVED: "down east" such as "basic country and lobster, beer." ADMISSION: varies by event, many free. ACCOMMODATIONS: motels and hotels, campgrounds, RV parks. RESTAURANTS: fast foods, family, elegant, seafood. CONTACT: International Festival, Inc., P. O. Box 367, St. Stephen, New Brunswick, E3L 2W9 or Sharon Frost in Calais, ME at (207) 454-3531.

WINTER HARBOR LOBSTER FESTIVAL *second Saturday in August,* Winter Harbor, Hancock Co., throughout town and at Acadia National Park, to honor the wonders of succulent lobster caught in the Winter Harbor area. Lobster boat races in fourteen categories feature "some of the fastest lobster boats around" and include a boat-builders class, Maine crafts, Fisherman's Tug of War with competition between towns, Kids Whacky Water Walk, 15 k Road Race Scenic Run, Marine Trade Show, softball tournament, karate demonstration, parade down Main Street, entertainment featuring lots of Maine humorists like Tim Sample, Humble Farmer Robert Skoglund, singer-songwriter Dave Mallett, the Danny Harper Band. FOODS SERVED: lobster feed and other seafoods. ADMISSION: free, charge for Lobster Feed $7.00–$8.00. ACCOMMODATIONS: motels and hotels, B&B's, campgrounds, RV parks. RESTAURANTS: family, seafood. CONTACT: Winter Harbor Chamber of Commerce, P. O. Box 459, Winter Harbor, ME 04693, (207) 963-5561. 10,000

MAINE FESTIVAL OF THE ARTS *third weekend in August,* Portland, Cumberland Co., to honor both the performing and visual arts. "The largest arts festival in the Northeast" includes exhibitions of crafts, Maine-made products and folk arts such as pine tree quilters, decoy carvers, Native American basketmakers, quillworkers and canoebuilders, Ukrainian Pysanky, fish smokehouse, wooden boatbuilding, and Shaker herb lore, including more than 800 participating artists each year; six continuously operating performance stages feature jazz, rock, classical, traditional folk and ethnic music such as Oi Gongen Daiko from Japan, Ghana's Talking Drums, Los Lobos, Leo Kottke, The Roches, Tiny Moore and hundreds more; dance; Maine Storytellers' Convention, Maine Songwriters' Convention, and world premieres of festival-commissioned works by contemporary choreographers and performers. FOODS SERVED: gourmet with emphasis on Maine's ethnic groups such as French, Southeast Asian, Greek, and Italian. ADMISSION: adults $7.00 per day, $12.00 per day and evening, children half price. ACCOMMODATIONS: motels and hotels, B&B's, campgrounds, RV parks. RESTAURANTS: fast foods, family, elegant, international, Cajun, Maine seafood. CONTACT: Maine Arts, Inc., 29 Forest Ave., Portland, ME 04101, (207) 772-9012. 30,000

FALL FOLIAGE COUNTRY FAIR *Columbus Day weekend (near October 12th),* Boothbay, Lincoln Co., at the Boothbay Railway Village, in recognition of the end of "summer season." More than 120 booths featuring arts and crafts. FOODS SERVED: Maine products and foods, baked goods, live entertainment. ADMISSION: free. ACCOMMODATIONS: motels and hotels, B&B's, campgrounds, RV parks. CONTACT: Mrs. Ellen Morrisette, Kenniston Hill Inn, or the Boothbay Chamber of Commerce, P.O. Box 161, Boothbay, ME 04537, (207) 633-4743 (seasonal). 5,000

NEW YEAR'S/PORTLAND *December 31,* Portland, Cumberland Co., downtown, to recognize the performing and visual arts. More than 100 performances at ten locations throughout "intown" Portland including classical, jazz, rock, reggae, traditional folk, Franco-American, Latin, bluegrass, ethnic, and folk music, and dance, mime, juggling, contemporary performance arts, participatory dancing, gala midnight parade and fireworks. FOODS SERVED: concessions. ADMISSION: adults $7.00, children and seniors $3.00. ACCOM-

MODATIONS: motels and hotels, B&B's. RESTAURANTS: fast foods, family, elegant, international, Cajun, Maine seafood. CON-TACT: Maine Arts, Inc., 29 Forest Ave., Portland, ME 04101, (207) 772-9012. 15,000

MASSACHUSETTS

DAFFODIL FESTIVAL *fourth weekend in April,* Brewster, Barnstable Co., on Cape Cod. More than 40,000 daffodils planted in the 1980's bloom, craft shows, floral displays, bike race, golf and tennis tournaments, films, tours of inns and historic tours, Classic Sport Cars Exhibit, herb demonstration, open houses, all coinciding with the herring run. FOODS SERVED: chowder, food booths. ADMISSION: free. ACCOMMODATIONS: motels and hotels, B&B's, campgrounds nearby. RESTAURANTS: family, elegant. CONTACT: Cape Cod Chamber of Commerce, Hyannis, MA 02601, (617) 362-3225.

ROCKPORT MUSIC FESTIVAL *month of June,* Rockport, Essex Co., at the Rockport Art Association. Each week two existing chamber groups collaborate for concerts running Thursday through Sunday featuring composer-in-residence and co-artistic director David Alpher and artists who have included the Annapolis Brass Quintet, Manhattan String Quartet, An Die Musik, Jubal Trio, Alexander String Quartet, Emmanuel Wind Quintet, Trio dell'arte, and guest narrator Robert J. Lurtsema. ADMISSION: adults $10.00, senior citizens and students $7.50, subscription plans available. ACCOMMODATIONS: motels and hotels, campgrounds nearby. RESTAURANTS: family, elegant. CONTACT: David Alpher, Box 312, Rockport, MA 01966, (617) 546-7391, or the Cape Ann Chamber of Commerce, 128 Main St., Gloucester, MA 01930, (617) 283-1601. 3,300

ST. PETER'S FIESTA AND BLESSING OF THE FLEET *last weekend in June,* Gloucester, Essex Co., to recognize the Gloucester fishing fleet and fishermen. Seine boat races, Blessing of the Fleet by Cardinal Law, sporting events, fireworks. FOODS SERVED: Italian. ADMISSION: free. ACCOMMODATIONS: motels and hotels, campgrounds. RESTAURANTS: fast foods, family, elegant, seafood. CONTACT: Cape Ann Chamber of Commerce, 128 Main St., Gloucester, MA 01930, (617) 283-1601.

WHALING CITY FESTIVAL *weekend after July 4th,* New Bedford, Bristol Co., at Buttonwood Park and Zoo. Craft show and flea market, children's entertainment. FOODS SERVED: "vendors." ADMISSION: free. ACCOMMODATIONS: motels and hotels, B&B's, campgrounds. RESTAURANTS: fast foods, family, elegant, international. CONTACT: City of New Bedford, Office of Tourism, New Bedford, MA 02740, (617) 991-6200. 50,000

NATIONAL FOLK FESTIVAL *fourth weekend in July,* Lowell, Essex Co., downtown, "the oldest multi-ethnic festival in (the) country." Showcase for ethnic talents, ethnic music and dancing, crafts, cultural exhibits, photo contests, evening concerts. FOODS SERVED: Asian, Irish, Greek, Spanish, Black. ADMISSION: free. ACCOMMODATIONS: motels and hotels, B&B's, campgrounds. RESTAURANTS: fast foods, family, elegant, Greek, Asian, Indian. CONTACT: The Chambers of Commerce and Industry, 45 Palmer St., Lowell, MA 01852, (617) 454-5633. 40,000

FEAST OF THE BLESSED SACRAMENT *first weekend in August,* New Bedford, Bristol Co., at Madeira Field, to celebrate the "Portuguese community from the Madeira Islands." Portuguese folkloric dancers and singers, Portuguese music, carnival. FOODS SERVED: Portuguese. ADMISSION: free. ACCOMMODATIONS: motels and hotels, B&B's, campgrounds. RESTAURANTS: fast foods, family, elegant, international. CONTACT: City of New Bedford, Office of Tourism, New Bedford, MA 02740, (617) 991-6200. 300,000

CENTER STREET FESTIVAL *second weekend in August,* New Bedford, Bristol Co., in the Waterfront Historic District, to celebrate its revitalization. Arts and crafts displays and demonstrations, music, street performers. FOODS SERVED: "vendors." ADMISSION: free. ACCOMMODATIONS: motels and hotels, B&B's, campgrounds. RESTAURANTS: fast foods, family, elegant, international. CONTACT: City of New Bedford, Office of Tourism, New Bedford, MA 02740, (617) 991-6200. 50,000

WATERFRONT FESTIVAL *third weekend in August,* Gloucester, Essex Co., on Cape Ann. Handmade crafts, military reenactment, live entertainment, fish fry. ADMISSION: free. ACCOMMODATIONS: motels and hotels, campgrounds. FOODS SERVED: pancake breakfast, fish fry. RESTAURANTS: fast foods, family, elegant. CONTACT: Waterfront Festivals, Ltd., P.O. Box 6159, Newburyport, MA 01950, (617) 462-1333, or the Cape Ann Chamber of Commerce, 128 Main St., Gloucester, MA 01930, (617) 283-1601.

FESTIVAL BY THE SEA *third weekend in August,* New Bedford, Bristol Co., at Piers 3 and 4, to salute New Bedford fishermen. Crafts, live entertainment, seafood tasting, FOODS SERVED: seafood, concessions. ADMISSION: free. ACCOMMODATIONS: motels and hotels, B&B's, campgrounds. RESTAURANTS: fast foods, family, elegant, international. CONTACT: City of New Bedford, Office of Tourism,

New Bedford, MA 02740, (617) 991-6200. 30,000

DENNIS FESTIVAL DAYS *last full week in August,* Dennis, Barnstable Co., on Cape Cod as "a party for all," to celebrate the "end of summer." Arts and crafts show, antique car exhibit and motorcade, band concert, Blueberry Recipe Contest, beer races, children's creative art show, flea market, Handicap Awareness Day, canoe race, cruise of Bass River, yacht races, 3–D Film Festival, Family Film Festival, puppets, Teen Dance, golf tournaments including grandmothers and grandfathers tournaments, book sale, bike tour, Kite Flying Contest, 40's Night, antique show and sale, magic show, Old Sound Show, road race, miniature golf. FOODS SERVED: blueberry baked goods, barbecue, Jazz Festival Cook-Out, smorgasbord, concessions. ADMISSION: free, charges to $5.00 for some events. ACCOMMODATIONS: motels and hotels, B&B's, campground, RV parks. RESTAURANTS: fast foods, family, elegant. CONTACT: Dennis Chamber of Commerce, P.O. Box 275, South Dennis, MA 02660, (617) 398-3573. 10,000

LOWER CAPE ARTS FESTIVAL *throughout September,* Provincetown, Truro, and Wellfleet, Barnstable Co., to highlight local ·artists. Theatrical and musical performances featuring local entertainers and artists. FOODS SERVED: Portuguese. ADMISSION: free. ACCOMMODATIONS: motels and hotels, B&B's, campgrounds, RV parks. RESTAURANTS: fast foods, family, elegant, Italian, Greek, Portuguese, French. CONTACT: Provincetown Chamber of Commerce, P.O. Box 1017, Provincetown, MA 02657, (617) 487-3424. 30,000

WORLD KIELBASA FESTIVAL *weekend after Labor Day (early September),* Chicopee, Hampden Co., on the grounds of Fairfield Mall, to recognize and celebrate Polish culture. Kielbasa cooking and eating contests, display of King Kielbasa, arts and crafts exhibits, amusement rides, midway, clowns, family fun, continuous entertainment by "top-name Polish and pop bands" including Jimmy Sturr, the Rymanowski Brothers, Dick Pillar, and the Crescents. FOODS SERVED: Polish kielbasa, golumbki, pierogis, Italian and Chinese foods. ADMISSION: adults $3.00, children 12 and under when accompanied by adult $2.00, advance adult tickets $2.00. ACCOMMODATIONS: motels and hotels. RESTAURANTS: fast foods, family, Polish, Italian, Chinese. CONTACT: Chicopee Chamber of Commerce Fireball Club, 93 Church St., Chicopee, MA 01020, (413) 594-2101. 60,000

CRANBERRY HARVEST FESTIVAL *second Friday through third Sunday in September,* Harwich, Barnstable Co., on Cape Cod. Cranberry Ball begins the celebration on the second Friday, followed by hundreds of events over nine days, including an arts and crafts show, fireworks, Country-Western Jamboree, and a "huge parade" on the final Sunday. FOODS SERVED: cranberries in many forms, concessions. ADMISSION: free. ACCOMMODATIONS: motels and hotels, B&B's, campgrounds nearby. RESTAURANTS: fast foods, family, elegant. CONTACT: Harwich Chamber of Commerce, Box 34, Harwich Port, MA 02646, summer: (617) 432-1600.

BOURNE SCALLOP FESTIVAL *second weekend in September,* Buzzards Bay, Barnstable Co., on Cape Cod at Buzzards Bay Park. Sixty craft, gift, and specialty booths, live entertainment daily. FOODS SERVED: scallop dinners. ADMISSION: free, charge for scallop dinners. ACCOMMODATIONS: motels and hotels, B&B's, campgrounds nearby. RESTAURANTS: family, elegant. CONTACT: Greater Bourne–Sandwich Chamber of Commerce, P. O. Box 304, Buzzards Bay, MA 02532, (617) 888-6202.

GREEK FOOD FESTIVAL *September,* Brockton, Plymouth Co. Greek hand-

crafts, children's games, Greek music, Macedonian dancers, Greek dancers and bands. FOODS SERVED: Greek shish kebob, moussaka, pastichio, dolmathas, pilaf, salads, and pastries. ADMISSION: free. ACCOMMODATIONS: motels and hotels, B&B's, campgrounds, RV parks nearby. RESTAURANTS: fast foods, family, elegant, international. CONTACT: Brockton Regional Chamber of Commerce, 1 Legion Parkway, Brockton, MA 02401, (617) 586-0500. 10,000

NORTHERN BERKSHIRE FALL FOLIAGE FESTIVAL *first weekend in October,* North Adams, Berkshire Co., in the Berkshires, to welcome autumn. "Mammoth parade," art show, dances, pet show, bicycle race, children's races and children's parade, crafts fair. FOODS SERVED: Italian and Polish. ADMISSION: varies by event, many free. ACCOMMODATIONS: motels and hotels, B&B's, campgrounds, RV parks. RESTAURANTS: fast foods, family, elegant, Mexican, Chinese, French, Italian. CONTACT: Northern Berkshire Chamber of Commerce, 69 Main St., North Adams, MA 01247, (413) 663-3735. 70,000

FIRST NIGHT NEW BEDFORD *December 31,* New Bedford, Bristol Co., to celebrate the New Year. Art shows, ice sculptures, continuous entertainment beginning midafternoon until midnight including jazz, folk music, storytelling, First Night Festival Orchestra, Your Theatre, James Puppet Theatre, Sippican Choral Society, fireworks display over New Bedford Harbor. FOODS SERVED: concessions. ADMISSION: $2.00 button admits to all events. ACCOMMODATIONS: motels and hotels, B&B's. RESTAURANTS: fast foods, family, elegant, international. CONTACT: City of New Bedford, Office of Tourism, New Bedford, MA 02740, (617) 991-6200. 15,000

NEW HAMPSHIRE

LAKES REGION FINE ARTS AND CRAFTS FESTIVAL *Labor Day weekend (early September)*, Meredith, Belknap Co., in the Lakes Region. More than ninety juried artists and craftspeople display and sell their works, musical entertainment. FOODS SERVED: "culinary delights." AD-MISSION: free. ACCOMMODATIONS: motels and hotels, B&B's, campgrounds. RESTAURANTS: fast foods, family, elegant. CONTACT: Meredith Chamber of Commerce, Box 732, Meredith, NH 03253, (603) 279-6121.

NEW JERSEY

THOMPSON PARK DAY *May 17*, Lincroft, Monmouth Co., in the Shore Region at Thompson Park. Arts and crafts, fine arts show, races, participation games, clowns, mimes, bands, folk singers. FOODS SERVED: concessions. ADMISSION: free. ACCOMMODATIONS: motels and hotels, campgrounds, RV parks. RESTAURANTS: fast foods, family. CONTACT: Monmouth Co. Park System, Newman Springs Rd., Lincroft, NJ 07738, (201) 842-4000. 12,000

FISHAWACK *second Saturday in June, even-numbered years*, Chatham, Morris Co., to celebrate the arts and crafts of American Indians and colonial heritage. Arts and crafts show and sale, Block Dance, giveaways, street festival, musical performances by local bands and choral groups, disc jockey with oldies, and the Quality Children's Musical Theatre. FOODS SERVED: ribs, hamburgers, hot dogs. ADMISSION: free. ACCOMMODATIONS: (nearby) motels and hotels, B&B. RESTAURANTS: family, elegant. CONTACT: Chatham Chamber of Commerce, P. O. Box 231, Chatham, NJ 07928, (201) 377-2750. 10,000

VICTORIAN PLAINFIELD FESTIVAL OF ART *second Saturday in July*, Plainfield, Union Co. More than 400 artists and craftspeople vie for thousands of dollars in prizes and display and sell their works. FOODS SERVED: concessions. ADMISSION: free. ACCOMMODATIONS: motels and hotels. RESTAURANTS: fast foods, family, elegant. CONTACT: Central Jersey Chamber of Commerce, 120 W. Seventh St., Plainfield, NJ 07060, (201) 754-7250.

FROGTOWN FROLIC *third Saturday in September (rain date fourth Saturday)*, Lincroft, Monmouth Co., at Thompson Park. Arts and crafts, pet show and competition, games, and races. FOODS SERVED: concessions. ADMISSION: $2.00 per person. ACCOMMODATIONS: motels and hotels, campgrounds, RV parks. RESTAURANTS: fast foods, family. CONTACT: Monmouth Co. Park System, Newman Springs Rd., Lincroft, NJ 07738, (201) 842-4000. 12,000

FESTIVAL ON THE GREEN *third Sunday in September (rain date fourth Sunday)*, Union, Union Co. Display and sale of art work, crafts, and photography, judged by professionals with cash prizes, performances by dance groups, puppeteers, and the Union Municipal Band. FOODS SERVED: all-American concessions. ADMISSION: free. ACCOMMODATIONS: motels and hotels. RESTAURANTS: fast foods, family, elegant, Italian, German. CONTACT: Union Township Chamber of Commerce, 2165 Morris Ave., Union, NJ 07083, (no phone calls). 12,000

TURKEY SWAMP PARK DAY *October 18*, Freehold, Monmouth Co., in the Shore Region at Turkey Swamp Park. Arts and crafts, fine art show, races, participation games, clowns, mimes, folk singers, and bands. FOODS SERVED: concessions. ADMISSION: free. ACCOMMODATIONS: motels and hotels, campgrounds, RV parks. RESTAURANTS: fast foods, family. CONTACT: Monmouth Co. Park System, Newman Springs Rd., Lincroft, NJ 07738, (201) 842-4000. 7,000

NEW YORK

WINTER CARNIVAL *second weekend in February*, Saranac Lake, Franklin Co., "the oldest winter carnival in the United States." Inner-tube races (on snow), snowshoe softball, ice golf, rugby, skiing and skating races, SnoBall, Gala Parade, torchlight skiing and snowmobiling, broom hockey, woodsmen's exhibition, ice diving, Ice Palace slide show, fireworks, entertainment featuring local talent. FOODS SERVED: concessions. ADMISSION: free. ACCOMMODATIONS: motels and hotels, B&B's. RESTAURANTS: fast foods, family, elegant, Mexican. CONTACT: Saranac Lake Area Chamber of Commerce, 30 Main St., Saranac Lake, NY 12983, (518) 891-1990.

INTERNATIONAL FESTIVAL *first Sunday in May*, Peekskill, Westchester Co., at River Front Green Park, as a fundraiser for the Community Ambulance Corps. "Potpourri of international foods, music, dance, crafts, and art with the entire park trimmed with flowers," variety of entertainment. FOODS SERVED: "international culinary delights from selected countries throughout the world." ADMISSION: $5.00 advance, $5.00 at the gate; supervised children under 12 free. ACCOMMODATIONS: motels and hotels. RESTAURANTS: fast foods, family, elegant. CONTACT: Peekskill/Cortlandt Chamber of Commerce, One S. Division St., Peekskill, NY 10566, (914) 737-3600.

TULIP FESTIVAL *Mother's Day weekend (early May)*, Albany, Albany Co., to celebrate spring and the Dutch heritage of many Albany residents. Tulip flower show, children's fair, arts and crafts, old world tradition of scrubbing the streets, crowning the Tulip Queen, music, dance, and theatre. FOODS SERVED: Dutch and other ethnic foods. ADMISSION: free. ACCOMMODATIONS: motels and hotels, B&B's. RESTAURANTS: fast foods, family, elegant, Chinese, Indonesian, Greek, French, Italian. CONTACT: Albany Co. Convention and Visitors Bureau, 52 S. Pearl St., Albany, NY 12207, (518) 434-1217.

CATSKILLS IRISH FESTIVAL *Memorial Day weekend (late May)*, East Durham, Greene Co., "Imported Irish entertainers, music, dancing, imported Irish merchandise, beers." Entertainers have included Dermott Henry, Paddy Noonan, Martin Flynn, and Pat Roper. FOODS SERVED: Irish foods and beer. ADMISSION: $4.00–$5.00. ACCOMMODATIONS: motels and hotels, B&B's, campgrounds, RV parks. RESTAURANTS: fast foods, family, elegant, Irish, Chinese, continental. CONTACT: East Durham Vacationland Festival Committee, Box 67, East Durham, NY 12423, (518) 634-7100, or The Greene County, Box 467, Catskill, NY 12414, (518) 943-3223. 10,000

WOODSTOCK FESTIVAL OF THE ARTS *June through October,* Woodstock, Ulster Co., in the Catskill Mountains. In a renowned center for the arts, the summer program includes the Dance Festival at the Playhouse, touring Broadway musicals, new plays series, and Sunday Maverick Concerts. ADMISSION: charges vary. ACCOMMODATIONS: motels and hotels, B&B's, campgrounds. RESTAURANTS: nearby fast foods, family, elegant. CONTACT: Woodstock Playhouse Association, Box 396, Woodstock, NY 12498, (914) 679-6000 or 679-2436. 100,000

ALLENTOWN ART FESTIVAL AND JUNETEENTH FESTIVAL *second or third weekend in June,* Buffalo, Erie Co. Allentown Art Festival features more than 500 exhibitors of arts and crafts including historic and contemporary disciplines in "one of the nation's largest preservation districts." Juneteenth celebrates the freedom of slaves in the 1870s and includes a big parade. FOODS SERVED: variety of concessions including ethnic delicacies. ADMISSION: free. ACCOMMODATIONS: motels and hotels, B&B's, campgrounds and RV parks nearby. RESTAURANTS: fast foods, family, elegant, international. CONTACT: Buffalo Area Chamber of Commerce, 107 Delaware Ave., Buffalo, NY 14202, (716) 852-7100.

STRAWBERRY FESTIVAL *third weekend in June,* Owego, Tioga Co., near Binghamton, to celebrate the strawberry harvest. Crafts, parade, fireworks, concession booths, clowns, mimes, and musical entertainment. FOODS SERVED: strawberry concoctions, Italian, Greek. ADMISSION: free. ACCOMMODATIONS: motels and hotels, campgrounds, RV parks. RESTAURANTS: fast foods, family. CONTACT: Tioga Co. Chamber of Commerce, 188 Front St., Owego, NY 13827, (607) 687-2020. 20,000

BACH ARIA FESTIVAL *third and fourth weeks in June,* Stony Brook, L.I., at the State University of New York Campus. Musicians from throughout the United States perform, study, and participate in symposia. ADMISSION: charge. ACCOMMODATIONS: motels and hotels, campgrounds nearby. RESTAURANTS: fast foods, family, elegant. CONTACT: Carol Baron, State University of New York, Stony Brook, NY 11794, (516) 689-6000.

SUMMERSCAPE ARTS FESTIVAL *late June through August,* Huntington, Long Island. Musical programs in Huntington's Heckscher Park featuring music, dance theatre ballet, choral performances, musicals, jazz, and some children's matinees on the Chapin Rainbow Stage. Entertainers have included Carmen McRae, the Long Island Philharmonic, the Paris Boys' Choir, North Carolina Dance Theatre, Oliver, American Ballroom Theatre, and the Jubilation Dance Co. ADMISSION: free to most events. ACCOMMODATIONS: motels and hotels, B&B's, campgrounds nearby. RESTAURANTS: fast foods, family, elegant. CONTACT: Arts Council, 213 Main St., Huntington, NY 11743, (516) 271-8442. 100,000

WEDNESDAYS AND SUNDAYS AT THE PLAZA *every Wednesday and Sunday from July 1 through September 13,* Albany, Albany Co., at Empire State Plaza, to recognize and feature "various ethnic cultures." "Thirty free public outdoor events on the Empire State Plaza" including ethnic and cultural family-oriented activities, such as Children's Day, International Bazaar, Black Arts and Cultural Festival, Irish Day, Italian Festa, arts and crafts show, and a senior showcase. FOODS SERVED: in accord with country featured each day. ADMISSION: free. ACCOMMODATIONS: motels and hotels, B&B's. RESTAURANTS: fast foods, family, elegant, Chinese, French, Italian, Indonesian, Greek. CONTACT: Albany Co. Convention and Visitors Bureau, 52 S. Pearl St., Albany, NY 12207, (518) 434-1217.

ITALIAN FESTIVAL *July 4th weekend,* Hunter, Greene Co., in the Catskills. Italian crafts, gifts, singing, dancing, and "top entertainment," which in the past has included Sergio Franchi, Frankie Avalon, Bobby Rydell, and Fabian. FOODS SERVED: Italian. ADMISSION: $7.50. ACCOMMODATIONS: motels and hotels, B&B's, campgrounds, RV parks. RESTAURANTS: fast foods, family, elegant, Northern Italian, Irish, continental, Chinese. CONTACT: Don Conover, Exposition Planners, Bridge St., Hunter, NY 12442, (518) 263-3800, or The Greene County, Box 467, Catskill, NY 12414, (518) 943-3223. 8,000

HARBOR FESTIVAL *July 4th,* New York, New York Co., hosted by the Port Authority of New York and New Jersey. Stars and Stripes Regatta, Liberty Cup, and Celebrity Regatta, fireworks, parades, crafts festivals and many ethnic festivals. ADMISSION: free. ACCOMMODATIONS: motels and hotels. RESTAURANTS: fast foods, family, elegant, international. CONTACT: Harbor Festival Foundation, Inc., World Trade Center, Suite 68W, New York, NY 10048, (212) 432-0998. 700,000

CORN HILL ART FESTIVAL *weekend after July 4th,* Rochester, Monroe Co. More than 500 artists and craftspeople display a variety of arts and crafts along twenty blocks of Rochester's historic district, entertainment including wide range of American and ethnic music. FOODS SERVED: multi-ethnic and American. ADMISSION: free. ACCOMMODATIONS: motels and hotels, B&B's. RESTAURANTS: fast foods, family, elegant, international. CONTACT: Convention and Visitors Bureau, 120 E. Main St., Rochester, NY 14604, (716) 546-3070. 150,000

TASTE OF BUFFALO *early July,* Buffalo, Eric Co. An outdoor epicurean festival featuring the specialities of Buffalo's ethnic restaurants, prepared and served outdoors on Main Street, continuous entertainment. FOODS SERVED: wide variety of ethnic delicacies. ADMISSION: free. ACCOMMODATIONS: motels and hotels, B&B's, campgrounds, RV parks nearby.

RESTAURANTS: fast foods, family, elegant, international. CONTACT: Buffalo Area Chamber of Commerce, 107 Delaware Ave., Buffalo, NY 14202, (716) 852-7100.

CHRISTMAS IN JULY *second Friday and Saturday in July,* Bath, Steuben Co., in the Finger Lakes region. Christmas decorations are hung in July to raise money for new decorations and other downtown projects. Teddy Bear Contest, parade, Bathtub races, crafts, entertainment by "none you have ever heard of," sidewalk sales. FOODS SERVED: "all kinds." ADMISSION: free. ACCOMMODATIONS: motels and hotels, B&B's, campgrounds, RV parks. RESTAURANTS: fast foods, family, elegant. CONTACT: Greater Bath Chamber of Commerce, P. O. Box 425, Bath, NY 14810, (607) 776-4031. 10,000

POTSDAM SUMMER FESTIVAL *second weekend in July,* Potsdam, St. Lawrence Co., in northern New York, to celebrate summer. Craft show and fair, Antique Car Show, BMX Race, Sportsmen's Show, sidewalk sales. Teen Dance, open air concert, Strawberry Festival, and big band sounds of the Stardusters. FOODS SERVED: strawberries, concessions. ADMISSION: free. ACCOMMODATIONS: motels and hotels, B&B's, campgrounds. RESTAURANTS: fast foods, family, elegant, Mexican, French, Chinese. CONTACT: Potsdam Chamber of Commerce, P. O. Box 717, Potsdam, NY 13676, (315) 265-5584. 5,000

LAKE GEORGE OPERA FESTIVAL *mid-July through mid-August,* Queensbury, Warren Co. Repertory productions in English, Opera On The Lake cruises each Sunday evening. FOODS SERVED: wine, champagne, soda, hors d'oeuvres. ADMISSION: charge. ACCOMMODATIONS: motels and hotels, B&B's, campgrounds, RV parks. RESTAURANTS: fast foods, family, elegant, international. CONTACT: Opera Festival, Box 425, Glens Falls, NY 12801, (518) 793-3858.

GERMAN ALPS FESTIVAL *three weeks in July*, Hunter, Greene Co. Goebelfest, "imported German entertainment such as Stadtkapelle Kempten," German dancing and dance lessons, singing, German crafts and gifts. FOODS SERVED: German foods and imported German beer. ADMISSION: $14.00. ACCOMMODATIONS: motels and hotels, B&B's, campgrounds, RV parks. RESTAURANTS: fast foods, family, elegant, continental, Chinese, Irish. CONTACT: Don Conover, Exposition Planners, Bridge St., Hunter, NY 12442, (518) 263-3800, or The Greene County, Box 467, Catskill, NY 12414, (518) 943-3223. 8,000

JULYFEST *third weekend in July*, Binghamton, Broome Co., to celebrate summer. Downtown Binghamton is filled with arts and crafts, antiques and collectibles, puppet show, concerts, and a farmers' market. FOODS SERVED: variety of ethnic foods. ADMISSION: free. ACCOMMODATIONS: motels and hotels, B&B's. RESTAURANTS: fast foods, family, elegant. CONTACT: Business and Professional Association, Box 995, Binghamton, NY 13902, (607) 772-8860.

INTERNATIONAL SEAWAY FESTIVAL *third weekend through fourth week in July*, Ogdensburg, St. Lawrence Co., across the St. Lawrence River from Ontario, Canada. Fishing derby, canoe race, bicycle race, 10,000m Run, Battle of Drums, tug of war, arts and crafts show, Antique Car Show, amusement rides, International Seaway Parade, big name entertainers such as Mel Tillis, Box Car Willie, Pointer Sisters, Janie Fricke, Chubby Checker, Tommy Hunter, Brenda Lee, and Mickey Gilley. FOODS SERVED: French Canadian, Italian, American. ADMISSION: free to some events, $8.00–$10.00 for others. ACCOMMODATIONS: motels and hotels, B&B's, campgrounds. RESTAURANTS: fast foods, family, elegant. CONTACT: Ogdensburg Chamber of Commerce, Community Center, Riverside Ave., Ogdensburg, NY 13669, (315) 393-3620. 50,000

COUNTRY MUSIC FESTIVAL Parts I and II *last weekend in July through first weekend in August, and third or fourth weekend in August*, Hunter, Greene Co. Commercial wares and gifts sales, beerfest, dancing, and "top entertainment" which has included the Oak Ridge Boys, Loretta Lynn, Crystal Gale, Ricky Skaggs, Waylon Jennings, Sweethearts of Rodeo, Forester Sisters, Mel Daniel, Tammy Wynette, Brenda Lee, Eddie Rabbitt, the Legends of Bluegrass, and Joe Stampley. FOODS SERVED: concessions, beerfest. ADMISSION: $14.00. ACCOMMODATIONS: motels and hotels, B&B's, campgrounds, RV parks. RESTAURANTS: fast foods, family, elegant, Irish, continental, Chinese. CONTACT: Don Conover, Exposition Planners, Bridge St., Hunter, NY 12442, (518) 263-3800, or The Greene County, Box 467, Catskill, NY 12414, (518) 943-3223.

INTERARTS FESTIVAL *month of August*, Palenville, Greene Co., near the town of Catskill, to celebrate the visual and performing arts. Chinese Golden Dragon Acrobats, Throne Dance Theatre, Yun Yung Tsuai Dancers, On The Lam Dixieland Band, Dave Brubeck and Laverne Trio, circus arts workshop and circus, children's shows, Great Australian Boomerang Meet, workshops. FOODS SERVED: ethnic and concessions. ADMISSION: varies by performance. ACCOMMODATIONS: motels and hotels, B&B's, campgrounds, RV parks. RESTAURANTS: fast foods, family, elegant, Irish, continental, Chinese. CONTACT: Palenville Interarts Colony, P. O. Box 59, Palenville, NY 12463, (518) 678-3332, or The Greene County, Box 467, Catskill, NY 12414, (518) 943-3223.

COXSACKIE RIVERSIDE FESTIVAL *first Saturday in August*, Coxsackie, Greene Co., to celebrate the arts. Arts and crafts displays and sales, riverboat rides, regional musical performances, dancing. FOODS SERVED: "variety." ADMISSION: free. ACCOMMODATIONS: motels and hotels, B&B's, campgrounds, RV parks.

RESTAURANTS: fast foods, family, elegant, Irish, continental, Chinese. CONTACT: Coxsackie Council on the Arts, Box 1, Coxsackie, NY 12051, (518) 731-2666, or The Greene County, Box 467, Catskill, NY 12414, (518) 943-3223.

NATIONAL POLKA FESTIVAL *first or second long weekend in August,* Hunter, Greene Co. Polka dancing and bands, polka dance lessons and contests, National Polka Queen Contest, crafts, "top entertainment including Bobby Vinton." FOODS SERVED: Polish foods and beers. ADMISSION: $7.50. ACCOMMODATIONS: motels and hotels, B&B's, campgrounds, RV parks. RESTAURANTS: fast foods, family, elegant, Irish, continental, Chinese. CONTACT: Don Conover, Exposition Planners, Bridge St., Hunter, NY 12442, (518) 263-3800, or The Greene County, Box 467, Catskill, NY 12414, (518) 943-3223.

SAUERKRAUT FESTIVAL *early August,* Phelps, Ontario Co., the "Sauerkraut Capital of the World." Parade, live entertainment, and special sauerkraut events. FOODS SERVED: loads of sauerkraut in everything, others to unpucker your mouth. ADMISSION: free. ACCOMMODATIONS AND RESTAURANTS in nearby Geneva. CONTACT: Finger Lakes Association, Lake St., Penn Yan, NY 14527, (315) 536-7488.

HARLEM WEEK *part of second week and third full week in August,* New York, New York Co. Large street fair including crafts, sightseeing tours, gospel, jazz and rhythm and blues concerts, and a basketball tournament. FOODS SERVED: concessions. ADMISSION: free. ACCOMMODATIONS: motels and hotels. RESTAURANTS: fast foods, family, elegant, international. CONTACT: New York Convention and Visitors Bureau or Michelle Scott, 310 Lennox Ave., Rm. 304, New York, NY 10027, (212) 427-7200 or 427-3306. 2,500,000

FESTIVAL OF NORTH COUNTRY FOLKLIFE *second Saturday in August,* Massena, St. Lawrence Co., at Barnhart Island. Displays and demonstrations of early traditions including lifestyles, crafts and music by families and individuals of French Canadian, Indian, Hungarian, Italian, and other origins; music includes fiddlers, banjo players, dancers, and family bands. FOODS SERVED: French Canadian, Italian, Hungarian, Indian, American. ADMISSION: free. ACCOMMODATIONS: motels and hotels, campgrounds, RV parks. RESTAURANTS: fast foods, family, elegant. CONTACT: Massena Chamber of Commerce, Inc., Town Hall, P. O. Box 387, Massena, NY 13662, (315) 769-3525. 7,000

ATHENS STREET FESTIVAL *second or third Saturday in August,* Athens, Greene Co., at Riverside Park, to celebrate "historic Athens on the Hudson River." Bus tours of historic Athens, riverboat tours on the Hudson River, crafts, gift sales, flea market, balloons, jugglers, fireworks, foot race, entertainment such as bluegrass, reggae, and the Mark Black Band. FOODS SERVED: "variety." ADMISSION: free. ACCOMMODATIONS: motels and hotels, B&B's, campgrounds, RV parks. RESTAURANTS: fast foods, family, elegant, Irish, continental, Chinese. CONTACT: Norman Benjamin, c/o Van Schaak, 25 Church St., Athens, NY 12015, or the Village and Town of Athens Chamber of Commerce, 2 First St., Athens, NY 12015, (518) 945-1551.

ITALIAN AMERICAN FESTIVAL *second or third Saturday in August,* Watkins Glen, Schuyler Co., in the Finger Lakes region, to celebrate the Feast of the Assumption. Mass at St. Mary's Church, parade, games, socializing, dancing, fireworks, lots of Italian dance music. FOODS SERVED: "delicious Italian" and American. ADMISSION: free. ACCOMMODATIONS: motels and hotels, B&B's, campgrounds, RV parks. RESTAURANTS: fast foods, family, elegant, Italian. CONTACT: Frank Chiacchearine, 804 Magee St., Watkins Glen, NY 14891, (607) 535-4550, or the Schuyler Co. Chamber of Commerce, 1000 N. Franklin, Watkins Glen, NY 14891, (607) 535-4300.

NEW YORK STATE WOODSMEN'S FIELD DAYS *third weekend in August,* Boonville, Oneida Co., to salute the timber industry and logging. "Large parade," loader and skidder competition, New York State Open Woodsmen's Competition, greased pole climb, entertainment. FOODS SERVED: "full dinners and fast foods." ADMISSION: $5.00 for full weekend, $3.00 per day. ACCOMMODATIONS: motels and hotels, B&B's, campgrounds, RV parks. RESTAURANTS: fast foods, family. CONTACT: New York State Woodsmen's Office, Box 123, Boonville, NY 13309, or the Boonville Area Chamber of Commerce, P.O. Box 163, Boonville, NY 13309, (315) 942-5512. 8,000

INTERNATIONAL CELTIC FESTIVAL *third weekend in August,* Hunter, Greene Co. Highland games, 200 bagpipes and bagpipes competition, Irish, Scottish, and Welsh crafts and gifts, Celtic entertainment by the Amerscot Highland Band, Breton Celts, Irish Wolfe Tones. FOODS SERVED: Guinness Stout, traditional Irish and Scottish soda breads, meat pies. ADMISSION: $7.50. ACCOMMODATIONS: motels and hotels, B&B's, campgrounds, RV parks. RESTAURANTS: fast foods, family, elegant, Irish, continental, Chinese. CONTACT: Don Conover, Exposition Planners, Bridge St., Hunter, NY 12442, (518) 263-3800, or The Greene County, Box 467, Catskill, NY 12414, (518) 943-3223.

GOLDEN OLDIES FESTIVAL *last weekend in August,* Hunter, Greene Co. A festival to enjoy the music of the 40's and 50's including Pat Boone, the Four Lads, Four Freshmen, Four Aces, the big bands of Tommy Dorsey, Harry James, Guy Lombardo, Glenn Miller, and Xavier Cugat. FOODS SERVED: concessions. ADMISSION: $7.50. ACCOMMODATIONS: motels and hotels, B&B's, campgrounds, RV parks. RESTAURANTS: fast foods, family,

elegant, Irish, continental, Chinese. CONTACT: Don Conover, Exposition Planners, Bridge St., Hunter, NY 12442, (518) 263-3800, or The Greene County, Box 467, Catskill, NY 12414, (518) 943-3223.

IROQUOIS INDIAN FESTIVAL *Labor Day weekend (early September),* Cobleskill, Schoharie Co., at Bouck Hall, SUNY Cobleskill on Route 7, to celebrate the creativity of the Iroquois Indians. Demonstration and sales of Iroquois arts, films and video on the Iroquois, archeology and art exhibits, special children's activities, native speakers, traditional Iroquois dance and musical performances including the Jim Sky Iroquois Dancers who perform and explain their dances and culture, Oneida comedian Charlie Hill, and the Six Nations Country Western Trio. FOODS SERVED: traditional Iroquois, such as corn soup, corn bread, ghost bread, and strawberry drink. ADMISSION: adults $3.50, seniors $2.50, students 14–18 $1.50, under 14 with parents free. ACCOMMODATIONS: motels and hotels, B&B's, campgrounds, RV parks. RESTAURANTS: fast foods, family, elegant. CONTACT: Schoharie Museum of the Iroquois Indian, Box 158, Schoharie, NY 12157, (518) 295-8553 or 234-2276. 3,000

NATIVE AMERICAN FESTIVAL *Labor Day weekend (early September),* Hunter, Greene Co., to celebrate local Indian heritage. Native American ritual dancing, Native American crafts, jewelry, pottery, sculpture, leathercrafts, Indian dance competition, hoop dancers, drama group, Indian storyteller, the Aztec Firedancers, and Indian drum group. FOODS SERVED: Native American tribal specialties and beverages. ADMISSION: $4.00. ACCOMMODATIONS: motels and hotels, B&B's, campgrounds, RV parks. RESTAURANTS: fast foods, family, elegant, Irish, continental, Chinese. CONTACT: Don Conover, Exposition Planners, Bridge St., Hunter, NY 12442, (518) 263-3800, or The Greene County, Box 467, Catskill, NY 12414, (518) 943-3223.

IRISH FESTIVAL *Labor Day weekend (early September),* Leeds, Greene Co., to celebrate the Irish heritage of many Leeds residents. Irish singing and dancing, step dancing, Irish entertainers such as Dermot Henry, Jerry Finley, The Rutherfords, Pat Roper. FOODS SERVED: Irish foods, Guinness and Harp beers. ADMISSION: $4.00. ACCOMMODATIONS: motels and hotels, · B&B's, campgrounds, RV parks. RESTAURANTS: fast foods, family, elegant, Irish, continental, Chinese. CONTACT: Leeds Chamber of Commerce, Box 6, Leeds, NY 12451.

POLKA HOLIDAYS OF THE FINGER LAKES *Labor Day weekend (early September),* Watkins Glen, Schuyler Co., in the Finger Lakes region, to perpetuate Polish music and customs. Dancing, eating and socializing, several Polish bands. FOODS SERVED: Polish and American. ADMISSION: "about $8.00." ACCOMMODATIONS: motels and hotels, B&B's, campgrounds, RV parks. RESTAURANTS: fast foods, family, elegant, Italian. CONTACT: Eugene Martin, 1201 N. Main St., Elmira, NY 14902, (607) 734-5738, or the Schuyler Co. Chamber of Commerce, 1000 N. Franklin, Watkins Glen, NY 14891, (607) 535-4300. 5,000

GOLDEN HARVEST FESTIVAL *first weekend after Labor Day (early September),* Baldwinsville, Onondaga Co., in central New York, to celebrate the end of summer and the beginning of autumn. More than 120 artists and craftspeople, horse-drawn hayrides, pony rides, petting zoo, canoe tours, hawktalks, wandering entertainers, guided nature walks, nature contests, games for children, Critter Call Contest, Pie Eating Contest, continuous entertainment such as "variety of bluegrass, folk, clogging," and other upstate New York entertainment. FOODS SERVED: "country." ADMISSION: adults $2.00, children $1.00. ACCOMMODATIONS: motels and hotels, campgrounds, RV parks. RESTAURANTS: fast foods, family, elegant. CONTACT: Beaver Lake Nature Center, 8477 E. Mud

Lake Rd., Baldwinsville, NY 13027, (315) 638-2519, or the Greater Baldwinsville Chamber of Commerce, 18 W. Genesee St., Baldwinsville, NY 13027, (315) 638-0550. 16,000

FINGER LAKES DIXIELAND JAZZ FESTIVAL *Sunday after Labor Day (early September),* Hector, Schuyler Co., in the Finger Lakes region, to benefit Schuyler Hospital. At least ten dixieland bands perform for listening and dancing, picnics invited, bring your own chairs. FOODS SERVED: barbecued chicken, wines. ADMISSION: $8.00. ACCOMMODATIONS: motels and hotels, B&B's, campgrounds, RV parks. RESTAURANTS: fast foods, family, elegant, Italian. CONTACT: Ann Meehan, RD 1, Box 151, Watkins Glen, NY 14891, (607) 535-4791, or the Schuyler Co. Chamber of Commerce, 1000 N. Franklin, Watkins Glen, NY 14891, (607) 535-4300. 3,500

OLD TIME GAS AND STEAM SHOW *second weekend in September,* Constableville, Lewis Co., in New York's "North Country," on Route 26, to recognize "past home and farm activities." Lumber sawing, shingle making mills, oat threshing, rock crushing, clothes washing, antique tractor show, gas engine display, Quilt Show and tying demonstrations, craftspeople, pie eating contests, sky divers, flea market, Friday night auction, lots of country entertainment such as yodler Elvira Lemon, fiddler Alice Clemons, the Tryon County Militia, and the Saturday Night Band for dancing. FOODS SERVED: pancake breakfast, "beefalo burgers," fried dough, chicken barbecue. ADMISSION: $1.00 to park, donations appreciated. ACCOMMODATIONS: motels and hotels, B&B's, campgrounds, RV parks. RESTAURANTS: fast foods, family, elegant. CONTACT: Charles Miller, Box 125, West Leyden, NY 13489, (315) 942-5102 after 5:00 p.m. 5,000

FESTIVAL OF GRAPES *third week and weekend in September,* Silver Creek,

Chautauqua Co., to celebrate the grape harvest. Vineyard tours, grape stomping, wine tasting, Grape Queen Pageant, arts and crafts show, parade. FOODS SERVED: food booths. ADMISSION: free. ACCOMMODATIONS: motels and hotels, B&B's, campgrounds, resorts. RESTAURANTS: fast foods, family, elegant. CONTACT: Chautauqua Co. Vacationland Association, Inc., 2 N. Erie St., Mayville, NY 14757, (716) 753-4304.

AUTUMN HARVEST FESTIVAL *third weekend in September,* Cooperstown, Otsego Co., at The Farmers' Museum to celebrate the harvest season. Craftspeople working at traditional 19th-century skills display and demonstrate their crafts including weaving, woodworking, soapmaking, basketmaking, paper marbling and wall stenciling; entertainment including music, song, dance, 19th-century fiddle music, storytelling, square and contra dancing, juggling, puppetry, games, horse-drawn wagon rides, fishing for children, hot air balloon ascensions. FOODS SERVED: homemade pies, local cheeses, maple products, fruits of the harvest. ADMISSION: varies by event. ACCOMMODATIONS: motels and hotels, B&B's, campgrounds, RV parks. RESTAURANTS: family, elegant. CONTACT: Farmers' Museum, P.O. Box 800, Cooperstown, NY 13326, (607) 547-2534. 3,500

ADIRONDACK BALLOON FESTIVAL *third weekend in September,* Glens Falls, Warren Co. More than 100 balloons fly in the "oldest meet in the state" of New York, art show, exhibits at Civic Center, airport, and Community College. FOODS SERVED: concessions. ADMISSION: free. ACCOMMODATIONS: motels and hotels, B&B's, campgrounds, RV parks. RESTAURANTS: fast foods, family, elegant, international. CONTACT: Warren Co. Tourism, Municipal Center, Lake George, NY 12845, (518) 761-6371. 150,000

FALL FESTIVAL *fourth weekend in September,* Plattsburgh, Clinton Co., downtown and at the County Fairgrounds. Children's parade; the Beaudoin Family performs traditional French Canadian country music; Theatre Grottesco incorporates techniques of European circuses, street performers, mask mime, and the Italian Commedia dell'arte, unicyclists, mimes; vaudeville; children's songs and games; Tom Chapin; the Adirondack Youth Orchestra, the Wildwood Marionettes, high school jazz band; U.S. Air Force Band of New England; Willsboro Bay Steel Drum Band; crafts show and sale, Shriner's clowns, face painting; old-fashioned fall harvest fair with hayrides, vintage farm equipment, farm animal petting zoo, farmers' market, contests, apple bobbing, pie eating contests, dressing contest, egg toss, antique boats display, horseshoe toss, evening dances, helicopter rides, skydiving demonstrations. FOODS SERVED: concessions. ADMISSION: button admits to all events, adults $3.00, children 10 and under $1.50. ACCOMMODATIONS: motels and hotels, B&B's, campgrounds, RV parks. RESTAURANTS: fast foods, family, elegant. CONTACT: Plattsburgh and Clinton Co. Chamber of Commerce, P. O. Box 310, Plattsburgh, NY 12901, (518) 563-1000. 15,000

SALAMANCA FALLING LEAVES FESTIVAL *fourth weekend in September,* Salamanca, Cattaraugus Co., to celebrate fall. "Giant parade," craft show, antique show, Seneca Indian dancing, Festival Dance, Photo Contest, art show, carnival, car show. FOODS SERVED: Italian, Polish, Indian. ADMISSION: free, charges for car show and antique show. ACCOMMODATIONS: motels and hotels, campgrounds, RV parks. RESTAURANTS: fast foods, family, elegant. CONTACT: Salamanca Area Chamber of Commerce, Inc. 636 Wildwood Ave., Salamanca, NY 14779, (716) 945-2034. 20,000

OYSTER FESTIVAL *last weekend in September,* Oyster Bay, Nassau Co., L.I. Arts and crafts, juried art show, Oyster Eating Contest and Oyster Shucking Contest aiming to get into the Guinness Book of

Records, Marine Midland Cycling Classic criterium which has been won by Eric Heiden and Davis Phinney, 5mi Run, local entertainment. FOODS SERVED: more than 60,000 oysters on the half shell, oyster stew and chowder, oysters in other forms, chicken. ADMISSION: free. ACCOMMODATIONS: motels and hotels, B&B's. RESTAURANTS: family, elegant. CONTACT: Oyster Bay Chamber of Commerce, Box 61, Oyster Bay, NY 11771, (516) 624-8082 or (516) 922-2100. 100,000

FALL FOLIAGE FESTIVAL *first weekend in October,* Cohocton, Steuben Co., in the Finger Lakes region. Tree Sitting Contest, King and Queen Contest, antique flea market on Village Green, arts and crafts, historical exhibit, sidewalk sales, Corning Area Community Band Concert, parade, fireworks, hiking meet, Helicopter Drop, horse and wagon rides around town, well-marked foliage tours, entertainment by the Hornell Maple City Barbershoppers, dances. FOODS SERVED: community groups offer luncheon and bake sales, chicken barbecue, beef luncheon, ham dinner. ADMISSION: free. ACCOMMODATIONS: motels and hotels, campgrounds. RESTAURANTS: fast foods, family, elegant. CONTACT: Mrs. Pauline Thorp, 5 S. Main St., Cohocton, NY 14826, (716) 384-5468. 12,000

FESTIVAL OF LIGHTS *November 28 through January 10,* Niagara Falls, Niagara Co., in western New York, to welcome the holiday season. Fabulous lights displays throughout town featuring more than 200 individual animated-characters in dozens of decorated scenes, including the Nabisco "Fantasy of Lights" at its Shredded Wheat Plant, Christmas Tree Festival at Factory Outlet Mall benefiting United Cerebral Palsy, arts and crafts show, oxy crafts show, toy train collector's show, and loads of local and internationally known entertainers such as Mel Tillis and Minnie Pearl, gospel music, U.S. Air Force's Tops in Blue blues band, jazz, minstrels, bell choir, Rainbow Square USA Square Dance Festival, Dundee Steel Drum Band, Retired Men's Service Club Chorus, high school musical performances, a flute ensemble, magicians, boxing matches, mime, boat show, doll show and sale, juried art show, Festival of Fashions, ecumenical concert. (Niagara Falls' factories whose products are represented at the Factory Outlet Mall include Bass shoes, Corning Glass, Royal Doulton, Benetton, Van Heusen, Pfaltzgraff, Polo Ralph Lauren, Jaegar, Campus, Jaymar slacks, and Windsor shirts.) FOODS SERVED: concessions. ADMISSION: free, except for events at Convention and Civic Center. ACCOMMODATIONS: motels and hotels, B&B's, campgrounds, RV parks. RESTAURANTS: fast foods, family, elegant, Greek, Italian, Chinese. CONTACT: SPUR/Chamber of Commerce Alliance, 345 Third St., Niagara Falls, NY 14303, (716) 285-9141. 850,000

SPARKLE OF CHRISTMAS *first Saturday in December,* Corning, Steuben Co., in the Finger Lakes region, to welcome the beginning of the holiday season. Christmas Tree Fair, East High Happening, Twin Tier Amateur Hockey Association exhibition, ice show, "A Christmas Story" in words and music, opening ceremonies, community caroling, Sparkle Snow Park, three shows by the Catskill Puppet People, pony rides and children's games, Mrs. Santa, petting zoo, craft booths, continuous music, costume contest. FOODS SERVED: concessions. ADMISSION: free. ACCOMMODATIONS: motels and hotels, B&B's, campgrounds, RV parks. RESTAURANTS: fast foods, family, elegant. CONTACT: Corning Intown Promotions, 42 E. Market St., Corning, NY 14830, (607) 936-4686. 15,000

PENNSYLVANIA

PENNSYLVANIA MAPLE FESTIVAL *late March or early April*, Meyersdale, Somerset Co., in Laurel Highlands area, to celebrate the "maple season." Old and new crafts including stained glass, ceramics, woodworking, wool spinning, quilling, chair caning, wheat weaving, wooden roses, tole painting, leather working, tin smithing, quilts, dolls, rope making, hickory goods, furniture, rug hooking, antiques and collectibles; Old Time Maple Sugar Camp, maple product sales; Grand Feature Parade, Horse Pulling Contest, antique–classic auto show, street and rod auto show, Costume Contest, Queen's Coronation and Ball, Oldies But Goodies Dance, Maple Producer's Contest, tree tapping, Maple Run race; live entertainment including bluegrass, cloggers, jazz, rock 'n' roll; window displays, antique cobbler's shop, antique doctor's office, country store. FOODS SERVED: all-you-can-eat pancake house, Dutch fries, country sausage, homemade soups, sugar cakes, spotza, funnel cakes, mountain pies, maple candy, and taffy. ADMISSION: $3.00 to park area, $4.50 for entertainment outside park. ACCOMMODATIONS: motels and hotels, B&B's, campgrounds. RESTAURANTS: family. CONTACT: Pennsylvania Maple Festival, Inc., P. O. Box 222, Meyersdale, PA 15552, (814) 634-0213. 75,000

PULASKI FESTIVAL *last weekend in April*, Bethlehem, Northampton Co., in the Lehigh Valley in downtown Bethlehem and South Bethlehem, to "honor General Casimir Pulaski, Revolutionary War hero who visited Bethlehem, PA," Krakow Café, reenactment of the General's visit, parade, Polish musical concert by renowned artists. FOODS SERVED: Polish. ADMISSION: free. ACCOMMODATIONS: motels and hotels, B&B's, campgrounds, RV parks. RESTAURANTS: fast foods, family, elegant. CONTACT: The Pulaski Foundation, Center for Polish-American Arts, P.O. Box 1201, Bethlehem, PA 18018, (215) 838-6858. 5,000

SHAD FESTIVAL *first Sunday in May*, Bethlehem, Northampton Co., to celebrate the shad runs and catches in colonial times. Arts and crafts, early Moravian colonial crafts demonstrations, lectures and exhibits, tours of historic buildings in Bethlehem's 18th-century industrial area. FOODS SERVED: "dinner of planked shad cooked over charcoal pit and served with colonial accompaniments." ADMISSION: $7.00. ACCOMMODATIONS: motels and hotels, B&B's. RESTAURANTS: fast foods, family, elegant. CONTACT: Bethlehem Area Chamber of Commerce, 459 Old York Rd., Bethlehem, PA 18018-5870, (215) 867-3788.

APPLE BLOSSOM FESTIVAL *first full weekend in May*, Gettysburg, Adams Co., at the South Mountain Fairgrounds on Route 234, as a salute to the apple industry and 21,000 blossoming trees. Bus and walking tours of orchards, pie eating and apple bobbing contests, Bakery in the Barn, arts and crafts displays, helicopter rides, old-time gasoline engines and antique car display, Apple Stitchery Contest, Apple Poster Contest, crowning of Apple Queen ceremony, country and bluegrass music, petting barnyard, livestock and agricultural exhibits, apple butter boil. FOODS SERVED: apple desserts, funnel cakes, apple goodies, chicken barbecue, pork roast, free fruit baskets, more apple products. ADMISSION: adults $1.00, children under 12 free. ACCOMMODATIONS: motels and hotels, B&B's, campgrounds, RV parks. RESTAURANTS: fast foods, family, elegant. CONTACT: Gettysburg-Adams Co. Chamber of Commerce, 33 York St., Gettysburg, PA 17325, (717) 334-8151. 10,000

BACH FESTIVAL *second and third Fridays and Saturdays in May*, Bethlehem,

Northampton Co., in the Lehigh Valley at Packer Memorial Church of Lehigh University. A series of choir and full orchestral performances of Bach's "Mass in B Minor" and other works, featuring guest artists such as soprano Arlene Auger, mezzo Janice Taylor, tenor Douglas Robinson, and bassist Jan Opalach. ADMISSION: $20.00–$36.00. ACCOMMODATIONS: motels and hotels, B&B's, campgrounds, RV parks. RESTAURANTS: fast foods, family, elegant. CONTACT: Bach Choir Office, 423 Heckewelder Place, Bethlehem, PA 18018, (215) 866-4382. 6,000

NATIONAL PIKE FESTIVAL *third weekend in May*, Ligonier, Hopwood and other communities, Somerset, Fayette and Washington counties "along the eighty-nine-mile stretch of Route 40," to recognize and remember "19th-century travel on the national road." "Dozens of communities and historic sites . . . hold special tours, exhibits, programs," old-time crafts demonstrations and shows, pioneer wagon train travels part of the eighty-nine-miles, old-time fiddlers, country bands, square dancers, cloggers, storytellers, banjoists, fife and drum corps, and several reenactment groups perform. FOODS SERVED: "traditional food." ADMISSION: free, charges to some historical sites. ACCOMMODATIONS: motels and hotels, campgrounds. RESTAURANTS: fast foods, family, elegant. CONTACT: Laurel Highlands Tourism, P. O. Box 63, Hopwood, PA 15445, (412) 238-5277, or Washington County Tourism, 59 N. Main St., Washington, PA 15301, (412) 222-8130.

PITTSBURGH FOLK FESTIVAL *third weekend in May*, Pittsburgh, Allegheny Co., at the David L. Lawrence Convention Center, as a "celebration of the ethnic origins within the city" and presented by Robert Morris College. Twenty-five countries exhibit crafts and displays, costumes, ethnic dancing, children's shows and presentations, and living customs. The printed program for this festival is worth the trip since it includes descriptions of customs and dances, history, menus, and recipes for each country featured. FOODS SERVED: specialties of all twenty-five nations prepared by local residents from those countries. ADMISSION: adults $5.00, children $2.00. ACCOMMODATIONS: motels and hotels. RESTAURANTS: fast foods, family, elegant, international. CONTACT: Robert Morris College, Center for Leadership, Narrows Run Rd., Coraopolis, PA 15108-1189, (412) 262-8407. 35,000

GREATER UNIONTOWN ALL ETHNIC FESTIVAL *third or fourth weekend in May*, Uniontown, Fayette Co., downtown in the Laurel Highlands area. This celebration of residents' ethnic heritage includes continuous entertainment, ethnic arts and crafts, children's rides, and a parade. FOODS SERVED: Italian, Polish, Greek, Syrian, American. ADMISSION: free. ACCOMMODATIONS: motels and hotels, campgrounds. RESTAURANTS: fast foods, family, elegant. CONTACT: Uniontown Downtown Business District Authority, Room 216, City Hall, 20 N. Gallatin Ave., Uniontown, PA 15401, (412) 438-4408. 100,000

ITALIAN FESTIVAL *late May*, Allentown, Lehigh Co., in the Lehigh Valley at Dorney Park/ Wildwater Kingdom, to celebrate the Italian heritage of local residents. Italian pageant, car show, Italian music and entertainment. FOODS SERVED: lots of Italian. ADMISSION: free. ACCOMMODATIONS: motels and hotels, B&B's, campgrounds, RV parks. RESTAURANTS: fast foods, family, elegant. CONTACT: Dorney Park/Wildwater Kingdom, 3830 Dorney Park Rd., Allentown, PA 18104, (215) 398-7955. 15,000

MAYFAIR *Memorial Day weekend (late May)*, Allentown, Lehigh Co., in the Lehigh Valley. A festival of the performing and visual arts including fine arts exhibits, workshops, theatre and dance which has included performers such as the late Buddy Rich and his band, folk singer John

Hartford, and the Dance Exchange from Washington, D.C. FOODS SERVED: concessions. ADMISSION: free. ACCOMMODATIONS: motels and hotels, B&B's, campgrounds, RV parks. RESTAURANTS: fast foods, family, elegant. CONTACT: Mayfair, 2020 Hamilton St., Allentown, PA 18104, (215) 437-6900. 300,000

THREE RIVERS ARTS FESTIVAL *first Friday through third Sunday in June,* Pittsburgh, Allegheny Co., at Gateway Center, Point State Park, to celebrate the arts. Artists' market and art exhibits featuring 400 artists from throughout the United States, Film Festival, video, indoor and outdoor sculpture, painting and graphics, photography, Artists in Action; 300 live performances on three stages and around the festival, including the Chamber Music Company, strolling entertainers and big name stars which have included Smokey Robinson, Roberta Flack, Sergio Mendez, Nitty Gritty Dirt Band, and Judy Collins. FOODS SERVED: international. ADMISSION: free. ACCOMMODATIONS: motels and hotels, B&B's, campgrounds, RV parks. RESTAURANTS: fast foods, family, elegant, international. CONTACT: Three Rivers Arts Festival, 5 Gateway Center, Pittsburgh, PA 15222, (412) 481-7040. 700,000

PORTUGUESE HERITAGE DAYS *first weekend in June,* Bethlehem, Northampton Co., downtown, to celebrate the heritage of Bethlehem's Portuguese population. Arts and crafts, a parade, Portuguese dance performances, soccer games, marathon run, Portuguese folklore groups and bands perform. FOODS SERVED: Portuguese. ADMISSION: free. ACCOMMODATIONS: motels and hotels, B&B's. RESTAURANTS: fast foods, family, elegant. CONTACT: Armindo Sousa at (215) 867-1847 or write the Bethlehem Area Chamber of Commerce, 459 Old York Rd., Bethlehem, PA 18018-5870, (215) 867-3788.

WESTERN PENNSYLVANIA LAUREL FESTIVAL *third week in June,* Brookville, Jefferson Co., in the "Magic Forest," to celebrate western Pennsylvania's natural beauty and the blooming of its laurel trees. Street carnivals, car shows, fiddlers' contests, parade, fashion shows, street dances, big-name country music stars. FOODS SERVED: concessions. ADMISSION: free, charge for big show. ACCOMMODATIONS: motels and hotels, B&B's, campgrounds, RV parks. RESTAURANTS: fast foods, family, elegant. CONTACT: Western Pennsylvania Laurel Festival, Inc., P. O. Box 142, Brookville, PA 15825, (814) 849-2024, or the Brookville Area Chamber of Commerce, 194 Main St., Brookville, PA 15825, (814) 849-8448. 7,000

MONESSEN'S CULTURAL HERITAGE FESTIVAL *third week in June,* Monessen, Westmoreland Co., to salute the many nationalities of the people who settled in Monessen. Entertainment typical of nations represented, including polka bands, big band sounds, Italian and Greek musicians, Tamburitzans, orchestral concerts, barbershop singers, gospel singers, rock groups, and many ethnic food booths. FOODS SERVED: Syrian, Greek, Russian, Mexican, English–pioneer, Italian. ADMISSION: free. ACCOMMODATIONS: motels and hotels, campgrounds. RESTAURANTS: fast foods, family, Chinese, Italian. CONTACT: Monessen Chamber of Commerce, 125 Sixth St., Monessen, PA 15062, (412) 684-3200. 35,000

SUSQUEHANNA BOOM FESTIVAL *fourth weekend in June,* Williamsport, Lycoming Co., in the Susquehanna Valley, to celebrate "the lumber heritage of the area." Hot air balloon rally, lumberjack contest, Prince Farington Great Race Triathlon, historical displays, rides, games, concerts and entertainment which has included the Four Tops, Tammy Wynette, Rare Earth, Happy Together Tour, Randy Travis, Care Bears, Shirttails, and the Smurfs. FOODS SERVED: concessions. ADMISSION: free, charges for some events. ACCOMMODATIONS: motels and hotels, B&B's, campgrounds, RV parks. RESTAU-

RANTS: fast foods, family, elegant. CON-
TACT: Lycoming Co. Tourist Promotion
Agency, 454 Pine St., Williamsport, PA
17701, (717) 326-1971. 75,000

ELLWOOD CITY ARTS, CRAFTS, AND FOOD FESTIVAL *July 4th weekend*, Ellwood City, Lawrence Co., at Ewing Park.

More than 100 arts and craft
displays, juried art show, antique car
show, continuous entertainment from
country to pop, choral groups, and big
bands. FOODS SERVED: Greek, Italian,
Mexican, Siberian, American. ADMISSION:
free. ACCOMMODATIONS: motels and hotels, campgrounds, RV parks. RESTAU-
RANTS: family. CONTACT: Ellwood City
Chamber of Commerce, P. O. Box 308,
Ellwood City, PA 16117, (412) 758-0216.
60,000

LEHIGH RIVER CANAL FESTIVAL *second Saturday in July*, Easton, Northampton Co., at Hugh Moore Park in the Lehigh Valley, to recognize the canal system's history.

Arts and crafts, canal boat
rides, historical displays, canal boatsmen's
reunion, canal pub, folk and jazz music.
FOODS SERVED: concessions. ADMISSION:
$3.00 per car. ACCOMMODATIONS: motels
and hotels, B&B's, campgrounds, RV
parks. RESTAURANTS: fast foods, family,
elegant. CONTACT: Canal Museum, P. O.
Box 877, Easton, PA 18042-0877, (215)
250-6700. 12,000

CENTRAL PENNSYLVANIA FESTIVAL OF THE ARTS *second full weekend after July 4th*, State College, Centre Co., on the campus of the Pennsylvania State University, to celebrate the arts.

Annual
sidewalk sale and exhibition representing
350 artists from thirty-six states, ten indoor arts and crafts exhibitions, Artists-
in-Action, poetry competition and readings for poets ranging in age from 4–100
in different categories, Art in the Parklet
children's participatory art activities,
young artists' sidewalk show and sale; 250
performing-arts events on six indoor and
outdoor stages including the Fred Waring

Elderhostel Chorus, Organ Interlude,
Penn State Jazz Ensemble, the Allegheny
String Band, The Chestnut Brass Company, madrigal singers, fiddlers' competition, aerobic dancing, handbell choir, puppets, the festival film series, and much
more! Entertainers who have performed
at this arts festival of arts festivals include
Gordon and Susan from "Sesame Street,"
Taj Mahal, Tom Chapin, John Sebastian,
Queen Ida, pianist Kathleen Roach, jazz
group Fast Tracks, John Jackson, Wade
and Julia Mainer, and The Fairfield Four.
This festival produces one of the most
beautiful programs anywhere, which includes the winning poetry from the festival's poetry competition, as well as a strik-
ing calendar. FOODS SERVED: local food
booths. ADMISSION: free. ACCOMMODA-
TIONS: motels and hotels, B&B's, campgrounds, RV parks. RESTAURANTS: fast
foods, family, elegant, Asian, Indian, Italian, Mexican. CONTACT: Central Pennsylvania Festival of the Arts, Box 1023, State
College, PA 16804, (814) 237-3682.
250,000

CHRISTMAS CITY FAIR *third weekend in July*, Bethlehem, Northampton Co., in the Lehigh Valley.

A community celebra-
tion of ethnic arts and crafts, displays, and
entertainment. FOODS SERVED: multi-ethnic. ADMISSION: free. ACCOMMODATIONS:
motels and hotels, B&B's, campgrounds,
RV parks. RESTAURANTS: fast foods, family, elegant. CONTACT: Richard Szulborski,
669 Atlantic St., Bethlehem, PA 18015,
(215) 865-3751, or the Lehigh Valley Convention and Visitors Bureau, Inc., P. O.
Box 2605, Lehigh Valley, PA 18001, (215)
266-0560. 40,000

MARLBORO MUSIC FESTIVAL *third Saturday in July through third Sunday in August*, Marlboro, Windham Co., at Marlboro College.

Twelve weekend concerts
of works for varied chamber music ensembles, featuring exceptionally gifted young
professional musicians in concert with distinguished master artists from the Marlboro School of music, Rudolf Serkin, artis-

tic director. ADMISSION: Tickets range from $3.50–$14.00. ACCOMMODATIONS: motels and hotels, B&B's, campgrounds. RESTAURANTS: family, elegant, international. CONTACT: June 16–August 20 Marlboro Music, Marlboro, VT 05344, (802) 254-2394 and from August 21–June 15 Marlboro Music, 135 S, 18th St., Suite 101A–103A, Philadelphia, PA 19103, (215) 569-4690. 15,000

LEHIGH VALLEY BALLOON FESTIVAL *fourth weekend in July,* Allentown, Lehigh Co., in the Lehigh Valley. Morning and evening balloon flights, model cars, hang gliders, arts and crafts, continuous live entertainment. FOODS SERVED: concessions. ADMISSION: $2.00 per person. ACCOMMODATIONS: motels and hotels, B&B's, campgrounds, RV parks. RESTAURANTS: fast foods, family, elegant. CONTACT: Bob Sparks, P. O. Box 9190, Allentown, PA 18105, (215) 867-2076, or the Lehigh Valley Convention and Visitors Bureau, Inc., P. O. Box 2605, Lehigh Valley, PA 18001, (215) 266-0560. 80,000

FORT ARMSTRONG FOLK FESTIVAL *last weekend in July,* Kittanning, Armstrong Co., at Riverfront Park, to "celebrate traditions that were practiced long ago in this area during the French and Indian War. Craftspeople demonstrate skills such as loom-weaving, stenciling, quilting, fine arts shows, continuous music and entertainment including pop, folk, country-western bands, storytelling, puppet shows. FOODS SERVED: ethnic foods such as Dutch funnel cakes, hot sausages. ADMISSION: free. ACCOMMODATIONS: motels and hotels, campgrounds, RV parks. RESTAURANTS: fast foods, family, elegant. CONTACT: Fort Armstrong Folk Festival Committee, N. Water St., Kittanning, PA 16201, (412) 543-6363 or (412) 543-1045. 90,000

THE PITTSBURGH THREE RIVERS REGATTA *last weekend in July,* Pittsburgh, Allegheny Co., at Point State Park, to recognize the recreational and indus-

trial uses of the Three Rivers. Speed Boat Race, water sports, water activities and performances, air shows, land events, musical performances from strolling entertainers to big-name stars. FOODS SERVED: "all types and kinds." ADMISSION: free. ACCOMMODATIONS: motels and hotels, B&B's, campgrounds, RV parks. RESTAURANTS: fast foods, family, elegant, international. CONTACT: Bill Roberts, 450 The Landmarks Bldg., One Station Square, Pittsburgh, PA 15219, (412) 261-5808. 700,000

DAS AWKSCHT FESCHT (The August Festival) *first weekend in August,* Macungie, Lehigh Co., in the Lehigh Valley. Antique car show, antique toys, arts and crafts, flea market, children's programs. FOODS SERVED: Pennsylvania Dutch, such as funnel cakes, chicken pies, chicken corn soup, and shoofly pie. ADMISSION: adults $2.00, children $1.00. ACCOMMODATIONS: motels and hotels, B&B's, campgrounds, RV parks. RESTAURANTS: fast foods, family, elegant. CONTACT: Musselman Advertising, 601 Hamilton Mall, Allentown, PA 18101, (215) 435-5102. 90,000

MUSIKFEST *nine days including the third week in August,* Bethlehem, Northampton Co., in the Lehigh Valley in the Historic Bethlehem section of town. More than 400 free concerts including performances by a band from Germany, others such as The Stadtkapelle Perg, the town band of Perg, Austria, vesper concerts, participatory art for children, cabaret, folk, rock, country/western, blues, bluegrass, jazz, colonial craftsmen and colonial musical instrument demonstrations; American stars have included Lionel Hampton, Arlo Guthrie, Carlos Montoya, and Judy Collins. FOODS SERVED: "various ethnic." ADMISSION: free. ACCOMMODATIONS: motels and hotels, B&B's, campgrounds, RV parks. RESTAURANTS: fast foods, family, elegant. CONTACT: Bethlehem Musikfest Association, 556 Main St., Bethlehem, PA 18108, (215) 861-0678. 400,000

DANKFEST *fourth weekend in August,* Harmony, Butler Co., at the Harmony Museum and Mennonite Meeting Haus, to preserve the Harmonist history and celebrate the harvest. Demonstrations of pioneer and Mennonite crafts and life skills such as antique kitchen utensils, chair caning, colonial guns and tools, corn cob items, corn husk mats, English smocking, flax preparation and spinning, log trimming and wood shingles, hand-carved water fowl, hickory brooms, rag rugs, rug hooking, whistle making, wooden flowers, rakes, and others, black powder demonstrations, butter churning, rope making, farmers' market, face painting, antique cars, tours of National Historic Landmark District, entertainment by local bands and singing groups. FOODS SERVED: "full homemade dinners, homemade root beer, hot dogs, sausages," barbecued chicken, shoofly pie, switchel, funnel cakes. ADMISSION: "about $3.00 per person." ACCOMMODATIONS: motels and hotels, campgrounds, RV parks. RESTAURANTS: fast foods, family, elegant, German, Italian. CONTACT: Harmony Museum, P. O. Box 524, Harmony, PA 16037, (412) 452-7341. 4,000

SPRINGS FOLK FESTIVAL *first Friday and Saturday in September,* Springs, Somerset Co., at the Festival Grounds on Rt. 669, to recognize and honor the arts and crafts of the pioneers, and the Pennsylvania Dutch heritage. Pioneer crafts demonstrations include painting and pottery-making, wheat weaving, basket making, grandfather-clock making, candle dipping, maple sugaring, apple butter boiling, log hewing, sauerkraut making, wool dyeing, spinning and weaving, tin smithing, fungus painting, apple cider making, bake oven breadmaking; live music includes banjos and fiddles, dulcimers, "a cappella" singing by local Mennonites. FOODS SERVED: Pennsylvania Dutch meals including sausage, Dutch-fried potatoes, corn, sausage burgers, bean soup, homemade baked goods, funnel cakes and apple butter on homemade bread. ADMISSION: adults $3.00. children under 12 $1.00, children

under 6 free. ACCOMMODATIONS: motels and hotels, campgrounds, RV parks. RESTAURANTS: fast foods, family, elegant, German. CONTACT: Springs Folk Festival, Box 293, Springs, PA 15562, (301) 895-5985 or (814) 662-4158. 15,000

THE GREAT ALLENTOWN FAIR *first week in September,* Allentown, Lehigh Co., in the Lehigh Valley. Crafts and agricultural exhibits, free entertainment, two midways, "superstar grandstand shows" have included performers such as Wayne Newton, the Beach Boys, Kenny Rogers, Hank Williams, Jr., and Kenny Loggins. FOODS SERVED: concessions. ADMISSION: adults $3.00, children $1.00. ACCOMMODATIONS: motels and hotels, B&B's, campgrounds, RV parks. RESTAURANTS: fast foods, family, elegant. CONTACT: Allentown Fair, 17th and Chew Sts., Allentown, PA 18102, (215) 433-7541. 585,000

PHILADELPHIA CEILI GROUP'S IRISH MUSIC AND DANCE FESTIVAL *second Saturday in September,* Lansdale, Montgomery Co., to celebrate traditional Irish music and dance. Traditional Irish crafts exhibited and demonstrated, workshops and concerts in dancing, fiddle, flute, harp, mini concerts, sligo music, songs and ballads, children's programs, evening concert and ceili. FOODS SERVED: Irish and traditional. ADMISSION: all festival adults $16.00, advance $12.00; children $5.00, advance $4.00; evening adults $10.00, advance $8.00; children $3.00, advance $2.00; family admission $30.00 available day of the festival only) ACCOMMODATIONS: motels and hotels. CONTACT: The Philadelphia Ceili Group, 6815 Emlen St., Room 2, Philadelphia, PA 19119, (215) 849-8899. 2,500

KEYSTONE COUNTRY FESTIVAL *third weekend in September,* Altoona, Blair Co., at Boyertown U.S.A. in the southern Alleghenies, as the end of summer "last chance." Arts and crafts, loads of music including the Jaffa String Band, Rockin'

Robin, Stardust, light and sound display, The Vicksburgs, Brush Mountain Strings, Boxcar Willie, juggler Bill King, B. J. Rock and the country Rockets; auto show including antiques, classic stock, sports car stock, mustang stock, special interest stock, street rods, street modification, trucks and vans. FOODS SERVED: Town Square Cafe sandwiches, country chicken, Bavarian tent, Italian tent, funnel cake tent, the Melon Patch, pizza tent, "Dutch Delites," gingerbreads, other food centers. ADMISSION: $5.00 per person. ACCOMMODATIONS: motels and hotels, campgrounds. RESTAURANTS: fast foods, family, elegant. CONTACT: Convention and Visitors Bureau of Blair Co. and Altoona Chamber of Commerce, 1212 Twelfth Ave., Altoona, PA 16601, (814) 943-8151. 30,000

FORT LIGONIER DAYS *second full weekend in October,* Ligonier, Westmoreland, Co., in Laurel Highlands, to commemorate the Battle of Fort Ligonier during the French and Indian War in 1755. Crafts, antique window displays, parade, sidewalk sales, battle reenactment, antique show, miniature train display, "flee market," Budweiser Clydesdales, and live entertainment. ADMISSION: free, charges for some displays and events. ACCOMMO-DATIONS: motels and hotels, B&B's, campgrounds, RV parks. RESTAURANTS: family, elegant. CONTACT: Ligonier Valley Chamber of Commerce, 120 E. Main St., Ligonier, PA 15658, (412) 238-4200. 60,000

AUTUMN LEAF FESTIVAL *early October,* Clarion, Clarion Co., in "The Magic Forest" of western Pennsylvania to celebrate the gorgeous colors of fall foliage. Crafts shows, golf and tennis tournaments, 10k run, car show, carnival, talent pageant, parades, flea market, art exhibits, auto driving competition, model railroad club exhibit, electronics festival, glass factory tour, fire truck rides, Kids' Parade, petting zoo, sidewalk sales, health fair, merchants' window decorating contest, dance, motorcycle show, local entertainers. FOODS SERVED: 20 concessionaires sell American, Oriental, and Mexican foods. ADMISSION: free to most events, reserved parade seating $3.00, beauty pageant $3.50 per evening. ACCOMMODATIONS: motels and hotels, B&B's, campgrounds, RV parks. RESTAURANTS: fast foods, family, elegant. CONTACT: Clarion Chamber of Commerce, 517 Main St., Clarion, PA 16214, (814) 226-9161. 100,000

RHODE ISLAND

PROVIDENCE FESTIVAL OF HISTORIC HOMES *first weekend in May,* Providence, Providence Co., to celebrate "Providence's wealth of restored private homes from the 18th and 19th centuries." Evening candlelight tours and day-long house and garden tour of more than two dozen beautifully-restored houses, guitar, piano, and flute music, jazz and other combos such as the Mac Crupcala Jazz Quintet and the Dixie All Stars. FOODS SERVED: "festive." ADMISSION: $15.00 per tour. ACCOMMODATIONS: motels and hotels, B&B's. RESTAURANTS: fast foods, family, elegant, international. CONTACT: Providence Preservation Society, 24 Meeting St., Providence, RI 02903, (401) 831-7440, or the Greater Providence Chamber of Commerce, 30 Exchange Terrace, Providence, RI 02903, (401) 521-5000. 3,500

NEWPORT JAZZ FESTIVAL *second or third weekend in August,* Newport, Newport Co., at Fort Adams State Park on the ocean. Two afternoons of outstanding jazz outdoors, which has included Ella Fitzgerald, Jerry Mulligan, and Spyro Gyra. Bring your blankets. FOODS SERVED: local concessions. ADMISSION: $21.00 per afternoon. ACCOMMODATIONS: motels and hotels, B&B's, campgrounds. RESTAURANTS: fast foods, family, elegant, continental. CONTACT: Newport Co. Chamber of Commerce, 10 America's Cup Ave., Newport RI 02840, (401) 847-1600. 30,000

FALL HARVEST FESTIVAL *fourth weekend in September,* Cranston, Providence Co., in front of the City Hall Complex. Arts and crafts, rides, amusements, Festival Road Race, live entertainment including B. Willie Smith, jazz fusion, country band Caribou, top 40 bands Ryme and Reason and Ronnie Rose and Friends, bluegrass by the Dixie All Stars, and the Rhode Island Symphonic Band. FOODS SERVED: local booths. ADMISSION: free. ACCOMMODATIONS: motels and hotels,

B&B's. RESTAURANTS: fast foods, family, elegant. CONTACT: Executive Chamber, City Hall, Cranston, RI 02910, (401) 461-1000. 20,000

AUTUMN FEST *Columbus Day weekend (near October 12),* Woonsocket, Providence Co., at World War II Memorial Park. Arts and crafts, carnival rides, trade show, exhibits, superstars athletic events, tennis tournament, military exhibits featuring U.S. Air Force Presidential Drill Team, petting zoo, two stages featuring continuous entertainment for three days including 1st Army Concert Band, Boston University Band, and the Royal Canadian Artillery Band of Montreal. FOODS SERVED: French, Canadian, Greek, Polish, Jewish, Armenian, Italian, Chinese. ADMISSION: free. ACCOMMODATIONS: motels and hotels. RESTAURANTS: fast foods, family, elegant, international. CONTACT: Greater Woonsocket Chamber of Commerce, P. O. Box 209, Woonsocket, RI 02895, (401) 762-1730. 300,000

VERMONT

MAPLE SUGAR FESTIVAL *fourth Friday and Saturday in April,* St. Johnsbury, Caledonia Co., in the Northeast Kingdom "to welcome spring and honor sugarmakers everywhere." Sugar-on-Snow, craft fair, cooking and art contests, Maple Sap Run including 2 mi and 6.2 mi foot races, street festival, judging of maple syrup, maple sugar, and maple fudge, maple sugar exhibits and demonstrations, sugar house tours, live entertainment. FOODS SERVED: maple sugar products, pancake breakfast, baked ham supper, luncheon. ADMISSION: free with charges to breakfast, luncheon, and supper, and for indoor entertainment. ACCOMMODATIONS: motels and hotels, B&B's, RV parks. RESTAURANTS: fast foods, family, elegant. CON-

TACT: St. Johnsbury Chamber of Commerce, 30 Western Ave., St. Johnsbury, VT 05819, (802) 748-3678. 4,000

FESTIVAL OF THE ARTS *early June through Columbus Day (October 12),* Manchester, Bennington Co., at the Southern Vermont Art Center, to celebrate the arts. Art exhibition of center's members and invited artists' work, films, special events, study classes, sculpture garden, botany trail, concerts including classical and jazz musicians, the Manchester Music Festival, Susanna McCorkle, and the WAZ. ADMISSION: exhibition free, charges for other events vary. ACCOMMODATIONS: B&B's, campgrounds. RESTAURANTS: fast foods, family, elegant. CONTACT: Southern Vermont Art Center, P.O. Box 617, Manchester, VT 05254 or the Manchester and the Mountains Chamber of Commerce, P. O. Box 928, Manchester, VT 05255, (802) 362-2100. 20,000

DISCOVER JAZZ FESTIVAL *mid-June,* Burlington, Chittenden Co., to salute jazz artists and Vermont's jazz talent, at many sites around Burlington and centered at the Flynn Theatre for the Performing Arts. Jazz at local clubs and gathering places, including abstract expressionist jazz, commercial jazz, contemporary jazz, mainstream, standards, originals, swing, blues, percussion, vocal standards, big band style, bebop, Latin, Brazilian, fusion jazz, Afro-Latin, Bronx funk, jazz videos, a jazz worship service, Jazz with a View, and a pre-school Pee Wee Jazz Band. Performers have included Sarah Vaughan, Modern Jazz Quartet, Lionel Hampton, Ella Fitzgerald, Patty Carpenter Trio, The Over The Hill Gang, and several Vermont groups, Jazz on Parade, a Jazz Picnic, and Jazz Afloat on the Ferry. ADMISSION: varies by event. ACCOMMODATIONS: motels and hotels, B&B's, campgrounds, RV parks. RESTAURANTS: fast foods, family, elegant, French, Mexican, Italian, Indian. CONTACT: Discover Jazz Festival, The Mayor's Council on the Arts, City Hall, Burlington, VT 05401, (802) 658-9300. 25,000

VERMONT MOZART FESTIVAL *last two weeks in July through first week in August,* Burlington, Chittenden Co., and surrounding communities in "some of the most spectacular settings in northern Vermont." Sixteen concerts at sites including Shelburne Farms South Porch and Coachyard, Basin Harbor at Bergennes, Lake Champlain ferry cruise, McCarthy Arts Center at St. Michael's College, the Trapp Family Lodge Meadow at Stowe, and Champlain College's Lola Aiken Hall Lawn. Performers have included the Vermont Mozart Festival Orchestra, pianist Menahem Pressler, a Safe Harbor, Beethoven concert by Festival Winds flautist

Paul Dunkel, Melvin Kaplan, Edward Carroll directing "Classy Brass," "Children's Caravan" with Paul Dunkel conducting the Festival Orchestra and storyteller Robert J. Lurtsema, New York Sousa Band, New York Chamber Soloists, and the prize winner of the Lionel Hampton Jazz Festival Competition, violinists Helen Kwalwasser and Katsuko Esaki, clarinetist Anand Devendra, the McGill Chamber Orchestra, and much more. Three one-week workshops for "musicians of many levels." FOODS SERVED: catered "gourmet meals" for workshop participants, picnics welcome. ADMISSION: $10.50–$18.00. ACCOMMODATIONS: motels and hotels, B&B's, campgrounds, RV parks. RESTAURANTS: fast foods, family, elegant, French, Mexican, Italian, Indian. CONTACT: Vermont Mozart Festival, Box 512, Burlington, VT 05402, (802) 862-7352. 13,000

STRATTON ARTS FESTIVAL *first Sunday after Labor Day (early September) through Columbus Day (October 12),* Stratton Mountain, Windham Co., at the Base Lodge, to celebrate the work of Vermont artists, craftspeople, and performing artists. Rotating exhibition of works of 300 outstanding painters, photographers, sculptors, and craftspeople of international and national renown, has included paintings, ceramics, baskets, quilts and wall hangings, pottery, handmade paper, and blown glass. Each weekend craftspeople demonstrate techniques in making one-of-a-kind pottery, functional baskets, jewelry, hand-blown glass, wooden pitchforks, printmaking, wrought iron, raku pottery, children's programs; performing artists have included the New England Bach Festival and Soviet Emigre Orchestra, a jazz concert, a dramatization of women's lives in 18th-century Vermont, and humorous anecdotes of country living, The Mystic Paper Beast masked theatre, folk songs and traditional instruments, the Musical Theatre Voice Ensemble, readings by Noel Perrin, the Vermont Jazz Ensemble, and Margaret MacArthur and Family singing songs of Vermont and New England. ADMISSION: adults $2.50, students and senior citizens $1.00, children 6 and under free. ACCOMMODATIONS: motels and hotels, B&B's, condominiums. RESTAURANTS: fast foods, family, elegant, German, Chinese. CONTACT: Stratton Arts Festival, P. O. Box 576, Stratton Mountain, VT 05155, (802) 297-2200. 12,000

FESTIVAL OF VERMONT CRAFTS
third weekend in October, Montpelier,
Washington Co., at the high school. More than sixty Vermont craftspeople display and sell their original works. FOODS SERVED: homemade pies, cookies, sandwiches. ADMISSION: $2.00. ACCOMMODATIONS: motels and hotels, B&B's, campgrounds. RESTAURANTS: (nearby) fast foods, family. CONTACT: Central Vermont Chamber of Commerce, P. O. Box 336, Barre, VT 05641, (802) 229-5711. 4,000

MID-ATLANTIC

Delaware / 35

District of Columbia (D.C.) / 35

Maryland / 37

Virginia / 43

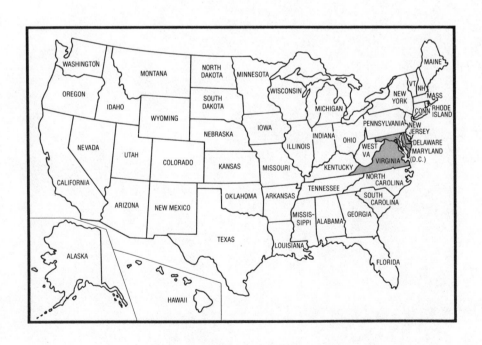

DELAWARE

SPRING FEST *Saturday of Memorial Day weekend (late May)*, Fenwick Island, Sussex Co., in the Bethany–Fenwick area known as "The Quiet Resorts" to celebrate spring. Craft show, flea market, games, raffle of a free weekend at the beach, lots of music such as the Dixieland Ramblers. FOODS SERVED: lots of seafood, sandwiches. ADMISSION: free. ACCOMMODATIONS: motels and hotels, campgrounds, RV parks. RESTAURANTS: fast foods, family, elegant. CONTACT: Bethany–Fenwick Area Chamber of Commerce, P. O. Box 881, Bethany Beach, DE 19930, (302) 539-2100. 5,000

DELMARVA CHICKEN FESTIVAL *second weekend in June*, Milford, Kent Co., in the Delmarva area, to recognize the local poultry industry. Parade, entertainment such as military and high school bands, country-western music, and jazz, magicians, clowns, dancers, trade show, concessions, giant fried chicken pan. FOODS SERVED: chicken and chicken products, drinks, candy. ADMISSION: free. ACCOMMODATIONS: motels and hotels, B&B's, campgrounds, RV parks. RESTAURANTS: fast foods, family, elegant, Chinese. CONTACT: Chamber of Commerce of Milford, River Park Offices, 204 N.E. Front St., Milford, DE 19963, (302) 422-3301. 30,000

RIVER AND HARVEST FESTIVAL *fourth weekend in September*, Milford, Kent Co., in recognition of outstanding contributions to agriculture. Flea markets, concessions, entertainment, politicians' Goat Milking Contest, Jail Bail sponsored by American Heart Association. FOODS SERVED: local food products such as chicken, concessions. ADMISSION: free. ACCOMMODATIONS: motels and hotels, B&B's, campgrounds, RV parks. RESTAURANTS: fast foods, family, elegant, Chinese. CONTACT: Chamber of Commerce of Milford, River Park Offices, 204 N.E. Front St., Milford, DE 19963, (302) 422-3301. 5,000

DISTRICT OF COLUMBIA (D.C.)

SMITHSONIAN KITE FESTIVAL *late March*, Washington, D. C., at the Washington Monument grounds. Kite flyers and kite makers of all ages gather to compete for prizes and trophies. ADMISSION: free. ACCOMMODATIONS: motels and hotels, B&B's, campgrounds, RV parks nearby. RESTAURANTS: fast foods, family, elegant, international. CONTACT: (202) 357-3030 or the Washington, D. C. Convention and Visitors Association, 1575 Eye St., N.W., Washington, D.C. 20005, (202) 789-7000.

CHERRY BLOSSOM FESTIVAL *second week in April*, Washington, D.C., to celebrate the blooming of the Japanese cherry blossoms. Parade with princesses, floats, and V.I.P.'s fashion show, Japanese lantern lighting ceremony, marathon run, lots of music. ADMISSION: free. ACCOMMODATIONS: motels and hotels, B&B's, campgrounds, RV parks nearby. RESTAURANTS: fast foods, family, elegant, international. CONTACT: Downtown Jaycees at (202) 293-0480 or the Washington, D.C.

Convention and Visitors Association, 1575 Eye St., N.W., Washington, D.C. 20005, (202) 789-7000.

POTOMAC RIVERFEST *every weekend in June*, Washington, D.C., in southwest D.C. Arts and crafts, tall ships, boat rides, water events, fireworks. ADMISSION: free. FOODS SERVED: ethnic. ACCOMMODATIONS: motels and hotels, B&B's, campgrounds, RV parks nearby. RESTAURANTS: fast foods, family, elegant, international. CONTACT: Washington, D.C. Convention and Visitors Association, 1575 Eye St., N.W., Washington, D.C. 20005, (202) 789-7000.

MOSTLY MOZART FESTIVAL *late June*, Washington, D.C., at the John F. Kennedy Center for the Performing Arts. A true festival of the works of Wolfgang Amadeus Mozart. ADMISSION: charge. ACCOMMODATIONS: motels and hotels, B&B's, campgrounds, RV parks nearby. RESTAURANTS: fast foods, family, elegant, international. CONTACT: (202) 254-3600 or the Washington, D.C. Convention and Visitors Association, 1575 Eye St., N.W., Washington, D.C. 20005, (202) 789-7000.

FESTIVAL OF AMERICAN FOLK-LIFE *last full weekend in June and long first weekend in July*, Washington, D.C., on the National Mall. Traditional crafts, music, occupational folklife, performances and demonstrations ranging from Appalachian fiddling to native American dancing and from quilting to coal mining. FOODS SERVED: native American, concessions. ADMISSION: free. ACCOMMODATIONS: motels and hotels, B&B's, campgrounds, RV parks nearby. RESTAURANTS: fast foods, family, elegant, international. CONTACT: (202) 357-2700 or the Washington, D.C. Convention and Visitors Association, 1575 Eye St., N.W., Washington, D.C. 20005, (202) 789-7000.

LATIN AMERICAN FESTIVAL *fourth weekend in July*, Washington, D.C., in the Adams–Morgan and Mt. Pleasant area of D.C. Arts and crafts, plays depicting Hispanic life, Latin music and dance. FOODS SERVED: Latin/Hispanic. ADMISSION: free. ACCOMMODATIONS: motels and hotels, B&B's, campgrounds, RV parks nearby. RESTAURANTS: fast foods, family, elegant. CONTACT: (202) 328-6533 or the Washington, D.C. Convention and Visitors Association, 1575 Eye St., N.W., Washington, D.C. 20005, (202) 789-7000.

NATIONAL FRISBEE FESTIVAL *Sunday of Labor Day weekend (early September)*, Washington, D.C., on the National Mall. "The largest competitive Frisbee festival featuring world-class Frisbee champions and disc-catching dogs." ADMISSION: free. ACCOMMODATIONS: motels and hotels, B&B's, campgrounds, RV parks. RESTAURANTS: fast foods, family, elegant, international. CONTACT: (301) 843-1800 or the Washington, D.C. Convention and Visitors Association, 1575 Eye St., N.W., Washington, D.C. 20005, (202) 789-7000.

WASHINGTON REGGAE FESTIVAL *third Saturday in September*, Washington, D.C., at Georgia Avenue and Bryant St., N.W. At least five reggae bands perform during the afternoon of music. ADMISSION: free. ACCOMMODATIONS: motels and hotels, B&B's, campgrounds, RV parks nearby. RESTAURANTS: fast foods, family, elegant, international. CONTACT: (202) 232-4602 or the Washington, D.C. Convention and Visitors Association, 1575 Eye St., N.W., Washington, D.C. 20005, (202) 789-7000.

MARYLAND

WINTERFEST *mid-March,* Deep Creek Lake and Oakland areas, Garrett Co., in Maryland's ski country. Ski races, sleigh rides, woodsmen contests, fireworks, torchlight parade, "zany Yakapah Parade," snowmobile hill-climb, live entertainment. FOODS SERVED: Bavarian food and beverages. ADMISSION: free. ACCOMMODATIONS: motels and hotels, cabins, campgrounds. RESTAURANTS: fast foods, family, elegant. CONTACT: Deep Creek Lake–Garret Co. Promotion Council, Courthouse, Oakland, MD 21550, (301) 334-1948.

SOUTHERN MARYLAND CELTIC FESTIVAL AND HIGHLAND GATH-ERING *last Saturday in April,* St. Leonard, Calvert Co., at Jefferson–Patterson Park, to celebrate the origins of many local citizens from Scotland, Ireland, and Wales. Southern Maryland Scottish Fiddling Championship, Highland Heptathalon, piping contests, living history exhibits, Parade of Clans and Nations, foot racing, Kilted Mile Race, rugby demonstrations, continuous music and dance performances including Sue Richards on the Celtic Harp, "Soda Bread," More or Les Morris Dancers, national fiddling champion John Turner, Kiltie Band of York. FOODS SERVED: meat pies, bridies, sausage rolls, fish and chips, British cookies and cakes. ADMISSION: adults 12 and over $5.00, children and seniors $2.00. ACCOMMODATIONS: motels and hotels, B&B's, campgrounds. RESTAURANTS: fast foods, family, elegant. CONTACT: Celtic Festival, P. O. Box 209, Prince Frederick, MD 20678, (301) 535-3274. 2,500

SALISBURY FESTIVAL *first weekend in May,* Salisbury, Wicomico Co., at the Downtown Plaza, Riverwalk Park, and at the City Dock and Marina, to celebrate the arrival of spring and the blooming of dogwood trees. Arts and crafts, giant block party, raft race, antiques displays and sales, 10k Run, bicycle race, children's rides, contests, local entertainers. FOODS SERVED: more than fifty food booths featuring local and ethnic specialties. ADMISSION: free. ACCOMMODATIONS: motels and hotels, campgrounds, RV parks. CONTACT: Salisbury Area Chamber of Commerce, P. O. Box 510, Salisbury, MD 21801, (301) 749-0144. 25,000

PREAKNESS STAKES AND FESTI-VAL WEEK *third week in May,* Baltimore, Baltimore Co., at the Inner Harbor and downtown, to celebrate the running of the "middle jewel of the Triple Crown" of horseracing, the Preakness. Balloon race, neighborhood competitions, frog hop, Hollywood Look-Alike Contest, road races, contests. FOODS SERVED: crabs, chili, "fun food." ADMISSION: free. ACCOMMODATIONS: motels and hotels, B&B's, campgrounds, RV parks. RESTAURANTS: fast foods, family, elegant, international, seafood (softshell crabs). CONTACT: Baltimore Office of Promotion and Tourism, 34 Market Place, Suite 310, Baltimore, MD 21202, (301) 837-INFO or (301) 752-8632. 40,000

CHESTERTOWN TEA PARTY *third weekend in May,* Chestertown, Kent Co., to commemorate the dumping of "tea from the 'Geddes' into the harbor in May of 1774 to protest British Port Act of 1774." Colonial Parade featuring the Tench Tilghman Fife and Drum Corps and the Maryland First Regiment, colonial working crafts exhibit from "candlemakers to scarecrow stuffers," tall ships, art show, walking tours of historic Chestertown, Children's Concert at the Children's Booth, Make Your Own instrument, Tea Party reenactment, entertainment including the Footloose Cloggers and a clogging workshop, Dance for Children Only, The Pepper Steppers, concert by the Sounding Brass Quintet, and square dancing, in addition to a performance by the Actor's

Community Theater. FOODS SERVED: Eastern Shore delicacies such as Maryland fried chicken, fish fry, crab cakes, chitlins. ADMISSION: free except for cocktail party $10.00, carriage rides $2.00. ACCOMMODATIONS: motels and hotels, B&B's, campgrounds. RESTAURANTS: fast foods, family, elegant, seafood. CONTACT: Kent Co. Chamber of Commerce, P. O. Box 146, Chestertown, MD 21620, (301) 778-0416. 7,000

HALFWAY PARK DAYS *fourth weekend in May,* Hagerstown, Washington Co., at Halfway County Park. Arts and crafts, softball tournaments, rides, variety of music. FOODS SERVED: "plenty." ADMISSION: free. ACCOMMODATIONS: motels and hotels, B&B's, campgrounds, RV parks. RESTAURANTS: fast foods, family, elegant. CONTACT: Steve Mountain, 228 Oak Forest Dr., Hagerstown, MD 21740, (301) 582-1337, or Washington Co. Tourism, Courthouse Annex, Hagerstown, MD 21740, (301) 739-2015. 50,000

CUMBERLAND HERITAGE DAYS *second weekend in June,* Cumberland, Allegany Co., at the Washington Street Historic District and Historic Downtown Mall. Arts and crafts, games, tours of historic buildings, trolley car rides, fiddle contest, entertainment such as local and regional bluegrass and country groups. FOODS SERVED: concessions. ADMISSION: free. ACCOMMODATIONS: motels and hotels, B&B's, campgrounds. RESTAURANTS: fast foods, family, elegant, international. CONTACT: Dave Williams at 127 Greene St., Cumberland, MD 21502, or the Greater Cumberland Chamber of Commerce, City Hall Plaza, Cumberland, MD 21502, (301) 722-2820. 25,000

POLISH FESTIVAL *third weekend in June,* Baltimore, Baltimore Co., to celebrate Polish heritage of many Baltimore residents. Polish costumes, Polish music and bands, Polish and handmade crafts and jewelry, cultural and educational exhibits. FOODS SERVED: Polish. ADMISSION: free.

ACCOMMODATIONS: motels and hotels, B&B's, campgrounds, RV parks. RESTAURANTS: fast foods, family, elegant, international, seafood (softshell crabs). CONTACT: Baltimore Office of Promotion and Tourism, 34 Market Place, Suite 310, Baltimore, MD 21202, (301) 837-INFO or (301) 752-8632. 35,000

POCOMOKE CITY CYPRESS FESTIVAL *first weekend of summer (late June),* Pocomoke City, "Friendliest Town on the Eastern Shore," Worcester Co. at Cypress Park to celebrate the beginning of summer. Craft show, water events, rides and games, a "sort of gigantic homecoming and reunion for families who still have relatives in the area combined with a fun-filled salute to summer." East Virginia Cloggers, Cypress Square Dancers, Sundance Rock Band, several country and bluegrass groups, local band competition. FOODS SERVED: "mostly good ole Eastern Shore–Southern." ADMISSION: free. ACCOMMODATIONS: motels and hotels, B&B, campgrounds. RV parks. RESTAURANTS: fast foods, family, elegant. CONTACT: Pocomoke City Chamber of Commerce, Inc., P. O. Box 356, Pocomoke City, MD 21851, (301) 957-1919. 10,000

FROSTBURG ITALIAN FESTIVAL *fourth weekend in June,* Frostburg, Allegany Co., on Main Street, to celebrate the Italian heritage of local residents. Arts and crafts, games, wine tasting, Italian dancing, entertainment including Italian tenor Mario Martinelli. FOODS SERVED: Italian. ADMISSION: free. ACCOMMODATIONS: motels and hotels. RESTAURANTS: fast foods, family, elegant, French, Italian. CONTACT: Elvis Jones, 222 McCulloh St., Frostburg, MD 21532 or the Frostburg Chamber of Commerce, P. O. Box 440, Frostburg, MD 21532, (301) 689-6000. 20,000

GRANTSVILLE DAYS *fourth weekend in June,* Grantsville, Garrett Co. Parade, fireworks, picnic in the park, craft booths, Coaster Derby, contests including fiddling, live bluegrass music, gospel music, dance. FOODS SERVED: chicken barbecue, homemade foods. ADMISSION: free. ACCOMMODATIONS: motels and hotels, campgrounds. RESTAURANTS: family. CONTACT: Deep Creek Lake–Garrett Co. Promotion Council, Courthouse, Oakland, MD 21550, (301) 334-2948.

OLD FASHIONED WEEKEND IN THE PARK *fourth weekend in June,* Western Port, Allegany Co., at the Westvaco Community Park. Arts and crafts, flea market, old-time contests such as tobacco spitting, banjo, and fiddle contests, "fun and games," North Carolina Cloggers. FOODS SERVED: variety. ADMISSION: free. CONTACT: Gary Galloway, Bloomington School, Bloomington, MD 21523, (301) 359-0331. 20,000

TIDEWATER MUSIC FESTIVAL *last week in June through second week in July,* St. Mary's City, St. Mary's Co., at St. Mary's College of Maryland. Performances of contemporary American music featuring guest composers and traditional musical offerings, summer music camp. Guest composers have included Aaron Copeland, Joseph Schwantner, and David Heinich and other musicians from throughout the United States. ADMISSION: varies. ACCOMMODATIONS: motels and hotels. RESTAURANTS: fast foods, family, elegant. CONTACT: William H. Street, Director, St. Mary's College of Maryland, St. Mary's City, MD 20686, (301) 862-0200. 3,000

PARK ARTS FESTIVAL *last weekend in June,* Hagerstown, Washington Co., at Doubs Woods County Park, to showcase the visual and performing arts. Arts and crafts, continuous entertainment, children's area. FOODS SERVED: Italian, Mexican, Chinese, French, German, and American. ADMISSION: "nominal." ACCOMMODATIONS: motels and hotels, B&B's, campgrounds, RV parks. RESTAURANTS: fast foods, family, elegant. CONTACT: Lieben Cohen, c/o Washington Co. Parks and

Recreation, 33 W. Washington St., Hagerstown, MD 21740, (301) 791-3125, or Washington Co. Tourism, Courthouse Annex, Hagerstown, MD 21740, (301) 739-2015. 50,000

TUCKAHOE STEAM AND GAS ENGINE SHOW *weekend after July 4th,* five miles north of Easton, Talbot Co., on the Eastern Shore, to preserve the heritage of steam and gas engines in agriculture. Working sawmills, wheat threshing, soap making, horse pulling, stone crushing, blacksmithing, grist mill, all operated by steam or gas; flea market including engine parts and equipment, parade of antique equipment daily, country-western music daily and evenings, dances, Sunday church service. FOODS SERVED: chicken, crab cakes, sub shop, concessions. ADMISSION: adults $2.00, under 16 free. ACCOMMODATIONS: motels and hotels, campgrounds, RV parks nearby. RESTAURANTS: (nearby) fast foods, family, elegant. CONTACT: Tuckahoe Steam and Gas Association, Inc., c/o Jean A. Bright, Rt 1, Box 123, Centreville, MD 21617, (301) 758-0462. 12,000

ITALIAN FESTIVAL *second weekend in July,* Baltimore, Baltimore Co., at Festival Hall to celebrate the Italian heritage of many Baltimore residents. Continuous Italian music, traditional costumes and bands, imported and handmade crafts and jewelry, cultural and educational exhibits. FOODS SERVED: traditional Italian. ADMISSION: $1.00. ACCOMMODATIONS: motels and hotels, B&B's, campgrounds, RV parks. RESTAURANTS: fast foods, family, elegant, international, seafood (softshell crabs). CONTACT: Baltimore Office of Promotion and Tourism, 34 Market Place, Suite 310, Baltimore, MD 21202, (301) 837-INFO or (301) 752-8632. 50,000

LOTUS BLOSSOM FESTIVAL *second weekend in July,* Buckeystown, Frederick Co., at Lilypons Water Garden, to celebrate the lovely lotus and water lily blossoms in this unique environment. Arts and crafts, entertainment. FOODS SERVED: concessions: ADMISSION: free. ACCOMMODATIONS: motels and hotels, B&B's, campgrounds, RV parks. RESTAURANTS: fast foods, family, elegant. CONTACT: Charles Thomas at (301) 874-5133 or the Chamber of Commerce of Frederick Co., P. O. Box 746, Frederick, MD 21701, (301) 662-4164. 12,000

AMERICAN INDIAN POW WOW
second weekend in July, McHenry, Garrett Co., at the County Fairgrounds. Tribal dances and singing with dance competitions each afternoon featuring participants from throughout the United States, native arts and crafts, traditional events and contests. FOODS SERVED: "native" (American Indian). ADMISSION: free. ACCOMMODATIONS: motels and hotels, campgrounds. RESTAURANTS: fast foods, family. CONTACT: Deep Creek Lake–Garrett Co. Promotion Council, Courthouse, Oakland, MD 21550, (301) 334-1948.

UNIVERSITY OF MARYLAND INTERNATIONAL PIANO FESTIVAL AND WILLIAM KAPELL COMPETITION *mid-July,* College Park, Prince George's Co., in the Washington, D.C. area. Major international piano competition is accompanied by a week-long festival featuring recitals by internationally renowned pianists, master classes, lecture–recitals, symposia on topics related to the piano and its artists, including some of the world's leading pianists. In the William Kapell Competition, forty young pianists vie for $40,000 in cash prizes. ADMISSION: single tickets available, $225.00 for entire week. ACCOMMODATIONS: motels and hotels, University dormitory. RESTAURANTS: fast foods, family, elegant, international. CONTACT: Piano Festival Coordinator, c/o Summer Programs, University of Maryland, College Park, MD 20742, (301) 454-3347. 4,000

J. MILLARD TAWES CRAB AND CLAM BAKE *third Wednesday in July,* Crisfield, Somerset Co., at Somers Cove Marina Grounds. Country music and all you can eat. FOODS SERVED: steamed crabs, steamed and raw clams, clam strips, fish, potatoes, sweet corn, watermelon, and drinks. ADMISSION: $19.50 per person. ACCOMMODATIONS: motels and hotels, campgrounds, RV parks. RESTAURANTS: family. CONTACT: Ruth Custis, Crisfield Area Chamber of Commerce, P.O. Box 292, Crisfield, MD 21817, (301) 968-2500. 4,000

OLD FASHIONED CORN ROAST FESTIVAL *first Saturday in August,* Westminster, Carroll Co., at the Union Mills Homestead, seven miles north of Westminster, and sponsored by the Union Mills Homestead Foundation, Inc., which exists to preserve and maintain the Shriver Homestead. Tours of the Grist Mill exhibiting the saw mill, cooper shop, blacksmith shop and tannery and the Homestead, all the roasted-in-the-husk corn you can eat, barbecued chicken and all the trimmings. Union Mills Homestead stone ground cornmeal, buckwheat and whole wheat flour are for sale. FOODS SERVED: corn-on-the-cob. ADMISSION: free to grounds, charges for tours of Grist Mill and museum. ACCOMMODATIONS: motels and hotels, B&B's, campgrounds, RV parks. RESTAURANTS: fast foods, family. CONTACT: Esther L. Shriver, Union Mills Homestead Foundation, 3311 Littlestown Pike, Westminster, MD 21157, (301) 848-2288.

FRONTIER CRAFT DAYS *first weekend in August,* Hagerstown, Washington Co., at Hager House on Key Street. More than sixty heritage craftspeople display and sell their works and demonstrate their skills, military encampment; bluegrass, traditional country, and German music. FOODS SERVED: German and American. ADMISSION: free. ACCOMMODATIONS: motels and hotels, B&B's, campgrounds, RV parks. RESTAURANTS: fast foods, family, elegant. CONTACT: Spring Ward, c/o Hager House, 19 Key St., Hagerstown, MD 21740 or Washington Co. Tourism, Courthouse Annex, Hagerstown, MD 21740, (301) 739-2015. 10,000

GERMAN FESTIVAL *second or third weekend in August,* Baltimore, Baltimore Co., to celebrate the German heritage of many Baltimore residents. Continuous music, imported and handmade arts and crafts, jewelry, cultural and educational exhibits, German costumes, oompah bands. FOODS SERVED: German. ADMISSION: free. ACCOMMODATIONS: motels and hotels, B&B's, campgrounds, RV parks. RESTAURANTS: fast foods, family, elegant, international, seafood (softshell crabs). CONTACT: Baltimore Office of Promotion and Tourism, 34 Market Place, Suite 310, Baltimore, MD 21202, (301) 837-INFO or (301) 752-8632. 35,000

C&O CANAL BOAT FESTIVAL *third weekend in August,* Cumberland, Allegany Co., at North Branch and Rt, 51, to recognize the importance of the C&O Canal. Tours of a canal boat, arts and crafts, horse and buggy rides, interpretive hikes of nature and canal structures in historic setting or original canal locks and restored lockhouse. FOODS SERVED: "old tyme food," including Canal Boat Bean Soup. ADMISSION: $1.00 per person. ACCOMMODATIONS: motels and hotels, campgrounds, RV parks. RESTAURANTS: fast foods, family. CONTACT: Sarah Mason, 1604 Frederick St., Cumberland, MD 21502 or the Greater Cumberland Chamber of Commerce, City Hall Plaza, Cumberland, MD 21502, (301) 722-2820. 25,000

NATIONAL HARD CRAB DERBY *Labor Day weekend, (early September),* Crisfield, Somerset Co., at Somers Cove Marina Grounds. Crab races, Boat Docking Contest, Crab Cooking Contest, Boat Parade, Crab Picking Contest, Miss Crustacean Beauty Pageant, fireworks, Religious Talent Show, 4-wheel Mud Hop, Governor's Cup Crab Race, Children's Plastic Bottle Boat Regatta, Crabbers' Ball, fishing tournament, 10k Marathon, tennis tournament, high school band concert, U.S. Navy Band, Army Drill Team, dock party, children's events. FOODS SERVED: mainly seafood such as crabs and oysters, oyster sandwiches. ADMISSION: adults $3.00, children under 12 $1.00. ACCOMMODATIONS: motels and hotels, campgrounds, RV parks. RESTAURANTS: family. CONTACT: Ruth Custis, National Hard Crab Derby, P. O. Box 215, Crisfield, MD 21817, (301) 968-2682. 10,000

BOONESBOROUGH DAYS *weekend after Labor Day (early September),* Boonsboro, Washington Co. Arts and crafts representative of Boonsboro's early days such as broommaking, candlemaking, log hewing, chair caning, antiques, bluegrass music. FOODS SERVED: "country." ADMISSION: free. ACCOMMODATIONS: motels and hotels, B&B's, campgrounds, RV parks. RESTAURANTS: family, elegant. CONTACT: Wanda Heyer, Rt. 1, Box 329, Boonsboro, MD 21713 or Washington Co. Tourism, Courthouse Annex, Hagerstown, MD 21740, (301) 739-2015. 100,000

HANCOCK LIONS APPLE CANAL FESTIVAL *second weekend in September,* Hancock, Washington Co., at Widmeyer Park. Arts and crafts, musical entertainment, wagon rides along the C&O Canal. FOODS SERVED: "homemade specialties." ADMISSION: free. ACCOMMODATIONS: motels and hotels, campgrounds, RV parks. RESTAURANTS: family. CONTACT: Washington Co. Tourism, Courthouse Annex, Hagerstown, MD 21740, (301) 739-2015. 10,000

BALTIMORE CITY FAIR *third weekend in September,* Baltimore, Baltimore Co., to celebrate life in Baltimore's diverse neighborhoods, and as a contribution to the revitalization of downtown Baltimore. Arts and crafts, rides, carnival, business exhibits, displays by non-profit organizations and neighborhood groups showing their ethnic and national origins with great color; five stages of continuous entertainment which has included major performers such as Melba Moore, Smokey Robinson, Miami Sound Machine, George Benson, Donny and Marie Osmond, and Ethel Ennis, in addition to many local entertainers. FOODS SERVED: "all types of food" including those of the many nationalities residing in Baltimore. ADMISSION: $3.00. ACCOMMODATIONS: motels and hotels, B&B's. RESTAURANTS: fast foods, family, elegant, international. CONTACT: Baltimore City Fair, P.O. Box 22359, Baltimore, MD 21203, (301) 547-0015. 500,000

SEAFOOD FESTIVAL *third weekend in September,* Cumberland, Allegany Co., at the County Fairgrounds in the Bowling Green area. Arts and crafts, musical entertainment, and seafood "of all types." FOODS SERVED: Chesapeake Bay seafood, crab soup, concessions. ADMISSION: free. ACCOMMODATIONS: campgrounds and RV parks. RESTAURANTS: fast foods, family, seafood. CONTACT: Greater Cumberland Chamber of Commerce, City Hall Plaza, Cumberland, MD 21502, (301) 722-2820. 25,000

MARYLAND WINE FESTIVAL *fourth weekend in September,* Westminster, Carroll Co., at the Carroll County Farm Museum. Two-day wine festival featuring all-day wine tasting, continuous entertainment and "top quality crafts." FOODS SERVED: "fine cuisine." ADMISSION: charge. ACCOMMODATIONS: motels and hotels, campgrounds. RESTAURANTS: fast foods, family. CONTACT: Carroll Co., Farm Museum, 500 So. Center St., Westminster, MD 21157, (301) 848-7775.

SUNFEST *fourth weekend in September,* Ocean City, Worcester Co., on the Eastern Shore. Four days of arts and crafts including ceramics and hand-painted porcelain, stuffed toys, pillows, driftwood, lobster tables, quilts, barrel-art painting, jewelry, leather goods; World Class Kite Festival, Indian Ceremonial Dancing by Chief Red Bird, Screaming Eagle, and Laughing Wolf of the Cherokee Nation and Frontiertown, Miss Sunfest Contest, Adeler Treasure Hunt for adults only on the beach for fifty leather pouches containing valuable gems, windsurfing competition, Miniature Golf Tournament. Seafood Day features demonstrations of how to shuck oysters, fillet fish, and pick hardshell crabs; wide range of music performed continuously all four days, including string bands, dixieland, country-western and bluegrass, big band, ragtime, country pickin', banjos, clogging, organ music, aerobic dancers, U.S. Army Band, jazz. FOODS SERVED: Maryland specialties such as oyster sandwiches, clam fritters, soft crabs, crab cakes, crab fluffs, smoked fish, Maryland cream of crab soup, clam strips, cannoli, open-pit beef, Philly-style cheese steaks, raw clams and oysters, Mexican, and Greek, concessions. ADMISSION: free. ACCOMMODATIONS: motels and hotels, B&B's. RESTAURANTS: fast foods, family, elegant, seafood. CONTACT: SUNFEST, Convention Center, 4001 Coastal Hwy., Ocean City, MD 21842, (301) 289-2800. 250,000

WESTMINSTER FALLFEST *last weekend in September,* Westminster, Carroll Co., in western Maryland. Arts and crafts, games, rides, parade, live bands. FOODS SERVED: "every kind of food imaginable." ADMISSION: free. ACCOMMODATIONS: motels and hotels, B&B's. RESTAURANTS: fast foods, family, elegant. CONTACT: City of Westminster, City Hall, Box 010, Westminster, MD 21157, (301) 848-9000. 12,000

FURNACE TOWN FALL FESTIVAL *first weekend in October,* Furnace Town, Snow Hill, Worcester Co., on the Eastern Shore, to celebrate life in a 19th-century industrial village that boasts "the site of earliest-known still-intact hot blast iron furnace in the United States." Arts and crafts, living history demonstrations of 1840s, interpretative tours of the village, bluegrass concerts featuring the dulcimer, folk harp, recorder, fiddle, and sacred harp, melody and other period music. FOODS SERVED: "1840s rural American and Eastern Shore home cooking." ADMISSION: $3.00 per person, $5.00 per family. ACCOMMODATIONS: (within 20 mi.) motels and hotels, B&B's, campgrounds. RES-

TAURANTS: (nearby) fast foods, family, elegant. CONTACT: Furnace Town Foundation, Inc., P. O. Box 207, Snow Hill, MD 21863, (301) 632-2032. 1,000

AUTUMN GLORY FESTIVAL *second weekend in October,* Oakland, Garrett Co., to celebrate "the beautiful fall foliage," held throughout the county with largest events in Oakland. Grand Feature Parade, Maryland State Five-String Banjo Championship, Maryland State Fiddle Championship, parades, antique show, arts and crafts, dancing, games. FOODS SERVED: Maryland turkey dinners sold throughout the festival weekend, concessions. ADMISSION: free. ACCOMMODATIONS: motels and hotels, campgrounds. RESTAURANTS: fast foods, family, elegant. CONTACT: Deep

Creek Lake–Garret Co., Promotion Council, Courthouse, Oakland, MD 21550, (301) 334-1948. 70,000

CATOCTIN COLORFEST *second weekend in October,* Thurmont, Frederick Co., at the foot of the Catoctin Mountains, to celebrate lovely fall foliage. More than 350 arts, crafts, and food booths feature handmade Maryland contemporary and traditional folk crafts, entertainment by local dance studio. FOODS SERVED: fried chicken, barbecue, concessions. ADMISSION: free. ACCOMMODATIONS: motels and hotels, campgrounds. RESTAURANTS: fast foods, family. CONTACT: Catoctin Color-Fest, Inc., P. O. Box 33, Thurmont, MD 21788, (301) 271-4333.

VIRGINIA

KITE FESTIVAL *second Sunday in March,* Lorton, Fairfax Co., at Gunston Hall Plantation. "Children through age 15 admitted free when accompanied by an adult to fly their kites in the field." Puppet shows, tours of 18th-century mansion house. FOODS SERVED: all-American. ADMISSION: adults $3.00, senior citizens $2.50. ACCOMMODATIONS: motels and hotels, campgrounds, RV parks nearby. RESTAURANTS: fast foods, family, elegant. CONTACT: Gunston Hall Plantation, Lorton, VA 22079, (703) 550-9220. 1,000

SPRING SEAPORT FESTIVAL *mid-April,* Alexandria, Fairfax Co. Free boat rides, waterfront displays throughout Old Town, waiters and waitresses races, costumes, live entertainment, demonstrations. FOODS SERVED: special seafood menus. ADMISSION: free. ACCOMMODATIONS: motels and hotels, B&B's, campgrounds, RV parks nearby. RESTAURANTS: fast foods, family, elegant, international. CONTACT: Old Town Business Association,

215 N. Washington St., Alexandria, VA 22314, (703) 549-1000 or the Alexandria Chamber of Commerce, 1454 Duke St., Alexandria, VA 22314, (703) 549-1000.

HEART OF VIRGINIA FESTIVAL *first weekend in May,* Farmville, Prince Edward Co. Arts and crafts show, educational exhibits, competitions, music including local country-music bands, folk bands, and performances by local college and community theatrical groups. FOODS SERVED: "all." ADMISSION: free. ACCOMMODATIONS: motels and hotels, B&B's, campgrounds. RESTAURANTS: fast foods, family, elegant. CONTACT: Farmville Chamber of Commerce, P. O. Box 361, Farmville, VA 23901, (804) 392-3939. 75,000

RIVERFAIR *second weekend in May,* Newport News, in the Tidewater area to celebrate spring. Marketplace, parade, 10k Run, golf and tennis tournaments, fashion show, Beach Music Dance, nationally known entertainers have performed a wide range of music including jazz, country, Top 40, rhythm and blues. Entertainers have included The Spinners, Reba McIntire, the late Rick Nelson, and the Marvellettes. FOODS SERVED: Latin American, German, Chinese, Greek, American. ADMISSION: free. ACCOMMODATIONS: motels and hotels. RESTAURANTS: fast foods, family, elegant. CONTACT: Cynthia F. Carter, Department of Parks and Recreation, 2400 Washington Ave., Newport News, VA 23607, (804) 247-8451. 30,000

VIRGINIA POULTRY FESTIVAL *third week in May,* Harrisonburg, Rockingham Co., in the Shenandoah Valley, to celebrate the poultry and egg industry. Chicken Pluckers Fun Day includes Battle of Chicken and Turkey Pluckers, Turkey Calling Contest, Poultry Judging Contest, antique car meet, Battle of the Plants, beauty pageant, Virginia Poultry Convention, bowling, tennis and golf tournaments, Ladies' Luncheon, banquet, dance, run, go-kart races, parade. FOODS SERVED: barbecued chicken, food booths. ADMISSION: free, charges for some events. ACCOMMODATIONS: motels and hotels, B&B's, campgrounds, RV parks. RESTAURANTS: fast foods, family, elegant. CONTACT: Virginia Poultry Federation, Jane Moss, Festival Coordinator, P. O. Box 552, Harrisonburg, VA 22801, (703) 433-2451.

VIVA! VIENNA! *Memorial Day weekend (late May),* Vienna, Fairfax Co. More than 300 crafts displays, entertainment for all ages, Memorial Day Ceremony, The Flagship Band and The Show Offs. FOODS SERVED: concessions. ADMISSION: free. ACCOMMODATIONS: motels and hotels. RESTAURANTS: fast foods, family, elegant, Asian, Mexican, French, Italian. CONTACT: ViVa! Vienna!, Greater Vienna Chamber of Commerce, 402 Maple Ave., W., Vienna, VA 22180, (703) 281-1333. 30,000

CELEBRATE SUMMER AT WOLF TRAP *June through August,* Vienna, Fairfax Co., at Wolf Trap Farm Park for the Performing Arts. Performances by artists representing many musical disciplines such as the Wolf Trap Opera Company, the Kirov Ballet from Leningrad, U.S.S.R., Anne Murray, Benny Goodman, Burl Ives, New York City Opera, Johnny Cash, Bonnie Raitt, Roy Orbison, Emmylou Harris, Smokey Robinson, Spyro Gyra, National Symphony Orchestra, Itzhak Perlman, Peter Nero, Joan Baez, Johnny Mathis, Windham Hill Summer Concert, Pete Seeger and Arlo Guthrie, Chuck Mangione, Natalie Cole, Judy Collins, Peter, Paul, and Mary, Preservaion Hall Jazz Band, Canadian Ballet Extravaganza, International Children's Festival, Kenny Loggins, and magician David Copperfield. FOODS SERVED: simple to elegant box lunches and Wolf Trap picnics available from $6.50–$23.95, American Cafe catering and dinner in a 200-seat tented-pavilion. ADMISSION: tickets from $10.00–$35.00. Shuttle bus departs from Washington, D.C., Chevy Chase, MD, National Place, and Tyson's Corner. ACCOMMODATIONS: motels and hotels. RESTAURANTS: fast foods, family, elegant, Asian, Mexican, continental. CONTACT: Wolf Trap Foundation for the Performing Arts, 1624 Trap Rd., Vienna, VA 22180, (703) 255-1860.

FREDERICKSBURG ART FESTIVAL *first weekend in June,* Fredericksburg, Spotsylvania Co. Outdoor festival featuring the fine arts and crafts of professional and amateur artists, nationally known judges, cash prizes and awards. ADMISSION: free. ACCOMMODATIONS: motels and hotels, B&B's, campgrounds, RV parks. RESTAURANTS: fast foods, family, elegant. CONTACT: Department of Tourism, 706 Caroline St., Fredericksburg, VA 22401, (703) 373-1776.

BEACH MUSIC FESTIVAL *June,* Stuart, Patrick Co., in the foothills of the Blue Ridge Mountains. Beach "music and eating." FOODS SERVED: concessions. ADMISSION: free. ACCOMMODATIONS: motels and hotels, B&B's, campgrounds, RV parks.

RESTAURANTS: fast foods, family. CONTACT: Patrick Co. Chamber of Commerce, P. O. Box 577, Stuart, VA 24171, (703) 694-6012. 3,000

HERITAGE FESTIVAL *July 4th weekend,* Fredericksburg, Spotsylvania Co., as a celebration of Fredericksburg's colonial, Revolutionary, and Civil War past. Great Rappahannock River Raft Race, arts and crafts shows, 5mi Race, riverside carnival, living history exhibits, fireworks, concerts. FOODS SERVED: concessions. ADMISSION: free. ACCOMMODATIONS: motels and hotels, B&B's, campgrounds, RV parks. RESTAURANTS: fast foods, family, elegant. CONTACT: Department of Tourism, 706 Caroline St., Fredericksburg, VA 22401, (703) 373-1776.

BLUEGRASS MUSIC FESTIVAL *July 4th weekend,* Stuart, Patrick Co., in the foothills of the Blue Ridge Mountains. Bluegrass "music and eating." FOODS SERVED: concessions. ADMISSION: free. ACCOMMODATIONS: motels and hotels, B&B, campgrounds, RV parks. RESTAURANTS: fast foods, family. CONTACT: Patrick Co. Chamber of Commerce, P. O. Box 577. Stuart, VA 24171, (703) 694-6012. 2,000

LAKEFEST *third weekend in July,* Clarksville, Mecklenburg Co., to celebrate life and recreational opportunities on "the lake," John S. Kerr Reservoir. Arts and crafts, pig pickin', sailing regatta, Pontoon Parade, jog-a-thon, street dance, flea market, Beach Music Festival. FOODS SERVED: fish fry, barbecue, concessions. ADMISSION: "separate costs for each function." ACCOMMODATIONS: motels and hotels, B&B's, campgrounds, RV parks. RESTAURANTS: fast foods, family. CONTACT: Clarksville Chamber of Commerce, P. O. Box 1017, Clarksville, VA 23927, (703) 374-2436.

HUNGRY MOTHER PARK ARTS AND CRAFTS FESTIVAL *third weekend in July,* Marion, Smyth Co., at Hungry

Mother State Park. Nearly 100 arts and crafts exhibitors display their works and many demonstrate their skills in mountain crafts, theatrical presentation by local performers, bluegrass music bands. FOODS SERVED: traditional foods, food booths. ADMISSION: free. ACCOMMODATIONS: motels and hotels, campgrounds. RESTAURANTS: fast foods, family, elegant, Chinese, continental. CONTACT: Marion Chamber of Commerce, P. O. Box 924, Marion, VA 24354, (703) 783-3161. 20,000

OLD FIDDLERS CONVENTION *second weekend in August,* Galax, Grayson, and Carroll Counties, in the Twin County Area of southern Virginia. Arts and crafts, old-time fiddlers contests, prizes totalling $10,000, folk music, dance. FOODS SERVED: "all kinds." ADMISSION: $5.00–$6.00. ACCOMMODATIONS: motels and hotels, B&B's, campgrounds, RV parks. RESTAURANTS: fast foods. CONTACT: Old Fiddlers Convention, c/o Galax Moose Lodge #733, P. O. Box 655, Galax, VA 24333-9655, (703) 236-8541, or the Galax–Carroll–Grayson Chamber of Commerce, 405 N. Main St., Galax, VA 24333, (703) 236-2184. 30,000

WINE FESTIVAL *last Saturday in August,* Middleburg, Fauquier Co., at the Valley View Vineyard in the Virginia Hunt Country, to celebrate Virginia wines. Wine auction, Waiter's Race, Grape Stompin' Contest, Barrel Rolling Race, Cork Throwing Contest, wine-judging demonstration, winegrowing seminar, jousting tournament, wine movies, Dixieland jazz all day. FOODS SERVED: "crepes and other appropriate foods to go with wine." ADMISSION: $10.00. ACCOMMODATIONS: motels and hotels, B&B's, campgrounds. RESTAURANTS: fast foods, family, elegant, French, Italian. CONTACT: Vinifera Wine Growers Association, P. O. Box P, The Plains, VA 22171, (703) 754-8564. 4,000

HAMPTON BAY DAYS *second weekend in September,* Hampton, Hampton Co., in downtown Old Hampton in Tidewater area, to celebrate the recreational, industrial, and ecological benefits of Chesapeake Bay. Art show, arts and crafts, tall ships, carnival rides, raft races, Yacht Race, professional bicycle race, Grand Prix 10k Run, Cycling Criterium, "world-class entertainment" which has included The Hooters, Eddie Kendrick, David Ruffin, Sha Na Na, Skitch Henderson, and the Virginia Symphony. FOODS SERVED: wide variety of ethnic foods. ADMISSION: free. ACCOMMODATIONS: motels and hotels, campgrounds. RESTAURANTS: fast foods, family, elegant. CONTACT: Hampton Bay Days, 22 Lincoln St., Hampton, VA 23669, (804) 727-6140. 500,000

CHILHOWIE APPLE FESTIVAL *third weekend in September,* Chilhowie, Smyth Co., to celebrate the apple. Crafts, flower and plant show, bake sale, demonstrations. FOODS SERVED: apple-baked goods, food booths. ADMISSION: free. ACCOMMODATIONS: motels and hotels. RESTAURANTS: fast foods, family, elegant, Chinese, continental. CONTACT: Marion Chamber of Commerce, P. O. Box 924, Marion, VA 24354, (703) 783-3161. 10,000

VIRGINIA BEACH NEPTUNE FESTIVAL *last weekend in September,* Virginia Beach, at the Oceanfront, to celebrate the end of the tourist season. Country Fair Day Hoedown and farmers' market, Chesapeake Light Sailing Race for monohulls, Trans-Virginia Beach Canoe Race, air show, triathlon including 2k swim, 10k bike ride and 10k run; King Neptune Surfing Classic, tennis and golf tournaments, Senior Citizens Golf Tournament, prayer breakfast, beach party, Neptune Ball, art show and oceanside creations; Boardwalk Celebration including sporting events, five stages of entertainment; Neptune Festival/East Coast Paddlesurfing Championships, volleyball tournament, Sandcastle Classic, Wheelchair Tennis Tournament, Youth Day with parade, Neptune Catamaran Ribbon Race, Windsurfing Regatta,

Grand Parade, fireworks, 8k Run, youth art show, King Neptune Luncheon and Fashion Show, Heritage Day; loads of music and entertainment. FOODS SERVED: ethnic and concessions. ADMISSION: free to most events, charges for some. ACCOMMODATIONS: motels and hotels, B&B's, campgrounds, RV parks. RESTAURANTS: fast foods, family, elegant, international. CONTACT: Virginia Beach Neptune Festival, Inc., 4512 Virginia Beach Blvd., Virginia Beach, VA 23462, (804) 490-1221. 1,500,000

POQUOSON SEAFOOD FESTIVAL *September,* Poquoson, York Co., at Poquoson City Park on the Virginia Peninsula, to celebrate the seafood industry. Juried art show, arts and crafts displays, Volkmarch, parade, fireworks, local entertainers such as Virginia Country, Sterling Ridge, First Class, Coastal Express, Hampton Jug Band, dancing by the Tidewater Dancers, Two-Stepping Panhandlers, and The Virginia Cloggers. FOODS SERVED: lots of seafood, barbecue, hot dogs. ADMISSION: free. ACCOMMODATIONS: motels and hotels, campgrounds, RV parks. RESTAURANTS: fast foods, family. CONTACT: City of Poquoson, Poquoson, VA 23362, at (804) 868-7151 or the Virginia Peninsula Tourism and Conference Bureau, Patrick Henry International Airport, Newport News, VA 23602, (804) 881-9777 or (800) 558-1818. 3,000

MEDLEY OF THE ARTS *October,* Hampton, on the Virginia Peninsula, as a celebration of the performing and visual arts. Arts and crafts exhibits, dancing, vocals, instrumentals, dramatic presentations, puppeteering, the Virginia Symphony Quintet, Virginia Opera, The York River Community Orchestra, The Virginia Choral Society, The Hampton University Theatre, The Heritage Dancers, and The Hampton Roads Civic Ballet. ADMISSION: free. ACCOMMODATIONS: motels and hotels, campgrounds, RV parks. RESTAURANTS: fast foods, family, Mexican, Polynesian, Asian. CONTACT: Ben DiSalvo at

(804) 461-7819 or the Virginia Peninsula Tourism and Conference Bureau, Patrick Henry International Airport, Newport News, VA 23602, (804) 881-9777 or (800) 558-1818. 5,000

NEWPORT NEWS FALL FESTIVAL *first weekend in October,* Newport News at City Park to celebrate fall and folklife. More than 200 traditional hand-crafters offer their works in a folklife marketplace and fifty in a juried show; lifeskill trades and demonstrations, folklife entertainment and folk music such as the Kingston Trio, The New Christy Minstrels, and Roy Bookbinder. FOODS SERVED: multi-ethnic. ADMISSION: free, parking fee $2.00 per car. ACCOMMODATIONS: motels and hotels, campgrounds, RV parks. RESTAURANTS: fast foods, family. CONTACT: Cynthia F. Carter, Department of Parks and Recreation, 2400 Washington Ave., Newport News, VA 23607, (804) 247-8451. 60,000

FALL FOLIAGE FESTIVAL *first and second weekends in October,* Waynesboro, Augusta Co., to celebrate the beautiful fall foliage in the area. Art and craft shows, 10k races, British car show, antique show, gem and mineral show, Apple Days saluting the apple industry, Grand Parade, tennis tournament, Doll Show, Run for Hospice. FOODS SERVED: barbecue, wide variety of others. ADMISSION: free. ACCOMMODATIONS: motels and hotels, B&B's, campgrounds. RESTAURANTS: fast foods, family, elegant. CONTACT: Marie Frye, P. O. Box 396, Waynesboro, VA 22980, (703) 943-3435 or the Waynesboro–East Augusta Chamber of Commerce, 1300 Chatham Rd., Waynesboro, VA 22980, (703) 949-8203. 30,000

OYSTER FESTIVAL *Saturday of Columbus Day weekend (near october 12),* Chincoteague Island, Accomack Co., on the Eastern Shore of Virginia, as a salute to the oyster industry. This is simply a celebration of the abundance of oysters in the area and is to be enjoyed as that. At the Maddox Family Campground you can feast on oyster fritters, raw oysters, steamed or fried oysters, cole slaw, potato salad, hush puppies, hot dogs and more. ADMISSION: $17.00 for all you can eat. ACCOMMODATIONS: motels, B&B's, ca.npgrounds. RESTAURANTS: fast foods, family, elegant, Italian, Chinese. CONTACT: Chincoteague Island Chamber of Commerce, P. O. Box 258, Chincoteague Island, VA 23336, (804) 336-6161. 2,000

HISTORIC APPOMATTOX RAILROAD FESTIVAL *second weekend in October,* Appomattox, Appomattox Co., in central Virginia. Arts and crafts, antique show, "Joe Sweeney Classic" 20k Foot Race, firemen's competition, petting zoo, street dance, puppet show, exhibits of Civil War memorabilia and miniature trains, Good Ole Days step back in time with exhibits, demonstrations, and products; Full Contact Karate Match, Railroad Willie Express; country, bluegrass, and gospel music including bands such as the Clark Family Band and Deborah Adair; politicians. FOODS SERVED: stews, barbecue, ribs, steaks, chicken, burgers, "variety." ADMISSION: free. ACCOMMODATIONS: motels and hotels, campgrounds. RESTAURANTS: fast foods, family. CONTACT: Historic Appomattox Railroad Festival, P. O. Box 513, Appomattox, VA 24522, (804) 352-5547. 20,000

SUFFOLK PEANUT FEST *second weekend in October,* Suffolk, Suffolk Co., to celebrate the harvest of peanuts and other crops. Arts and crafts, "World's Only Peanut Butter Sculpture Contest," Peanut Cooking Contest, horse show, children's activities, Shrimp Feast, commercial exhibits and military displays, continuous entertainment on three stages which has included Miss Virginia, local beach bands, Eddie Rabbitt, Mamas and Papas, Anheuser-Busch Clydesdales, and Mickey Mouse and Goofy from Disney World have served as parade Grand Marshalls. FOODS SERVED: Shrimp Feast, barbecue, southern fried chicken, Greek,

Asian, Mexican, Italian. ADMISSION: free, parking $3.00 per car. ACCOMMODATIONS: motels and hotels, campgrounds, RV parks. RESTAURANTS: fast foods, family. CONTACT: Suffolk Peanut Fest, P. O. Box 1852, Suffolk, VA 23434, (804) 539-5483. 150,000

YORKTOWN DAY *October 19,* Yorktown, York Co., on the Virginia Peninsula, to celebrate the surrender of General Cornwallis to General George Washington ending the American Revolutionary War. Parade along Main Street, costumed townspeople serve colonial lunch, memorial ceremonies, arts and crafts displays, military exhibitions and reenactments. FOODS SERVED: colonial foods such as Brunswick Stew, ham biscuits, homemade pies and desserts. ADMISSION: free. ACCOMMODATIONS: motels and hotels, campgrounds, RV parks. RESTAURANTS: fast foods, family, Asian, Italian, Greek. CONTACT: Ms. Ann Meyers at (804) 898-3400 or the Virginia Peninsula Tourism and Conference Bureau, Patrick Henry International Airport, Newport News, VA 23602, (804) 881-9777 or (800) 558-1818. 7,000

FALL FOLIAGE FESTIVAL *third weekend in October,* Clifton Forge, in the Alleghany Highlands, the "Mountain Playground of Virginia." Arts and crafts, flea market, 5k or 10k run, exhibits, local mountain entertainment and music. FOODS SERVED: Southern and traditional mountain foods. ADMISSION: free. ACCOMMODATIONS: (nearby) motels and hotels, campgrounds. RESTAURANTS: fast foods, family, elegant, French, Italian, Chinese. CONTACT: Clifton Forge Fall Foliage, P. O. Box 526, Clifton Forge, VA 24422 or the Greater Alleghany Highlands Chamber of Commerce, 403 E. Ridgeway St., Clifton Forge, VA 24422, (703) 862-4969. 30,000

MID-SOUTH

Kentucky / 51

North Carolina / 55

Tennessee / 62

West Virginia / 74

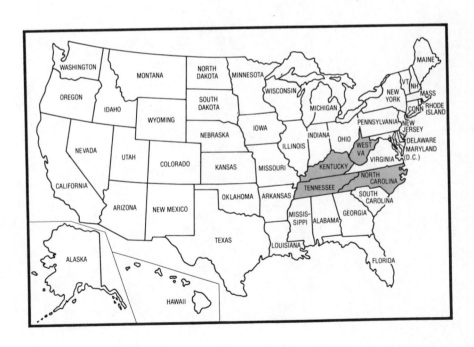

TATER DAY *first Monday in April,* Benton, Marshall Co., throughout the city of Benton, to honor the sweet potato and the old Benton custom of knife and dog trading. Arts and crafts, gun, coin, and knife show, parade, Miss Tater Day Contest, road races, horse and mule pull, Antique Car Show, cook-off, bake-off, flea market, motorcycle races, horse-drawn vehicle show, carnival, lots of "old-time gospel music." FOODS SERVED: sweet potato specialties, concessions. ADMISSION: "reasonable if not free." ACCOMMODATIONS: motels and hotels, B&B's, campgrounds, RV parks. RESTAURANTS: fast foods, family, elegant, Cajun, Kentucky Lake catfish. CONTACT: Marshall Co. Chamber of Commerce, Rt. 7, U.S. 68 at 641, Benton, KY 42025-8918, (502) 527-7665. 30,000

MOUNTAIN FOLK FESTIVAL *second weekend in April,* Berea, Madison Co., at the Berea College campus and at the Folk Center. Appalachian arts and literature, craft demonstrations and sales, college tours, folk dancing. FOODS SERVED: regional specialties. ADMISSION: free. ACCOMMODATIONS: motels and hotels, campgrounds. RESTAURANTS: fast foods, family, elegant. CONTACT: Folk Circle Association, 415 Estill St., Berea, KY 40403, (606) 986-9341 ext. 453.

INTERNATIONAL BAR-B-Q FESTIVAL *second weekend in May,* Owensboro, Daviess Co., to celebrate the "barbecue tradition in Catholic parishes." Each parish in the area enters a team to compete in cooking 500 chickens, 1,200 pounds of mutton, and a cauldron of burgoo, Backyard Cook Contest, arts and crafts, children's games, country-bluegrass music. FOODS SERVED: see above. ADMISSION: free. ACCOMMODATIONS: motels and hotels, campgrounds, RV parks. RESTAURANTS: fast foods, family, elegant, Chinese, Mexican. CONTACT: Owensboro Daviess Co. Tourist Commission, 326 St., Elizabeth, Owensboro, KY 42301, (502) 926-1100. 30,000

MAIFEST *third weekend in May,* Covington, Kenton Co., at MainStrasse Village, a "historic German village" in Kentucky. Arts and crafts, entertainment, "special events," games, carnival. FOODS SERVED: German. ADMISSION: free. ACCOMMODATIONS: motels and hotels. RESTAURANTS: fast foods, family. CONTACT: MainStrasse Village Association, 616 MainStrasse, Covington, KY 41011, (609) 491-0458. 100,000

THE GREAT INLAND SEAFOOD FESTIVAL *fourth weekend in June,* Covington, Kenton Co., in MainStrasse Village, a "historic German village" in Kentucky. Lots of seafood and entertainment. FOODS SERVED: Seafood in many forms. ADMISSION: free, charges for food. ACCOMMODATIONS: motels and hotels. RESTAURANTS: fast foods, family. CONTACT: MainStrasse Village Association, 616 Main Strasse, Covington, KY 41011, (609) 491-0458. 100,000

OWENSBORO SUMMER FESTIVAL *July 4th weekend,* Owensboro, Daviess Co., on the banks of the Ohio River and at the Amphitheatre in the Green River region. "Largest fireworks-and-symphony-orchestra extravaganza in the state of Kentucky," arts and crafts, Anything That Goes and Floats Race, Lighted Boat Parade, Food Festival, beer garden, children's plays and rides, dances, musical events such as the Owensboro Symphony Orchestra's Pops Concert on the river. ADMISSION: free. ACCOMMODATIONS: motels and hotels, campgrounds, RV parks. RESTAURANTS: fast foods, family, elegant. CONTACT: Kirk Kirkpatrick, Owensboro Summer Festival, Box 461, Owensboro, KY 42301, (502) 926-0008. 23,000

BEREA CRAFTS FESTIVAL *second weekend in July,* Berea, Madison Co., at the Indian Fort Theatre in the "Crafts Capital of Kentucky." More than "100 of the nation's finest" craftspeople "displaying, demonstrating, and selling quality handmade crafts," lots of entertainment. FOODS SERVED: local specialties. ADMISSION: adults $2.50, children $1.00, group rates available. ACCOMMODATIONS: motels and hotels, campgrounds. RESTAURANTS: fast foods, family, elegant. CONTACT: Berea Craft Festival, P. O. Box 508, Berea, KY 40403 or the Berea Tourism Commission, 105 Boone St., Berea, KY 40403, (606) 986-2450.

CORBIN NIBROC FESTIVAL *first full week in August,* Corbin, Whitley and Knox counties at the home of Kentucky Fried Chicken. Arts and crafts sale and show, beauty pageant, Street Rod Show, antique car show, street concessions, parade, moonlight races, Old Fashion Days, street dances, clogging, square dances, Sidewalk Days. FOODS SERVED: "everything from hot dogs to funnel cakes and elephant ears." ADMISSION: free. ACCOMMODATIONS: motels and hotels, campgrounds, RV parks. RESTAURANTS: fast foods, family, Chinese. CONTACT: Greater Corbin Chamber of Commerce, 401 S. Lynn Ave., Corbin, KY 40701, (606) 528-6390. 30,000

PIONEER DAYS FESTIVAL *fourth weekend in August,* Harrodsburg, Mercer Co., in Kentucky's bluegrass country to celebrate being "Kentucky's first permanent settlement west of the Allegany Mountains in 1774." Kentucky arts and crafts, antique and classic car show, hot air balloon race, 5k and 10k runs, flea market, square dancing, clogging, street dances, Top 40's, Street Dance for teens, Kids' Day, reenactment of attack on old Fort Harrod with militia group portraying 1774 pioneers, Pioneer Parade, two stages of entertainment including dramas of Daniel Boone's and Abraham Lincoln's lives. FOODS SERVED: Pioneer Pig-Out

Supper, Mercer County Cooking, regional southern cooking. ADMISSION: free, charges for some events. ACCOMMODATIONS: motels and hotels, B&B's, campgrounds, RV parks.. RESTAURANTS: fast foods, family, elegant, all southern. CONTACT: Harrodsburg–Mercer Co. Chamber of Commerce, 222 S. Chiles St., Harrodsburg, KY 40330, (606) 734-2365. 85,000

OKTOBERFEST *second weekend in September,* Covington, Kenton Co., in MainStrasse Village, a "historic German village" in Kentucky. Three-day street fair includes more than 100 arts and crafts exhibits, three entertainment and performance areas, games, carnival. FOODS SERVED: more than twenty-five food booths featuring German food. ADMISSION: free. ACCOMMODATIONS: motels and hotels. RESTAURANTS: fast foods, family. CONTACT: MainStrasse Village Association, 616 Main Strasse, Covington, KY 41011, (609) 491-0458. 175,000

LOUISVILLE BLUEGRASS FESTIVAL *second weekend in September,* Louisville, Jefferson Co., to honor bluegrass music and its traditions. Continuous bluegrass entertainment including Bill Monroe and the Bluegrass Boys, New Grass Revival, Green Grass Cloggers, Doc Watson, Ricky Skaggs, Emmylou Harris, Osborne Brothers, and Berline, Crary and Hickman. FOODS SERVED: "regular fare." ADMISSION: free. ACCOMMODATIONS: motels and hotels, campgrounds, RV parks. RESTAURANTS: fast foods, family, elegant, international. CONTACT: Director of Promotions and Public Relations, Louisville Central Area, 555 Brown & Williamson Tower, Louisville, KY 40202, (502) 583-1671. 150,000

BLACK GOLD FESTIVAL *third weekend in September,* Hazard, Perry Co., on Main Street, to recognize "coal—our major resource." Arts and crafts, auctions, parade, coal truck competition, carnival, beauty contests, style show, public-service booths, gospel and country music. Stars who have appeared include the cast of "The Dukes of Hazzard," B.J. Thomas, Waylon Jennings, and Jerry Reed. FOODS SERVED: "variety." ADMISSION: free. ACCOMMODATIONS: motels and hotels, B&B's, campgrounds. RESTAURANTS: fast foods, family, elegant. CONTACT: Hazard–Perry Co., Chamber of Commerce, 221 Memorial Dr., Hazard, KY 41701, (606) 439-2659. 110,000

GOLDEN ARMOR FESTIVAL *fourth week in September,* Radcliff, Hardin Co., to express appreciation for the quality of life in the Fort Knox military community. Bazaar, golf tournament, military displays, parachuting, balloon races, Sister City Observance with Munster, Germany, open house, Student Government Days, athletic events, receptions, parade. FOODS SERVED: "multinational." ADMISSION: free. ACCOMMODATIONS: motels and hotels, campgrounds, RV parks. RESTAURANTS: fast foods, family, German, Asian. CONTACT: Radcliff–North Hardin Chamber of Commerce, P. O. Box 912, Radcliff, KY 40160, (502) 351-4450. 20,000

INTERNATIONAL BLUEGRASS MUSIC FESTIVAL *fourth Wednesday through the weekend in September,* Owensboro, Daviess Co., at Peter B. English Park, with a Bluegrass Trade Show simultaneously at the Executive Inn Convention Center. Bluegrass With Class Festival, Bluegrass Fan Fair, musicians such as Bill Monroe and the Bluegrass Boys, The Osborne Brothers, Doyle Lawson and Quicksilver, Bluegrass Cardinals, Jim and Jesse and the Virginia Boys, Johnson Mountain Boys, The Whites and the ninety piece Owensboro Symphony Orchestra. FOODS SERVED: barbecue, catfish dinners, concessions. ADMISSION: free. ACCOMMODATIONS: motels and hotels, campgrounds, RV parks. RESTAURANTS: fast foods, family, elegant, Italian. CONTACT: Owensboro Daviess Co. Tourist Commission, 326 St. Elizabeth, Owensboro, KY 42301, (502) 926-1100. 20,000

FESTIVAL OF THE HORSE *last weekend in September,* Georgetown, Scott Co. Arts and crafts, horse parades, horse rides, games, balloon rides, music from the likes of Charley McClain, Jennifer Savidge, Bob Brown, and Patrick Duffee. FOODS SERVED: elephant ears, pork chops, concessions. ADMISSION: free. ACCOMMODATIONS: motels and hotels, B&B's, campgrounds. RESTAURANTS: fast foods, family. CONTACT: Georgetown–Scott Co. Chamber of Commerce, 100 S. Broadway, Georgetown, KY 40324, (502) 863-5424. 4,000

COUNTRY HAM DAYS *last weekend in September,* Lebanon, Marion Co., in Kentucky's bluegrass country, to celebrate "country pride." Arts and crafts, flea market, Pigasus Parade, 10k Pokey Pig Run, car show, bluegrass and country music. FOODS SERVED: "country ham breakfast served in the streets of downtown Lebanon and pork related food booths." ADMISSION: free. ACCOMMODATIONS: motels and hotels, campgrounds, RV parks. RESTAURANTS: fast foods, family, elegant. CONTACT: Lebanon–Marion Co. Chamber of Commerce and Economic Development Office, 107A W. Main St., Lebanon, KY 40033, (502) 692-2661. 60,000

BIG RIVERS ARTS AND CRAFTS FESTIVAL *first weekend in October,* near Owensboro, Daviess Co., at picturesque Audubon State Park. More than 200 of Kentucky's finest arts and crafts exhibitors, local musicians and food. FOODS SERVED: concessions. ADMISSION: free. ACCOMMODATIONS: (nearby) motels and hotels, campgrounds, RV parks. RESTAURANTS: fast foods, family, elegant, Italian. CONTACT: Green River Area Development District Tourism Committee, 3860 Highway 60 West, Owensboro, KY 42301, (502) 926-4433. 65,000

WASHINGTON COUNTY SORGHUM FESTIVAL *first weekend in October,* Springfield, Washington Co., to celebrate the sorghum harvest. Arts and crafts, Antique Car Show, golf tournament, road race, window displays, hot air balloon race, home tour, square dancing, country music show and contest, bluegrass music. FOODS SERVED: giant pizza and giant sorghum cookie, concessions. ADMISSION: free. ACCOMMODATIONS: motels and hotels. RESTAURANTS: fast foods, family. CONTACT: Springfield–Washington Co. Chamber of Commerce, Main St., Springfield, KY 40069, (606) 336-3810.

LINCOLN DAYS CELEBRATION *second weekend in October,* Hodgenville, LaRue Co., to recognize Hodgenville as Abraham Lincoln's birthplace. Art shows, local crafts, rail splitting contests, Lincoln Look-Alike Contest, pioneer games, antique costume contest, parade, storytelling, foot races, country and bluegrass music. FOODS SERVED: "outdoors country cooking." ADMISSION: free. ACCOMMODATIONS: motel, B&B's, campgrounds, RV park. RESTAURANTS: fast foods, family. CONTACT: Lincoln Day Celebration, Inc., P. O. Box 176, Hodgenville, KY 42748, (502) 358-3411. 30,000

POAGE LANDING DAYS CELEBRATION *third week in October,* Ashland, Boyd Co., to celebrate the settling of Ashland. Arts and crafts, Chili Cook-Off, children's activities, entertainment, professional lumberjack show including pole climbing, log rolling, sawing and chopping lumber. FOODS SERVED: chili. ADMISSION: free. ACCOMMODATIONS: motels and hotels. RESTAURANTS: fast foods, family, elegant. CONTACT: Ashland Area Tourism Center, P. O. Box 987, Ashland, KY 41101, (606) 329-1007.

AURORA COUNTRY FESTIVAL *third weekend in October,* Benton, Marshall Co., in the Aurora area to celebrate fall. Arts and crafts, flea market, antique car parade, molasses making, sorghum demonstrations, Strut Dance, parade, gospel and country music including big-name stars to be announced. FOODS SERVED: molasses and sorghum products, concessions. ADMISSION: free, concerts $4.00–$8.00. ACCOMMODATIONS: motels and hotels, B&B, campgrounds, RV parks. RESTAURANTS: fast foods, family, elegant, Cajun, Kentucky Lake catfish. CONTACT: Jonathan Aurora Action Committee (JAAC), c/o Carol Wilson, Lakeside Campground, Rt. 5, Benton, KY 42025, (502) 354-8157 or the Marshall Co. Chamber of Commerce, Rt. 7, U.S. 68 at 641, Benton, KY 42025-8919, (502) 527-7665. 15,000

BLOOMFIELD TOBACCO FESTIVAL *third weekend in October,* Bloomfield, Nelson Co., to recognize the tobacco industry in Kentucky. Queen selection, parades, antique and flea market, Tobacco Spitting Contest, Auctioneering Contest, pipe smoking and other contests, dances, auctions, tobacco judging for Future Farmers of America. FOODS SERVED: concessions. ADMISSION: free. ACCOMMODATIONS: motels and hotels, B&B, campgrounds, RV park. RESTAURANTS: fast foods, family, elegant, Italian. CONTACT: Mayor of Bloomfield, Bloomfield Tobacco Festival Committee, Bloomfield, KY 40008 (502) 252-8222, or the Bardstown–Nelson Co. Chamber of Commerce, P. O. Box 296, Bardstown, KY 40004, (502) 348-9545.

TRADITIONAL MUSIC FESTIVAL *last weekend in October,* Berea, Madison Co., to salute traditional country music in a pleasant atmosphere. Street and square dances, concerts, workshops and lectures. ADMISSION: free, charges for some events. ACCOMMODATIONS: motels and hotels, campgrounds. RESTAURANTS: fast foods, family, elegant. CONTACT: Berea Tourism Commission, 105 Boone St., Berea, KY 40403, (606) 986-2450.

CORN ISLAND STORYTELLING FESTIVAL *October,* Louisville, Jefferson Co., to recognize and preserve the art of storytelling. Storytelling, workshops, seminars, tale swapping, "other storytelling activities." FOODS SERVED: local. ADMISSION: $30.00 per weekend. ACCOMMO-

DATIONS: motels and hotels, campgrounds, RV parks. RESTAURANTS: fast foods, family, elegant, southern. CON- TACT: Lee Pennington of the International Order of Ears, 11905 Liliac Way, Diddli- town, KY 40243, (502) 245-0643. 20,000

NORTH CAROLINA

GRIFTON SHAD FESTIVAL *first week in April,* Grifton, Pitt Co. Parade, bass and hickory shad fishing contests, canoe races, 1mi, 2mi, and 10k Spring Shad Run, 23mi Bicycle Race, arts and crafts, queen pageant, tennis, horseshoe, archery and golf tournaments, "Fishy Tales" storytell- ing (or liar's) contest, games, kiddie rides, "Shad–O" bingo, flea market, historical museum with demonstrations of tradi- tional folk skills; entertainment including street dance, clogging, band concert, bar- bershop singing. FOODS SERVED: fish fry and fish stew, barbecue, others. ADMIS- SION: free. ACCOMMODATIONS: motels and hotels. RESTAURANTS: family. CONTACT: Mrs. Ruthanne Rhem, P. O. Box 928, Grifton, NC 28530, (919) 524-4356.

CAROLINA DOGWOOD FESTIVAL *second weekend in April,* Statesville, Ire- dell Co., "as a tribute to the natural beauty of Statesville and to the excellence of the area's high school marching bands." Parade through dogwood-lined streets, Dogwood Queen Pageant, track meet, arts and crafts, storytelling, golf and ten- nis tournaments, Carolina Dogwood Fes- tival 5k and 10k runs, 1mi Fun Run, Muz- zle-loader Shooting Match, The Bill Watt, Jr. Memorial Chess Tournament, Dog- wood Floral Arrangement Contest, sun- rise religious service, Senior Citizens Shuffleboard Tournament, Senior Citizens Walkathon, swim meet, Bass Tournament, half marathon, Table Tennis Tournament, softball and racquetball tournaments, gos- pel singing, Band Field Show, Jazz Festival and jazz band competition, Carolina Dog- wood Festival Bench Press and Southern Wrist Westling Championship, square dancing, Open Horseshoe Tournament for men, women, boys and girls. FOODS SERVED: pancake breakfasts, concessions, family picnics encouraged. ADMISSION: free, charges for some events. ACCOM- MODATIONS: motels and hotels, B&B's, campgrounds, RV parks. RESTAURANTS: fast foods, family, elegant. CONTACT: Ca- rolina Dogwood Festival, Box 653, States- ville, NC 28677 or the Greater Statesville Chamber of Commerce, P. O. Box 1064, Statesville, NC 28677, (704) 873-2892.

DOGWOOD FESTIVAL *second week in April,* Fayetteville, Cumberland Co., to celebrate the blooming of dogwood trees. Parade, arts and crafts, celebrity golf tournament, tours, street dance, prayer breakfast, beauty pageant, air shows, ten- nis and softball tournaments. FOODS SERVED: concessions. ADMISSION: free. ACCOMMODATIONS: motels and hotels, B&B's, campgrounds, RV parks. RESTAU- RANTS: fast foods, family, elegant. CON- TACT: Fayetteville Chamber of Com- merce, 519 Ramsey St., Fayetteville, NC 28301, (919) 483-8133.

NATIONAL WHISTLERS CONVEN- TION *fourth Friday and Saturday in April,* Louisburg, Franklin Co. Whistling concert and contests in classical and con- temporary categories for adult and chil- dren's national championships, museum heritage arts, whistling workshops, street dancing. ADMISSION: charge. ACCOMMO- DATIONS: motels and hotels, camp- grounds. RESTAURANTS: fast foods, fam- ily. CONTACT: Allen de Hart, College Box 845, Louisburg, NC 27549, (919) 496- 2521, or the Louisburg–Franklin Co.

Chamber of Commerce, P. O. Box 62, Louisburg, NC 17549, (919) 496-3056.

APPLE CHILL *fourth Sunday in April,* Chapel Hill, Orange Co., as a "coming out" for spring time. Community street fair featuring local crafts, children's activities, dancing, local musical groups and bands. FOODS SERVED: American, Chinese, Korean, Mexican. ADMISSION: free. ACCOMMODATIONS: motels and hotels. RESTAURANTS: fast foods, family, elegant. CONTACT: Parks and Recreation Dept., Town of Chapel Hill, 306 N. Columbia St., Chapel Hill, NC 27514-3699, (919) 968-2784. 20,000

ARTSPLOSURE SPRING FESTIVAL *last week in April through first week in May,* Raleigh, Wake Co. A true festival of the arts featuring performing, visual, and participatory activities. FOODS SERVED: concessions. ADMISSION: free, charges for some events. ACCOMMODATIONS: motels and hotels, B&B's, campgrounds, RV parks. RESTAURANTS: fast foods, family, elegant. CONTACT: ArtsPlosure, P. O. Box 590, Raleigh, NC 27602, (919) 890-3195.

WATAUGA COUNTY SPRING FESTI-VAL *first weekend in May,* Boone, Watauga Co., at Appalachian State University. Two days of continuous entertainment on two stages including Appalachian mountain music, more than 200 craftspeople demonstrating and selling traditional and contemporary crafts. FOODS SERVED: local concessions. ADMISSION: free. ACCOMMODATIONS: motels and hotels, B&B's, campgrounds, RV parks. RESTAURANTS: fast foods, family, elegant. CONTACT: Center for Appalachian Studies, Appalachian State University, Boone, NC 28608, (704) 262-4089. 7,000

PLEASURE ISLAND SPRING FESTI-VAL *second or third weekend in May,* Carolina and Kire Beaches, Pleasure Island, to celebrate spring at the beach. Craft shows, Pig Cook-off, road races, parade, live entertainment such as Bobby

McLamb. FOODS SERVED: pork and concessions. ADMISSION: free. ACCOMMODATIONS: motels and hotels, campground, RV park. RESTAURANTS: fast foods, family, elegant. CONTACT: Pleasure Island Chamber of Commerce, P. O. Box 1560, Carolina Beach, NC 28428, (919) 458-8434 or 1-800-982-1602.

WHITE LAKE WATER FESTIVAL *third weekend in May,* White Lake, Bladen Co., to celebrate the "beginning of the lake season." Art and photo shows, crafts exhibit and sale, Water Ski Show, beauty pageant, 10k Race and 1mi Fun Run, parade, golf tournament, fireworks, dance, live bands including The Fantastic Shakers and The Embers. FOODS SERVED: concessions. ADMISSION: free, dance $6.00–$10.00. ACCOMMODATIONS: motels and hotels, campgrounds, RV parks. RESTAURANTS: fast foods, family. CONTACT: Elizabethtown–White Lake Chamber of Commerce, P. O. Box 306, Elizabethtown, NC 28337, (919) 862-4368. 15,000

MAYFEST INTERNATIONAL FESTI-VAL *third weekend in May,* Winston–Salem, Forsyth Co. Multinational entertainment, crafts and children's entertainment, and foods. FOODS SERVED: multi-ethnic, and concessions. ADMISSION: free, some charges for food. ACCOMMODATIONS: motels and hotels, B&B. RESTAURANTS: fast foods, elegant. CONTACT: Urban Arts of the Arts Council, P. O. Box 10935, Winston–Salem, NC 27108, (919) 722-5293.

OLD-TIME FIDDLERS' AND BLUE-GRASS FESTIVAL *Memorial Day weekend (late May),* Union Grove, Iredell Co., annually for more than sixty years since its founding by Henry Price (H.P.) Van Hoy, father of the current coordinator. Old-time and bluegrass band competitions and contests for individuals, workshops in all major instruments, clog dancing, storytelling, shape-note singing, occasional visits and performances by Doc Watson, who lives nearby. FOODS SERVED: barbecued chicken, concessions. ADMISSION: free.

ACCOMMODATIONS: motel, campground on site. RESTAURANTS: family. CONTACT: Harper A. Van Hoy, P. O. Box 11, Union Grove, NC 28689, (704) 539-4417. 4,000

CHARLOTTE FOLK MUSIC FESTIVAL *second Saturday in June,* Charlotte, Mecklenburg Co., at Latta Plantation Park. Traditional music including old-time string bands, bluegrass, blues, shape-note hymns, concert performances and workshops. FOODS SERVED: concessions. ADMISSION: free. ACCOMMODATIONS: motels and hotels, campgrounds nearby. RESTAURANTS: fast foods, family, elegant. CONTACT: Charlotte Folk Music Society, P. O. Box 9007, Charlotte NC 28299–9007, (704) 866-1899.

NORTH CAROLINA BLUE CRAB DERBY AND FESTIVAL *second Friday and Saturday in June,* Morehead City, Carteret Co., to celebrate the harvest of blue crab from local waters. Crab races, games, auctions, arts and crafts exhibits, live entertainment. FOODS SERVED: lots of blue crab and other seafoods. ADMISSION: free. ACCOMMODATIONS: motels and hotels, B&B's, campgrounds, RV parks. RESTAURANTS: fast foods, family, elegant. CONTACT: Richard L. Evans, 4028 Arendell St., Morehead City, NC 28557, (919) 726-6340 or the Carteret Co. Chamber of Commerce, P. O. Box 1198, Morehead City, NC 28557, (919) 726-6831.

AMERICAN DANCE FESTIVAL *mid-June through late July,* Durham, Durham Co., at Duke University. "Spectacular performances by world's greatest dance companies," premieres of new works created for the festival, school, professional workshops, community projects, humanities series, daily tours. ADMISSION: charge. ACCOMMODATIONS: motels and hotels, B&B's, campgrounds, RV parks. RESTAURANTS: fast foods, family, elegant, international. CONTACT: Administrative Director, American Dance Festival, P. O. Box 6097, College Station, Durham, NC 28734, (919) 684-6402.

CULLOWHEE MUSIC FESTIVAL *last two weeks in June,* Cullowhee, Jackson Co., at Western Carolina University. Musicians and vocalists from throughout the country gather to perfrom in orchestral and "pops" concerts, young artists' competitions, musical and operatic performances in Cullowhee and several other western North Carolina locations. ADMISSION: charge to some events. ACCOMMODATIONS: motels and hotels, B&B's, campgrounds, RV parks. RESTAURANTS: fast foods, family, Italian, Mexican. CONTACT: Bert Wiley, Western Carolina University Music Dept., Cullowhee, NC 28723, (704) 227-7608 or the Cullowhee Chamber of Commerce, Rt. 67, Box 112-H, Cullowhee, NC 28723, (704) 293-9648.

RHODODENDRON FESTIVAL *third week in June,* Bakersville, Mitchell Co., near Roan Mountain, the site of the "largest natural rhododendron garden in the United States," to celebrate the blooming of rhododendrons. Beauty pageant, marathon race, Mountain Crafts Fair, golf tournament, street dances every night, "old-timey Appalachian entertainment" and music including clogging and dancing. FOODS SERVED: concessions. ADMISSION: free. ACCOMMODATIONS: motels and hotels, B&B's, campgrounds, RV parks. RESTAURANTS: fast foods, family, elegant. CONTACT: Rhododendron Festival, Town of Bakersville, Bakersville, NC 28705, (704) 688-3113. 10,000

FESTIVAL OF FESTIVALS *third weekend in June,* Franklin, Macon Co., at Nikwasi Park, "the Gem and Quilt Capital of the World," in western North Carolina to showcase the best of regional festivals of western North Carolina. More than 100 "of the finest juried craftsmen in the southeast exhibit and sell their work" from the "twenty leading festivals of the mountain region." Live entertainment includes bagpipes from the Highland Games, German Bavarian music from the Oktoberfest, champion fiddlers and cloggers, Indian dancers from the Cherokee Indian Reser-

vation, gospel and bluegrass music. FOODS SERVED: heritage and ethnic foods. ADMISSION: adults $3.00, children under 12 free. ACCOMMODATIONS: motels and hotels, B&B's, campgrounds, RV parks. RESTAURANTS: fast foods, family, Italian. CONTACT: Franklin Area Chamber of Commerce, P. O. Box 180, Franklin, NC 28734, (704) 524-3161. 16,000

BLUE RIDGE MOUNTAIN FAIR WEEK *last week in June through first weekend in July,* Sparta, Alleghany Co.

Music festival, horse shows, Mud Sling, traditional and contemporary mountain crafts sales, 10k Race, flea market, softball tournaments, entertainment for children and adults, parade. FOODS SERVED: multiple local apple products such as hard and plain cider, apple butter, apple sauce, southern specialties, concessions. ADMISSION: free. ACCOMMODATIONS: motels and hotels, B&B's, campgrounds, RV parks. RESTAURANTS: fast foods, family, elegant. CONTACT: Alleghany Co. Chamber of Commerce, P. O. Box 1237, Sparta, NC 28675, (919) 372-5473.

GRANDFATHER MOUNTAIN HIGHLAND GAMES AND GATHERING OF SCOTTISH CLANS *second full weekend in July,* Linville, Avery Co.,

at Grandfather Mountain on US 221 North. Colorful celebration of their heritage by 120 Scottish clans, that includes highland dancing, bagpipes, highland athletic competitions, parades, Scottish bazaar, called the "Best Highland Games in America" by *Better Homes and Gardens.* FOODS SERVED: Scottish. ADMISSION: charge. ACCOMMODATIONS: motels and hotels, B&B's, campgrounds, lodges. RESTAURANTS: fast foods, family, elegant. CONTACT: Harris Prevost, Grandfather Mountain, Box 995, Linville, NC 28646, (704) 733-2013. 20,000

EASTERN MUSIC FESTIVAL *last week in July through first week in August,* Greensboro, Guilford Co., at Guilford College. Classical music festival features

the Eastern Philharmonic Orchestra, summer institute for intensive classical music study, young artists' orchestra concert, and chamber music recitals. ADMISSION: charge. ACCOMMODATIONS: motels and hotels, B&B's, campgrounds, RV parks. RESTAURANTS: fast foods, family, elegant. CONTACT: Eastern Music Festival, 200 N. Davie St., Greensboro, NC 27401, (919) 373-4712.

SOURWOOD FESTIVAL *first weekend in August,* Black Mountain, Buncombe Co., in the Swannanoa Valley to showcase

local and area craftsmen and musicians. Large parade, 150 crafts displays, tennis, golf, and horseshoe tournaments, folk music, square dancing, big-name entertainer, and the international folk dancers of Folkmoot, International. FOODS SERVED: "country southern cooking, some Mexican and Italian." ADMISSION: free. ACCOMMODATIONS: motels and hotels, B&B's, campgrounds, RV park. RESTAURANTS: fast foods, family, elegant. CONTACT: Black Mountain–Swannanoa Chamber of Commerce, 201 E. State St., Black Mountain, NC 28711, (704) 669-2300. 5,000

MOUNTAIN DANCE AND FOLK FESTIVAL *first Thursday, Friday, and Saturday in August,* Asheville, Buncombe Co., at the Asheville Civic Center in west-

ern North Carolina to celebrate the musical and dance heritage of early settlers of the Southern Appalachian Mountains. Traditional mountain-style clog and figure dancing, old-time and bluegrass string bands, dulcimers, buck dancing, ballads, storytelling, audience participation encouraged. ADMISSION: Thursday and Friday $5.00, Saturday $7.00. ACCOMMODATIONS: motels and hotels, B&B's, campgrounds, RV parks. RESTAURANTS: fast foods, family, elegant. CONTACT: Asheville Convention and Visitors Bureau, P. O. Box 1011, Asheville, NC 28802, (704) 258-3916. 7,000

NORTH CAROLINA APPLE FESTIVAL *week before Labor Day weekend and*

Labor Day weekend (late August–early September), Hendersonville, Henderson Co., in western North Carolina to celebrate the apple harvest. Craft shows, golf tournaments, parades, square dancing and clogging. FOODS SERVED: apples galore, others. ADMISSION: varies by event. ACCOMMODATIONS: motels and hotels, B&B's, campgrounds, RV parks. RESTAURANTS: fast foods, family, elegant. CONTACT: North Carolina Apple Festival, c/o the Greater Hendersonville Chamber of Commerce, Inc., 330 N. King St., Hendersonville, NC 28739, (704) 692-1413. 50,000

PINEY WOODS FESTIVAL *Labor Day weekend (early September),* Wilmington, New Hanover Co., at Hugh MacRae Park in Lower Cape Fear country, as a heritage arts and crafts festival. More than sixty old-timey and contemporary arts and crafts exhibitors, jazz and bluegrass music. FOODS SERVED: international including thirteen European and Far Eastern countries. ADMISSION: free. ACCOMMODATIONS: motels and hotels, B&B's, campgrounds, RV parks. RESTAURANTS: fast foods, family, elegant. CONTACT: Arts Council of the Lower Cape Fear, P. O. Box 212, Wilmington, NC 28402, (919) 762-4223. 35,000

NORTH CAROLINA PICKLE FESTIVAL *second week in September,* Mount Olive, Wayne Co., to celebrate the pickle. Arts and crafts show, car show, street dance, parade, pageant. FOODS SERVED: pickles and others. ADMISSION: free. ACCOMMODATIONS: motel. RESTAURANTS: fast foods, family. CONTACT: Mount Olive Area Chamber of Commerce, Inc., 123 N. Center St., Mount Olive, NC 28365, (919) 658-3113.

CENTERFEST *third weekend in September,* Durham, Durham Co. Fine arts and crafts, wandering entertainers, children's area and children's stage featuring puppets, jugglers, cloggers, the Big Zucchini Washboard Bandits, mimes, children's musical parade; local and regional musical groups including the Durham Symphony, Durham Community Concert Band, and the Durham Savoyards; jazz, country, bluegrass, gospel, reggae, rock and roll, rhythm and blues. FOODS SERVED: variety. ADMISSION: free. ACCOMMODATIONS: motels and hotels, campgrounds. RESTAURANTS: fast foods, family, elegant, Asian, continental, Cajun, vegetarian. CONTACT: CenterFest, c/o Durham Arts Council, 120 Morris St., Durham, NC 27701-3282, (919) 489-8931, or the Greater Durham Chamber of Commerce, 201 N. Roxboro St., Durham, NC 27702, (919) 682-2133.

NATIONAL BALLOON RALLY *third or fourth weekend in September,* Statesville, Iredell Co. More than 125 hot air balloons lift off from Statesville Municipal Airport and participate in races, trajectory bean-bag drops, precision flying maneuvers, and two-by-two competition; arts and crafts, children's entertainment, model flyers, magic, comedy, pop and beach music, bluegrass; tethered balloon rides, balloon rides, corporate balloons, helicopter rides. FOODS SERVED: local concessions. ADMISSION: Friday $5.00 per car, Saturday and Sunday $15.00 per car. ACCOMMODATIONS: motels and hotels, B&B's, campgrounds, RV parks. RESTAURANTS: fast foods, family, elegant. CONTACT: Greater Statesville Chamber of Commerce, P. O. Box 1064, Statesville, NC 28677, (704) 873-2892. 52,000

MOUNTAIN HERITAGE DAY *last Saturday in September,* Cullowhee, Jackson Co., at Western Carolina University in the Appalachian or Smoky Mountains, to celebrate the "heritage of the mountain people." Tobacco Spitting and Hog Calling contests, mountain crafts, Country Run, dog and cat show, old truck show, chainsaw competition, Beard and Dress Contests, children's activities, Cherokee Indian crafts and dance, workshops and exhibits, traditional music and dancing including David Holt, Doc Watson's Medicine Show, regional bluegrass and string bands, championship cloggers and smooth square dancing, and the Appalachian Puppet Theatre. FOODS SERVED: Cherokee Indian fry breads, traditional foods indigenous to the region. ADMISSION: free. ACCOMMODATIONS: motels and hotels, B&B's, campgrounds, RV parks. RESTAURANTS: fast foods, family, Italian, Mexican. CONTACT: Mountain Heritage Day, 40 Western Carolina University, Cullowhee, NC 28723 or the Cullowhee Chamber of Commerce, Rt, 67, Box 112-H, Cullowhee, NC 28723, (704) 293-9648. 35,000

BRUSHY MOUNTAIN APPLE FESTIVAL *first Saturday in October,* North Wilkesboro, Wilkes Co., in northwestern North Carolina to celebrate the Brushy Mountain apple harvest. Old-timey crafts such as quilting, basketmaking, cider making and molasses boiling, steam tractors exhibit, 450 artists and craftspeople exhibit their work, antique cars, photo contest, almost continuous country and gospel music, Big Band Night with Big Band music performed by the Wilkes Community College Jazz Ensemble. FOODS SERVED: "apples, apples, apples" and "good country food and drink." ADMISSION: free, $2.00 to Big Band Night. ACCOMMODATIONS: motels and hotels, B&B's, campgrounds, RV parks. RESTAURANTS: fast foods, family, elegant. CONTACT: Brushy Mountain Apple Festival, Rt. 1, Box 65, Moravian Falls, NC 28654 or Brushy Mountain Ruritan Club, Rt. 1, Box 119, Moravian Falls, NC 28654, (919) 667-3322. 165,000

FALL FESTIVAL *first weekend in October,* Asheboro, Randolph Co., in the Piedmont Triad, to celebrate the arrival and beauty of fall. Arts and crafts, parade, wagon train, Antique Car Show, 10k Run, dance exhibitions, live entertainment by local and area talent. FOODS SERVED: barbecue, hush puppies, concessions. ADMISSION: free. ACCOMMODATIONS: motels and hotels, campgrounds. RESTAURANTS: fast foods, family, Asian. CONTACT: Randolph Arts Guild, P. O. Box 1033, Asheboro, NC 27204, (919) 629-0399. 200,000

CHEROKEE INDIAN FALL FESTIVAL *second week in October,* Cherokee, Swain Co., at the Ceremonial Grounds on the Cherokee Indian Reservation, to celebrate the ancient Cherokee Corn Festival. Traditional Cherokee dances and sports, demonstrations of Cherokee arts and crafts, mountain clog dancing, Miss Cherokee beauty contest, Miss Fall Festival, blowgun and archery contests, gospel singing in English and Cherokee languages, country music, and Indian Fancy Dance. FOODS SERVED: traditional Cherokee food, including corn. ADMISSION: adults $3.00, children and senior citizens $1.50. ACCOMMODATIONS: motels and hotels, campgrounds, RV parks. RESTAURANTS: fast foods, family. CONTACT: Marty Sinclair, P. O. Box 366, Cherokee, NC 28719, (704) 497-3028 or write to Cherokee Tribal Travel and Promotion, P.O. Box 465, Cherokee, NC 28719, (704) 497-9195. 15,000

MOUNTAIN GLORY FESTIVAL *second Saturday in October,* Marion, McDowell Co., to celebrate the mountain heritage of western North Carolina at harvest time "when color is peaking." As a regional art show and foodfest, more than 100 artists and craftspeople display their work, Mountain Glory heritage tours, the Appalachian Puppet Theatre performs, mimes, folk and mountain music. FOODS SERVED: Appalachian, Laotian, Chinese. ADMISSION: free. ACCOMMODATIONS: motels and hotels, B&B, campgrounds, RV parks. RESTAURANTS: fast foods, family, elegant, Chinese, Italian. CONTACT: McDowell Chamber of Commerce, 17 N. Garden St., Marion, NC 28752, (704) 652-4240, 20,000

NORTH CAROLINA OYSTER FESTIVAL *second weekend in October,* Ocean Isle Beach, Brunswick Co., at the South Brunswick Isles. North Carolina Oyster Shucking Contest featuring National Champion from the area, Fun Run, Bullshooting (tall-tale telling) Competition, more than eighty arts and crafts booths, entertainment by local church choral groups. FOODS SERVED: oysters fried, roasted, or cocktailed, fried flounder, hush puppies, coleslaw, clam chowder, hot dogs and other foods for landlubbers. ADMISSION: free. ACCOMMODATIONS: motels and hotels, B&B's, campgrounds, RV parks. RESTAURANTS: family. CONTACT: South Brunswick Islands Chamber of Commerce, P. O. Box 1380, Shallotte, NC 28459, (919) 754-6644. 10,000

AUTUMN LEAVES FESTIVAL *second weekend in October,* Mount Airy, Surry Co., to enjoy and celebrate the colorful leaves in the Mount Airy area. Down-home demonstrations of traditional crafts and lifestyles, making of apple butter, cider, and molasses, petting zoo, crafts for sale, horseshoe pitching, continuous country and bluegrass music. FOODS SERVED: ham biscuits, pinto beans, cornbread. ADMISSION: free. ACCOMMODATIONS: motels and hotels, B&B, campgrounds, RV parks. RESTAURANTS: fast foods, family. CONTACT: Mount Airy Chamber of Commerce, Inc., P. O. Box 913, Mount Airy, NC 27030, (919) 658-3113. 250,000

JOHN BLUE COTTON FESTIVAL *third Friday and Saturday in October,* Laurinburg, Scotland Co., at the John Blue House and grounds. Crafts sales, demonstrations of early homemaking skills and early farm tools, farm wagon rides, petting farm, engines, antique, and cotton exhibits, Games of Yesteryear, high-school poster-contest exhibit, Frog Jumpin' Contest, Ugly Face Contest, log cabins, Revolutionary War Encampment, Bald Head Men's Contest, entertainment including clogging and folk music, a roving clown and mime, jazz, square dancing, Big Zucchini Washboard Bandits Band; tours of John Blue House. FOODS SERVED: concessions. ADMISSION: adults $1.00. ACCOMMODATIONS: motels and hotels. RESTAURANTS: fast foods, family, Chinese. CONTACT: Scotland Co. Parks and Recreation, P. O. Box 1668, Laurinburg, NC 28352, (919) 276-0412, or the Laurinburg/ Scotland Co. Area Chamber of Com-

merce, P. O. Box 1025, Laurinburg, NC 28352, (919) 276-7420. 8,000

CHRYSANTHEMUM FESTIVAL *third weekend in October,* New Bern, Craven Co., at the Tryon Palace Restoration and Gardens Complex and downtown, to celebrate the exquisite blooming of chrysanthemums in the gardens and downtown. Military encampment at Tryon Palace, street dance, street entertainment, crafts, antiques. ADMISSION: charge for some events, others free. ACCOMMODATIONS: motels and hotels, B&B's, campgrounds, RV parks. RESTAURANTS: fast foods, family, elegant. CONTACT: Events Office, Tryon Palace Complex, P. O. Box 1007, New Bern, NC 28560, (919) 638-1560.

WOOLLY WORM FESTIVAL *third Saturday in October,* Banner Elk, Avery Co., to forecast the severity of the winter to come. The woolly worm is a black-and-brown caterpillar-like creature with a fuzzy coat. To enter the race one may hunt for one's own woolly worm along the side of the road or buy one from a young entrepreneur who may sell them from a shoe box. The stripes on the winner of the Woolly Worm Race forecast winter: the blacker they are, the heavier the winter (considered good for this ski area); the browner they are, the lighter the winter weather will be. Mountain music and traditional arts and crafts are offered. FOODS SERVED: southern and mountain specialties. ADMISSION: free. ACCOMMODATIONS: motels and hotels, B&B's, campgrounds, RV parks. RESTAURANTS: fast foods, family, elegant. CONTACT: Banner Elk Chamber of Commerce, P. O. Box 335, Banner Elk, NC 28604, (704) 898-5605.

OLD SALEM CHRISTMAS *third Friday and Saturday in December (date varies),* Winston–Salem, Forsyth Co., in Old Salem, to remember and celebrate a recreation of Christmas in the period from 1790–1830. Period music including choral and instrumental performances, period decorations on and in buildings of Old Salem, creches, horse-drawn wagon rides, entertainment by Paddy's Pals, Moravian brass bands, and others. FOODS SERVED: period foods including sugar cake, ginger cookies, and apples. ADMIS-SION: adults $8.00, children 3–14 $4.00. ACCOMMODATIONS: motels and hotels, B&B. RESTAURANTS: fast foods, elegant. CONTACT: Old Salem, Inc., Drawer F, Salem Station, Winston–Salem, NC 27108, (919) 723-3688. 5,000

TENNESSEE

STATE OF TENNESSEE OLD-TIME FIDDLERS' CHAMPIONSHIPS first Friday and Saturday in April, Clarksville, Montgomery Co., at the Clarksville Fairgrounds. More than 300 artists compete in the "offical state championships" in fourteen events with a total of $5,750 in prize money awarded; old-time musicians attend and participate in informal jam sessions, flatfoot dancing, old-time music, bluegrass, and "the big fiddle-off." FOODS SERVED: concessions. ADMISSION: charge. ACCOMMODATIONS: motels and hotels, campgrounds, RV parks. RESTAURANTS: fast foods, family, elegant, seafood, German, southern. CONTACT: Clarksville–Montgomery Co. Tourist Commission, P.O. Box 513, Clarksville, TN 37041-0513, (615) 647-2331.

MULE DAY COUNTRY LIVING first weekend in April, Columbia, Maury Co., at Maury County Park and downtown Columbia. Western Mule Show, crafts festival, knife and gun show, Checkers Contest, arm wrestling, Liars Contest, Mule Pulling Contest, parade, Mule Sale, square dance, Mule Day Dance. FOODS SERVED: pancake breakfast, concessions. ADMISSION: to park adults $2.00, children under 12 $1.00, includes Tennessee state amusement tax. ACCOMMODATIONS: motels, campground. RESTAURANTS: fast foods, family. CONTACT: Maury Co. Bridle and Saddle Club, P. O. Box 66, Columbia, TN 38402, (615) 381-9557 or the Maury Co. Chamber of Commerce, P. O. Box 1076, Columbia, TN 38402, (615) 388-2155.

DOGWOOD ARTS FESTIVAL second Friday in April and two weeks following, Knoxville, Knox Co., to celebrate the spring flowering of the dogwoods. More than 300 events and activities and 200 hours of live entertainment. Grand Band Parade, juried fine craft fair, juried area Art Show, photograph competition and exhibition, Arts Alive on Market Square, Master Furniture-Makers Show, Tennessee Artists Spring Show, quilt competition, Hot Air Balloon Rally, Chili Cook-off, Folk Arts Festival, children's activities, fireworks, Knoxville Embroiderers' Guild Exhibit, free bus tours, flower show, Craftsmen at Work, Outdoor Appalachian Square Dance, Tennessee State Handbell Festival, puppets, Knoxville Youth Symphony Concert, Dogwood Road Race, golf tournament, BMX Race, Kite Flying Derby, Super Run, Mayor's Fitness Walk, tennis and bass tournaments, River Parade, rock concert, bluegrass competition, jazz concerts and competitions, Clogging Contest, and a special performance by the Knoxville Opera Company, many camera sites and open gardens. FOODS SERVED: concessions and foods prepared by local restaurants. ADMISSION: free, charges for some events. ACCOMMODATIONS: motels and hotels, B&B's, campgrounds, RV parks. RESTAURANTS: fast foods, family, elegant. CONTACT: Dogwood Arts Festival, 901 E. Summit

Hill Dr., Knoxville, TN 37915 or the Greater Knoxville Chamber of Commerce, P. O. Box 2688, Knoxville, TN 37901, (615) 637-4550. 1,400,000

BLOUNT COUNTY DOGWOOD ARTS FESTIVAL *second weekend through fourth weekend in April,* Alcoa–Maryville, Blount Co., near Knoxville, to celebrate the blooming of the dogwoods in the area. Dogwood Drives, student art show, wildflower walks, square dancing, golf and softball tournaments, clogging competition, Five Mile Hike, performances by the ballet, the Blount County Community Playhouse, Bluegrass in the Greenbelt with Steve and Marty Womac, Festival of Voices, and stars such as Miss Tennessee, Razzy Bailey, and Minnie Pearl have appeared in the past. ADMISSION: free, charges for some events. ACCOMMODATIONS: motels and hotels, campgrounds, RV parks. RESTAURANTS: fast foods, family, Chinese. CONTACT: Blount Co. Chamber of Commerce, 309 S. Washington St., Maryville, TN 37801, (615) 983-2241.

WORLD'S BIGGEST FISH FRY *third or fourth week in April,* Paris, Henry Co., near Kentucky Lake. Arts and crafts show, car show, beauty pageant, 5k and 10k runs, Rock Jam, rodeo, soccer tournament, Small Fry Parade, junior fishing Rodeo, WAKQ catfish frying Cook-off, giant fish fry, Grand Parade, country music. FOODS SERVED: 8,500 pounds of catfish, golden hush puppies, coleslaw, soup beans. ACCOMMODATIONS: motels, resorts, campground. RESTAURANTS: fast foods, family. ADMISSION: $5.00. CONTACT: Fish Fry, P. O. Box 444, Paris, TN 38242 or the Paris and Henry Co. Chamber of Commerce, P. O. Box 82, Paris, TN 38242, (901) 642-3431. 50,000

MID-SOUTH JAZZ FESTIVAL *fourth Thursday and Friday in April,* Clarksville, Montgomery Co., at Clement Auditorium of the Austin Peay State University campus. "A well-known guest musician is featured each year at the festival along with

the Austin Peay State University Jazz Collegians, high school jazz groups, and other college jazz ensembles" as a showcase of southern jazz talent. ADMISSION: charge. ACCOMMODATIONS: motels and hotels, campgrounds, RV parks. RESTAURANTS: fast foods, family, elegant, seafood, German, southern. CONTACT: Clarksville–Montgomery Co. Tourist Commission, P.O. Box 513, Clarksville, TN 37041–0513, (615) 647-2331.

LAKE CHICKAMAUGA SPRING FESTIVAL *last weekend in April or first weekend in May,* Chattanooga, Hamilton Co., at the Chickamauga Lake Recreation Area to celebrate the beginning of spring. Arts and crafts, games, clogging, bluegrass music and other continuous live entertainment. FOODS SERVED: "international foods and beverages." ADMISSION: free. ACCOMMODATIONS: motels and hotels, B&B's, campgrounds, RV parks. RESTAURANTS: fast foods, family, elegant, Mexican, Italian, Asian, French. CONTACT: Chattanooga Area Chamber of Commerce, 1001 Market St., Chattanooga, TN 37402, (615) 756-2121. 60,000

MEMPHIS IN MAY INTERNATIONAL FESTIVAL *month of May,* Memphis, Shelby Co., to celebrate springtime and local foreign cultures. Five weekends of free events including 10k and 2mi Fun Run, cultural events of honored country; International Children's Festival on Mud Island theme and amusement park on a sandbar in the Mississippi River includes the Smurfs, Russian folk music group Troika Balalaikas, Japanese Minyo Dancers, a taiko drum troupe, storytellers, dancers and musicians; The Great Mississippi Canoe and Kayak Race with more than 200 canoes, International Business Conference, International Barbecue Cooking Contest in which more than 500 potential competitors from the U. S. and five foreign countries apply for 200 contestant spots to cook in three categories: ribs, shoulder, and whole hog; Miss Piggy Contest, hog-calling contests, holiday rock honoring rock music's Memphis ori-

gins including the Beale Street Music Festival, triathlon including a 1.5k swim, 40k bike ride and 10k run; and the Sunset Symphony during which 250,000 people sit on blankets along the banks of the Mississippi, sip champagne and listen to classical and pop music by the Memphis Symphony Orchestra; Film Festival, Essay Contest, art exhibits, Great Wine Race. FOODS SERVED: those of the honored country, concessions. ADMISSION: most events free. ACCOMMODATIONS: motels and hotels, B&B's, campgrounds. RESTAURANTS: fast foods, family, elegant. CONTACT: Marketing Coordinator, Memphis in May Festival, Inc., 245 Wagner Place, Suite 220, Memphis, TN 38103, (901) 525-4611. 1,000,000

DOWNTOWN ARTS FESTIVAL *first weekend in May*, Chattanooga, Hamilton Co., at Miller Park, to celebrate the fine arts in the area. Juried art show, arts and crafts, children's activities, live performances such as the Brass Quintet, Blues Band, Swing Orchestra, Gospel Orchestra, Bach Choir, Boys Choir, Dixieland Band, Dance Theatre Workshop, Chattanooga Ballet, and puppet arts. FOODS SERVED: ethnic and cultural food booths. ADMISSION: free. ACCOMMODATIONS: motels and hotels, B&B's, campgrounds, RV parks. RESTAURANTS: fast foods, family, elegant, Mexican, Italian, Asian, French. CONTACT: Chattanooga Downtown Alliance, 1001 Market St., Chattanooga, TN 37402, (615) 756-2121. 10,000

FAIR ON THE SQUARE *first weekend in May*, Collierville, Shelby Co., at the Town Square, to celebrate local arts and crafts. Arts and crafts, pony rides, games, exhibits, live entertainment such as gospel groups and teenage pop bands. FOODS SERVED: "authentic southern pork" barbecue, baked goods, and other food stands. ADMISSION: free. ACCOMMODATIONS: motels and hotels. RESTAURANTS: fast foods, family, Chinese. CONTACT: Mrs. Pat Treadwell at (901) 853-4010 or the Collierville Area Chamber of Commerce, Depot Town Square, Collierville, TN 38017, (901) 853-1949. 12,000

TENNESSEE CRAFTS FAIR *first weekend in May*, Nashville, Davidson Co., at Centennial Park. Juried fine crafts show including 150 exhibitors, ongoing demonstrations, children's craft activities, live country music all on the lawn in front of "the historic Parthenon." FOODS SERVED: "fine food for picknicking in the park." ADMISSION: free. ACCOMMODATIONS: motels and hotels, B&B's, campgrounds, RV parks. RESTAURANTS: fast foods, family, elegant. CONTACT: Tennessee Crafts Fair, P.O. Box 150704, Nashville, TN 37215, (615) 383-2502. 60,000

AZALEA FESTIVAL *Mother's Day weekend (early May)*, Oak Ridge, Anderson Co., at the Civic Center Plaza, as a celebration of spring. Arts and crafts show, Tour d'Oak Ridge bike tour, road race, Garden Club Azalea Trail tour, Realtors' Relays, street dance, international food bazaar, children's activities, local and regional entertainment including bands, dancers, singers, and Senior Citizen Band. FOODS SERVED: Chinese, Greek, Mexican, Italian, American. ADMISSION: free, $5.00 for bike tour. ACCOMMODATIONS: motels and hotels, campgrounds and RV parks nearby. RESTAURANTS: fast foods, family, elegant, Chinese, Greek. CONTACT: John Collins, City of Oak Ridge, P.O. Box 1, Oak Ridge, TN 37831, (615) 482-8316, or Arts Council of Oak Ridge, P.O. Box 324, Oak Ridge, TN 37830, (615) 482-3395. 4,000

EAST MAIN STREET FESTIVAL *second Saturday in May*, Murfreesboro, Rutherford Co. Arts and crafts, parade by visiting dancers from International Folk Fest the previous week, theatrical productions, local groups performing popular, classical, and mountain music. FOODS SERVED: wide range of concessions. ADMISSION: free. ACCOMMODATIONS: motels and hotels, B&B's, campgrounds, RV parks. RESTAURANTS: fast foods, family.

CONTACT: The Arts and Humanities Council of Murfreesboro and Rutherford County, P.O. Box 1552, Murfreesboro, TN 37120, (615) 895-2787, or the Rutherford Co. Chamber of Commerce, P.O. Box 864, Murfreesboro, TN 37130, (615) 893-6565. 30,000

EAST TENNESSEE STRAWBERRY FESTIVAL *second week in May,* Dayton, Rhea Co., to salute the strawberry growers in east Tennessee. Crafts fair, art show, beauty pageant, parade, golf and tennis tournaments, carnival, theatrical presentation by the Tennessee Wesleyan Players. FOODS SERVED: strawberries and other concessions. ADMISSION: free, beauty pageant $5.00. ACCOMMODATIONS: motels and hotels, RV parks. RESTAURANTS: fast foods, family. CONTACT: Dayton Chamber of Commerce, 305 E. Main Ave., Dayton, TN 37321, (615) 775-0361. 25,000

ANDREW JACKSON DAYS *second or third weekend in May,* near Nashville, Davidson Co., at the Hermitage, site of President Jackson's birth on March 15, 1767, to remember and celebrate his life and presidency. Arts and crafts, antiques, "star entertainment." FOODS SERVED: "good food." ADMISSION: free, parking $1.00. ACCOMMODATIONS: motels and hotels, B&B's, campgrounds, RV parks. RESTAURANTS: fast foods, family, elegant. CONTACT: Donelson Hermitage Chamber of Commerce, 3051 Lebanon Rd., Donelson Medical Plaza, Suite 100, Nashville, TN 37214, (615) 883-7896. 20,000

GREAT SMOKEY MOUNTAIN–GATLINBURG HIGHLAND GAMES *third weekend in May,* Gatlinburg, Sevier Co., at Mills Park, to recognize and celebrate Scottish traditions and customs. Three-day festival of local Highland heritage including Scottish social events, traditional athletic competitions, kilt races, dancing contests, Highland music and special events which vary each year, parades, bagpipes and Scottish drummers. FOODS

SERVED: beef pies and other Scottish specialties. ADMISSION: to grounds, adults $6.00, children $3.00, additional charges to social events. ACCOMMODATIONS: motels and hotels, campgrounds, RV parks. RESTAURANTS: fast foods, family, elegant ("come as you are"). CONTACT: Gatlinburg Chamber of Commerce, P.O. Box 527, Gatlinburg, TN 37738, (800) 251-9868 outside Tennessee or (800) 824-4766 inside Tennessee. 15,000

SUMMER LIGHTS FESTIVAL *last weekend in May,* Nashville, Davidson Co., at Legislative Plaza and other downtown locations. Unusual round-the-clock hours during this four-day festival which is a tribute to top artists of many disciplines including culinary arts, country music, rock 'n' roll, ballet, theatre; special demonstrations and exhibits showcasing the visual arts, arts and crafts markets, urban tours, and culinary creations. FOODS SERVED: the best of southern and international delicacies. ADMISSION: free, charges for some indoor events. ACCOMMODATIONS: motels and hotels, B&B's, campgrounds, RV parks. RESTAURANTS: fast foods, family, elegant. CONTACT: Summer Lights Coordinator, Summer Lights Festival, c/o The Nashville Symphony, 1805 West End Ave., Nashville, TN 37201, (615) 329-3033. 500,000

TULLAHOMA FINE ARTS AND CRAFTS FESTIVAL *last weekend in May,* Tullahoma, Coffee Co., site of the George Dickel Distillery. More than 100 artists and craftspeople display and sell their works in this juried exhibition, fine arts. FOODS SERVED: traditional foods. ADMISSION: $1.00. ACCOMMODATIONS: motels and hotels, B&B's, campgrounds, RV parks. RESTAURANTS: fast foods, family, elegant. CONTACT: Tullahoma Fine Arts Center, 401 S. Jackson St., Tullahoma, TN 37388, (615) 455-1234, or the Tullahoma Chamber of Commerce, P.O. Box 1205, Tullahoma, TN 37388, (615) 455-5497. 10,000

GREAT RIVER CARNIVAL *month of June,* Memphis, Shelby Co. Art exhibits, masked balls, Grand Parade, River Pageant, Karnival for Kids, Music Festival, Stone Soul Weekend, fashion shows, Grand Krewe parties, educational seminars, Industry Salute and Awards Banquet. ADMISSION: $2.00–$7.00. ACCOMMODATIONS: motels and hotels, B&B's, campgrounds, RV parks. RESTAURANTS: fast foods, family, elegant, international. CONTACT: Great River Carnival Association, 1060 Early Maxwell Blvd., Memphis, TN 38104, (901) 278-0243, or the Memphis Area Chamber of Commerce, P.O. Box 224, Memphis, TN 38103, (901) 523-2322. 450,000

INTERNATIONAL COUNTRY MUSIC FAN FAIR *second week in June,* Nashville, Davidson Co., at the Tennessee State Fairgrounds, Opryland, and Vanderbilt University's Dudley Field, as a genuine "thank you" to country music fans. More than thirty-five hours of stage shows by the stars of country music who come home to Nashville for this week, other musical events, picture and autograph sessions with fans and stars, competitive events such as the All-American Country Games and The Grand Masters Fiddling Championship. ADMISSION: about $60.00, which includes all scheduled activities and concerts, some meals, the All-American Country Games, tickets to Opryland, Ryman Auditorium, and the Country Music Hall of Fame and Museum. ACCOMMODATIONS: motels and hotels, B&B's, campgrounds, RV parks. RESTAURANTS: fast foods, family, elegant. CONTACT: Fan Fair, 2804 Opryland Dr., Nashville, TN 37214 or the Nashville Area Chamber of Commerce, 161 Fourth Avenue North, Nashville, TN 37219, (615) 259-3900. 22,000

COVERED BRIDGE CELEBRATION *second week in June,* Elizabethton, Carter Co., to celebrate the birthday of the Covered Bridge. Arts and Crafts Festival, bike race, 10k Race, ice cream and pie eating contest, Little Miss Country and Little Mr. Hillbilly contests, parade, fireworks, nightly music including bluegrass, country, cloggers, square dancing. FOODS SERVED: concessions. ADMISSION: free. ACCOMMODATIONS: motels and hotels, campgrounds. RESTAURANTS: fast foods, family, elegant, seafood, Italian, "home cooking." CONTACT: Elizabethton–Carter Co. Chamber of Commerce, P.O. Box 190, Elizabethton, TN 37643, (615) 543-2122. 16,000

THE MARTHA WHITE–LESTER FLATT HOMETOWN MEMORIAL FESTIVAL *second Saturday in June,* Sparta, White Co., at the White County Fairgrounds, to honor Grand Ole Opry star Lester Flatt. Bluegrass and gospel music, Little Miss Martha White Contest, Lester Flatt Memorial Award and trophy to the best bluegrass band, best gospel, and best single instrument. FOODS SERVED: "Tennessee home cooking." ADMISSION: free. ACCOMMODATIONS: motels and hotels, campgrounds, RV parks. RESTAURANTS: fast foods, family, Italian. CONTACT: E. P. England, Rt. 5, Box 509, Sparta, TN 38583, (615) 761-2847 or the Sparta–White Co. Chamber of Commerce, P.O. Box 131, Sparta, TN 38583, (615) 836-3552. 2,000

DEFEATED/CORDELL HULL BLUEGRASS MUSIC FESTIVAL *second weekend in June,* near Brush Creek, Smith Co., at the Cordell Hull Lake-Defeated Campground. Craft fair, Bluegrass Music Competition featuring amateur musicians in individual competition at banjo, mandolin, guitar, and other instruments, square dancing. FOODS SERVED: traditional, concessions. ADMISSION: free. ACCOMMODATIONS: motels and hotels, campgrounds. RESTAURANTS: fast foods, family. CONTACT: Roger Glover, Rt. 1, Brush Creek, TN 38547 or the Smith Co. Chamber of Commerce, Inc., P.O. Box 70, Carthage, TN 37030, (615) 735-2093. 20,000

HIGH FOREST JAMBOREE *third weekend in June,* Hohenwald, Lewis Co., at the Lewis State Forest, to celebrate the settlement of Hohenwald and of Lewis County. Craft fair, beauty contests, flea market, games; musicals, gospel, and country music. FOODS SERVED: local mountain and other specialties. ADMISSION: free. ACCOMMODATIONS: motels, campgrounds, RV parks. RESTAURANTS: fast foods, family. CONTACT: Lewis Co. Chamber of Commerce, P.O. Box 182, Hohenwald, TN 38462, (615) 796-2731. 5,000

ROAN MOUNTAIN RHODODEN-DRON FESTIVAL *third weekend in June,* Roan Mountain, Carter Co., to celebrate the blooming of 600 acres of rhododendrons. Arts and crafts show, political-office holders, beauty pageants, Roan Mountain Cloggers, dancing, dulcimers, other mountain music. FOODS SERVED: apple butter, fried chicken, concessions. ADMISSION: free. ACCOMMODATIONS: motels and hotels, campgrounds, cabins. RESTAURANTS: fast foods, family. CONTACT: Durward Julian of the Roan Mountain Citizens Club at (615) 772-3264 or the Elizabethton–Carter Co. Chamber of Commerce, P.O. Box 190, Elizabethton, TN 37643, (615) 543-2122. 15,000

FOLK MEDICINE FESTIVAL *fourth Saturday in June,* Red Boiling Springs, Macon Co., in the Upper Cumberlands to "revive the town's historical significance." Folk arts representing early Red Boiling Springs traditions, booths and demonstrations of "alternative medicine, herbs, reflexology, and health foods," wagon rides, country music including Frazier Moss and Band. FOODS SERVED: "English, country-style food," health foods. ADMISSION: $1.00. ACCOMMODATIONS: hotels. RESTAURANTS: fast foods, family. CONTACT: Brenda Thomas, Rt. 3, Box 448A, Red Boiling Springs, TN 37150 or the Red Boiling Springs "Sulphur City Association," Red Boiling Springs, TN 37150, (615) 699-2011. 5,000

WINFIELD APPALACHIAN DUM-PLIN' FESTIVAL *fourth Saturday in June,* Winfield, Scott Co. Arts and crafts festival, dumplin' and other eating contests, games, live music which has included Buck Trent. FOODS SERVED: "dumplin's of all kinds." ADMISSION: free. ACCOMMODATIONS: motels and hotels, campgrounds, RV parks. RESTAURANTS: fast foods, family. CONTACT: Cecil Trunk, Mayor, c/o Appalachian Dumplin' Festival Committee, P.O. Box 39, Winfield, TN 37892, (615) 569-6139. 5,000

OLD TIME FIDDLERS' JAMBOREE AND CRAFTS FESTIVAL *first Friday and Saturday in July,* Smithville, DeKalb Co., at Courthouse Square, as a pure bluegrass festival and competition with cash prizes. Crafts, competitions in clogging, buck dancing, old-time fiddle band, dobro guitar, 5-string banjo, novelty event, fiddling for all ages, gospel singing, dulcimer, flat top guitar, country harmonica, folk singing, bluegrass band, mandolin; country music Beginners National Championships in fiddle, mandolin, five-string banjo, flat-top guitar, dobro guitar, senior cloggers (61 and over), senior fiddlers (51 and older), square dancing, Jr. and Sr. Fiddlers' Fiddle-off for Grand Championship. FOODS SERVED: country cooking such as beans and cornbread, barbecue, hamburgers. ADMISSION: free, $3.00 per person to compete. ACCOMMODATIONS: motels and hotels, B&B's, campgrounds, RV parks. RESTAURANTS: fast foods, family. CONTACT: Smithville Chamber of Commerce, P.O. Box 64, Smithville, TN 37166, (615) 597-4163. 75,000

HORSESHOE BEND FESTIVAL *weekend after July 4th,* Clifton, Wayne Co. Arts and crafts, horseshoe pitching, car show, USSSA State Class D Qualifying Slo-pitch Softball Tournament, street square dance, Bass Fishing Tournament. FOODS SERVED: fish fry. ADMISSION: free. ACCOMMODATIONS: motels and hotels, campgrounds, RV parks. RESTAURANTS: fast foods, family. CONTACT: Bill Willoughby at (615) 676-3764 or the Wayne Co. Chamber of Commerce, P.O. Box 107, Waynesboro, TN 38485, (615) 722-3418.

DOLLYWOOD NATIONAL MOUNTAIN MUSIC FESTIVAL *July 13–28,* Dollywood, Pigeon Forge, Sevier Co., in the Great Smoky Mountains to "officially ring in summer." A night-time music extravaganza including bluegrass, gospel, mountain, and country music, and happy music. FOODS SERVED: country delicacies such as funnel cakes, apple fritters, hickory-smoked meats, banana pudding. ADMISSION: cost admits to Dollywood and music festival; adults $13.50 plus tax, children 4–11 $9.95 plus tax, children under 4 free. ACCOMMODATIONS: motels, B&B's, cottages, campgrounds, RV parks. RESTAURANTS: fast foods, family, elegant, Italian, Chinese. CONTACT: Dollywood, 700 Dollywood Lane, Pigeon Forge, TN 37863-4101, (615) 428-9400. 350,000

CEDAR CITY SUMMER CELEBRATION *third weekend in July,* Lebanon, Wilson Co., at Baird Park, celebrating Tennessee and country music. Gospel music concert, Fiddlers Competition, bluegrass bands, buck dancing, banjo, square dance teams, craft booths; and in the past, Grand Ole Opry entertainers have performed in the open amphitheatre, as have local artists. FOODS SERVED: all-American food booths. ADMISSION: free. ACCOMMODATIONS: motels and hotels, campgrounds, RV parks. RESTAURANTS: fast foods, family, Chinese. CONTACT: Lebanon–Wilson Co. Chamber of Commerce, 105 W. Market St., Lebanon, TN 37087, (615) 444-5503. 6,000

FUN FEST *last Friday in July and following nine days,* Kingsport, Sullivan Co., in the Tri-Cities area. Hot Air Balloon Race, Crazy Boat Race, concerts which in the past have included the Four Tops, Atlanta, Osmond Brothers, Coasters, Lee Greenwood, Eddie Rabbitt, and Chubby Checker. FOODS SERVED: Taste of the Tri-Cities including specialties of locally owned restaurants. ADMISSION: free, "small" charge for some events. ACCOMMODATIONS: motels and hotels, B&B's, campgrounds. RESTAURANTS: fast foods,

family, elegant. CONTACT: Kingsport Area Chamber of Commerce, P.O. Box 1403, Kingsport, TN 37662, (615) 246-2010. 50,000

ARTS AND CRAFTS FAIR *fourth weekend in August,* Beersheba Springs, Grundy Co. More than 200 artists and craftspeople exhibit and sell their work including woodwork, stained glass, quilts, leather, painted china, honey, all hand- or homemade; music by local bands played at night for hotel and campground guests. FOODS SERVED: food booths. ADMISSION: free. ACCOMMODATIONS: hotel, campground, RV park nearby at Stone Door State Park. CONTACT: Maude Hunter, Box 5, Beersheba Springs, TN 37305, (615) 692-3753. 17,000

ITALIAN STREET FAIR *last weekend in August,* Nashville, Davidson Co., at the Gay Street Connector and Courthouse Plaza, as an annual fundraiser for the Nashville Symphony Orchestra. Extravaganza of food, Italian markets, carnival rides, games, arts and crafts, wine-making contest and grape stomping for the public; non-stop entertainment includes a Sunday-afternoon performance by the Nashville Symphony Orchestra. FOODS SERVED: Italian and lots of pasta. ADMISSION: adults $3.00 at gate, $2.00 advance; children under 12 $1.00. ACCOMMODATIONS: motels and hotels, B&B's, campgrounds, RV parks. RESTAURANTS: fast foods, family, elegant. CONTACT: Nashville Symphony Guild Office, 208 23rd Ave., N., Nashville, TN 37203-1502 at (615) 329-3033 or the Nashville Area Chamber of Commerce, 161 Fourth Avenue North, Nashville, TN 37219, (615) 259-3900. 50,000

THE MEMPHIS MUSIC FESTIVAL *Sunday of Labor Day weekend (early September),* Memphis, Shelby Co. More than thirty groups perform throughout the Beale Street area including blues, jazz, rhythm and blues, rock, and country music including star performers from Memphis such as Sam and Dave, Steve Cropper, Donald "Duck" Dunn, Albert King, and Rufus Thomas, who return home and jam with local bands. ADMISSION: $5.00 admits to all events. ACCOMMODATIONS: motels and hotels, B&B's, campgrounds. RESTAURANTS: fast foods, family, elegant. CONTACT: Davis E. Tillman, 203 Beale St., Suite 303, Memphis, TN 38103, (901) 522-9260. 3,600

OLD TIME MUSIC DAY *Labor Day (early September)*, Hendersonville, Sumner Co., at Drakes Creek Park, to celebrate "grass roots Tennessean music and crafts." Tennessee craftspeople, Buck Dancing Contest, flea market, crafts demonstrations, concessions, Tennessee music stars such as Patsy Sledd, Warner Mack, Billy Walker, and Skeeter Davis. FOODS SERVED: "grass roots Tennessee-style cooking" such as barbecue, country ham, white beans, cornbread, fish fry, watermelon, Chili cook-off, ice cream, baked goods. ADMISSION: adults $2.00, children $1.00. ACCOMMODATIONS: motels and hotels, campgrounds. RESTAURANTS: fast foods, family, Chinese. CONTACT: Hendersonville Arts Council, P.O. Box 64, Hendersonville, TN 37077-0064, (615) 822-0789. 8,000

OLD TIMER'S DAY *Labor Day (early September)*, Manchester, Coffee Co., on the Square, the home of the Jack Daniels distillery with the George Dickel distillery in nearby Tullahoma. Free Marksmanship BB Shooting contests, 10k Foot Race, Best Old-Timey Costume contests, parade, tennis tournament, Horseshoe Pitching Contest, Log Sawing Contest, bingo, Best Beard Contest, three beauty contests, children's games including Banana Eating Contest, sack and three-legged races, Big Wheel Race, balloon-toss and balloon batting race, live entertainment including Tennessee Sweetheart Cloggers and The Country Gentlemen, Maxwell Air Force Base Band, public square dancing in the street. FOODS SERVED: pancake breakfast, concessions. ADMISSION: free. ACCOMMODATIONS: motels and hotels, campgrounds, RV parks.

RESTAURANTS: fast foods, family, elegant. CONTACT: Manchester Area Chamber of Commerce, 305 Murfreesboro Hwy., Manchester, TN 37355, (615) 728-7635. 6,000

TENNESSEE APPLE FESTIVAL *second Saturday through third Saturday in September*, Sevierville, Sevier Co., at Courthouse Square, to salute apple and fruit growing in Tennessee. Arts and crafts, Apple Pie Contest, Apple Arrangements Contest, parade, beauty pageant, road race, local entertainers drawing from nearby attractions such as Dollywood and Smoky Mountain Jubilee, Bite of Sevier County. FOODS SERVED: twenty-five area-restaurants offer their specialties ranging from shrimp, sausage balls and homemade breads to desserts and "home cookin'."ADMISSION: free, charges for Bite of Sevier County" (only 300 tickets available). ACCOMMODATIONS: motels and hotels, B&B's, campgrounds, RV parks. RESTAURANTS: fast foods, family, elegant, Italian, Chinese. CONTACT: Ruby Fox, Sevierville Chamber of Commerce, P.O. Box 285, Sevierville, TN 37862, (615) 453-6411. 10,000

FOLKLIFE FESTIVAL *second Sunday in September*, Roan Mountain State Park, Carter Co., to celebrate fall foliage in the mountains. Arts and crafts, apple butter making, pig roast, bluegrass-style mountain music, clogging. FOODS SERVED: "home-cooked mountain food." ADMISSION: free. ACCOMMODATIONS: motels and hotels, campgrounds, cabins. RESTAURANTS: fast foods, family. CONTACT: Paul Cates at (615) 772-8272 or the Elizabethton–Carter Co. Chamber of Commerce, P.O. Box 190, Elizabethton, TN 37643, (615) 543-2122. 10,000

ARTFEST *third Friday in September through second Saturday in October*, Knoxville, Knox Co., as a celebration of the arts. Knoxville Symphony Orchestra Pops Concert at the Tennessee Amphitheatre World's Fair site; Riverfeast, a barbecue cook-off with entertainment; Brown-Bag-It with the Arts includes live music and entertainment with related food specialties at Market Square Mall; Saturday Night on the Town featuring the "largest street party in the southeast (with) food, music, dancing, clowns, fireworks on Downtown Gay Street"; Mayor's Art Auction and Awards Ceremony; Artfest Five 5k Run for the Arts, A Taste of Knoxville featuring specialties from visual and performing artists and local restaurants at the Knoxville Convention and Exhibition Center; Kids on the Town featuring unique arts activities for children; live entertainment including big bands and bluegrass. FOODS SERVED: barbecue and foods served daily by local restaurants on Market Square. ADMISSION: free, charges for a few events. ACCOMMODATIONS: motels and hotels, B&B's, campgrounds, RV parks. RESTAURANTS: fast foods, family, elegant. CONTACT: The Arts Council, P.O. Box 2506, Knoxville, TN 37901, (615) 523-7543. 100,000

TENNESSEE GRASS ROOTS DAYS *fourth weekend in September,* Nashville, Davidson Co., to remember the state's rich heritage of talent through traditional crafts, music, and folklore. More than 200 performers and folklife-demonstrators "show the grass roots culture of Tennessee's working people: black, white, and Native American." Folklife and old-time survival demonstrations include mule driving, grist milling, bee keeping, quilting, shingle riving and many medicine exhibits, marble making, apple-cider pressing, traditional country music. FOODS SERVED: "ole-time food." ADMISSION: free. ACCOMMODATIONS: motels and hotels, B&B's, campgrounds, RV parks. RESTAURANTS: fast foods, family, elegant. CONTACT: Southern Folk Cultural Revival Project, c/o Ms. Anne Romaine, 339 Valeria St., Nashville, TN 37210 or the Nashville Area Chamber of Commerce, 161 Fourth Avenue North, Nashville, TN 37219, (615) 259-3900. 15,000

DOLLYWOOD NATIONAL CRAFTS FESTIVAL *September 26–October 25 (closed Thursdays),* Dollywood, Pigeon Forge, Sevier Co., in the Great Smoky Mountains. Billed "The Largest Crafts Festival in the Smokies," this crafts festival features master craftspeople from throughout the United States who display unique mountain crafts, skills, traditions, and secrets passed down from generation to generation. FOODS SERVED: country delicacies such as funnel cakes, apple fritters, hickory-smoked meats, banana pudding. ADMISSION: adults $13.50 plus tax, children 4–11 $9.95 plus tax, under 4 free (these are Dollywood admission charges). ACCOMMODATIONS: motels and hotels, B&B's, cottages, campgrounds, RV parks. RESTAURANTS: fast foods, family, elegant, Italian, Chinese. CONTACT: Dollywood, 700 Dollywood Lane, Pigeon Forge, TN 37863-4101, (615) 428-9400. 150,000

PIGEON FORGE ROTARY CRAFT FESTIVAL *first three weeks in October,* Pigeon Forge, the home of Dollywood, Dolly Parton's amusement and folklore center, Sevier Co., in the Great Smoky Mountains, at what is truly the "action-packed resort city" as it calls itself. In a resort which boasts its own crafts village, traditional mountain crafts are displayed and featured during the festival. Guests are surrounded by games, rides, music, and food. FOODS SERVED: "homegrown, back-home cooking." ADMISSION: "donation." ACCOMMODATIONS: motels, B&B's, cottages, campgrounds, RV parks. RESTAURANTS: fast foods, family, elegant, Italian, Chinese. CONTACT: Pigeon Forge Department of Tourism, P.O. Box 209, Pigeon Forge, TN 37863-0209, (615) 251-9100 from outside Tennessee or (615) 453-8574.

MADISON HILLBILLY DAY *first Saturday in October,* Madison, Davidson Co., in the metropolitan Nashville area. Hillbilly parade, crafts, rides, exhibits, hillbilly dress and costumes. FOODS SERVED: "short order food—corn on the cob, barbecue, sweets." ADMISSION: free. ACCOMMODATIONS: motels and hotels, RV parks.

RESTAURANTS: fast foods, family. CON-TACT: Madison Chamber of Commerce, P.O. Box 97, Madison, TN 37115, (615) 865-5400. 100,000

FESTIVAL *first weekend in October,* Athens, McMinn Co., at Sunset Park, to celebrate the arts of the area. Juried and non-juried arts and crafts shows, Children's Festival including many hands-on projects such as pottery, soapmaking, weaving, and games; local and regional entertainers present the traditional music of the Cumberland Plateau such as fiddle as well as banjo tunes, folk songs, traditional dances, and Marily McMinn McCredie who is a storyteller, folklorist, and balladeer, Black Choir, local clown group, dulcimer players, and "World's #1 Fiddler" Frazier Moss, resulting in continuous entertainment. FOODS SERVED: traditional and international. ADMISSION: free. ACCOMMODATIONS: motels and hotels. RESTAURANTS: fast foods, family, Chinese, Mexican. CONTACT: Athens Area Council for the Arts, P.O. Box 95, Athens, TN 37303, (615) 745-8781, or the Athens Area Chamber of Commerce, 13 N. Jackson St., Athens, TN 37303, (615) 745-0334. 15,000

NILLIE BIPPER ART AND CRAFT FESTIVAL *first weekend in October,* Cleveland, Bradley Co., at the Red Clay State Historical Area. Juried arts and crafts displays and sales, local musicians and dance groups. FOODS SERVED: stews, soups, baked goods, hot dogs, cotton candy. ADMISSION: $1.00. ACCOMMODATIONS: motels and hotels, B&B's, RV parks. RESTAURANTS: fast foods, family. CONTACT: Cleveland Creative Arts Guild at (615) 478-3114 or the Cleveland–Bradley Chamber of Commerce, P.O. Box 2275, Cleveland, TN 37320-2275, (615) 472-6587. 11,000

FAYETTE COUNTY EGG FESTIVAL *first weekend in October,* Somerville, Fayette Co., in west Tennessee to honor the egg industry in the "Egg Capital of Tennessee." Bake-off, Garden Tractor Pull, parade, carnival, Egg Packing Championships, antique car show, Chicken Beauty Contest ("dress up your favorite chicken"); Boiled Egg Custard, Egg Custard Pie and Stuffed Deviled Egg Contest, The Great Egg Scramble, Egg Coloring Contest, Ice Cream Eating Contest; meringue-throwing at state, county, and city officials, crafts fair, Allegrezza International Folk Dancers, Coca-Cola Country Store, gospel and country singers. FOODS SERVED: barbecued chicken!, and baked goods. ADMISSION: free. ACCOMMODATIONS: (nearby) motels and hotels, B&B's, campgrounds, RV parks. RESTAURANTS: fast foods, family, elegant. CONTACT: Fayette Co. Chamber of Commerce, P.O. Box 411, Somerville, TN 38068, (901) 465-8690. 5,000

BLACK FOLKLIFE FESTIVAL *first Monday in October,* Nashville, Davidson Co., at the Fisk University Library. Black folk-artisans, music, performance by the Fisk Jubilee Singers, and an exhibit from the Fisk Collection. ADMISSION: free. ACCOMMODATIONS: motels and hotels, B&B's, campgrounds, RV parks. RESTAURANTS: fast foods, family, elegant. CONTACT: Dr. Jessie Carney Smith, University Library, 17th Ave., North, Nashville, TN 37203-4501, (615) 329-8730. 500

OCTOBERFEST *first Thursday and Friday in October,* Chattanooga, Hamilton Co., at the Market Center, to celebrate "hometown arts and crafts." Arts and crafts, live musical entertainment such as Bill Byrd's Bavarian Six playing oompah music, the University of Tennessee's Marching Band, and a local dance band. FOODS SERVED: German sausage platters, other food booths. ADMISSION: free. ACCOMMODATIONS: motels and hotels, B&B's, campgrounds, RV parks. RESTAURANTS: fast foods, family, elegant, Mexican, Italian, Asian, French. CONTACT: Chattanooga Downtown Alliance, 1001 Market St., Chattanooga, TN 37402, (615) 756-2121. 10,000

UNICOI COUNTY APPLE FESTIVAL
first weekend in October, Erwin, Unicoi
Co., as a salute to local apple growers.
"Handmade crafts of all types and materials," old-fashioned apple butter making
and sale, Apple Pie and Dish Baking Contest, Erwin Art League Exhibit and Sale,
10k Road Race, "Valley Choo Choo" train
ride for children, merchants sidewalk
sales, Blue Ridge Pottery Show and Sale,
farmer's market, apple festival exhibits,
beauty pageant, square dancing, bluegrass music. FOODS SERVED: apple butter,
pie and other apple products, concessions. ADMISSION: free. ACCOMMODATIONS: motels and hotels, campgrounds.
RESTAURANTS: fast foods, family. CONTACT: Unicoi Co. Chamber of Commerce,
Box 713, Erwin, TN 37650, (615) 743-
3000. 14,000

**OCTOBERFEST AND CARROLL
COUNTY PORK FESTIVAL** *first weekend in October,* McKenzie, Carroll Co., to
celebrate fall and the pork industry. Arts
and crafts show, Pork Barbecue Cook-Off,
the winners of which go on to the Memphis in May Barbecue Cook-off, Talent
Show, American Cancer Society 5k Run,
lots of local talent. FOODS SERVED: pork
barbecue from cook-off. ADMISSION: free.
ACCOMMODATIONS: motel. RESTAURANTS:
fast foods, family. CONTACT: Carroll Co.
Chamber of Commerce, P.O. Box 726,
Huntingdon, TN 38344, (901) 986-4664.

AUTUMN GOLD FESTIVAL *second
weekend in October,* Coker Creek, Monroe
Co., at Tellico Mountain Camp to celebrate east Tennessee's gold and fall colors. Arts and crafts, covered-wagon
rides, queen's contests in period dress,
working craftspeople demonstrate pioneer
skills such as log splitting and shingle
making, gold panning, syrup and soap
making, country and bluegrass music,
square dancing and clogging, magician,
and an "old-time medicine show." FOODS
SERVED: "Tennessee country cooking and
full meals." ADMISSION: adults $2.50, children 6–12 $1.00, groups and senior citizens, $2.00. ACCOMMODATIONS: B&B's,

campgrounds, others nearby. RESTAURANTS: family, others nearby. CONTACT:
Ralph Murphy, Coker Creek, TN 37314,
(615) 261-2242 or the Monroe Co. Chamber of Commerce, 110 Locust St., Madisonville, TN 37354, (615) 442-4588.
20,000

NATIONAL STORYTELLING FESTIVAL *second weekend in October,* Jonesborough, Washington Co., to celebrate and
preserve storytelling traditions in America
and abroad in "the oldest town in the state
of Tennessee." Sponsored by the National
Association for the Preservation and Perpetuation of Storytellers (NAPPS), features local and guest tellers in the town
"considered by many as the birthplace of
the revival of storytelling in America," has
included Alex Haley, folktellers Barbara
Freeman and Connie Regan-Blake, Doc
McConnell, Donald Davis, Elizabeth Ellis,
Linda Goss, Ray Hicks, Norman Kennedy, Gayle Ross, Laura Simms, Ed Stivender, Jackie Torrence, and Kathryn
Windham. FOODS SERVED: international.
ADMISSION: $30.00 for NAPPS members
for weekend, $35.00 for nonmembers.
ACCOMMODATIONS: motels and hotels,
B&B's, campgrounds. RESTAURANTS: fast
foods, family, elegant. CONTACT: National
Association for the Preservation and Perpetuation of Storytelling, P.O. Box 309,
Jonesborough, TN 37659, (615) 753-
2171. 4,000

**MICHELOB TRADITIONAL JAZZ
FESTIVAL** *second weekend in October,*
Memphis, Shelby Co., in the historic
Beale Street district, to celebrate the history of Beale Street and dixieland jazz.
Jazz Ball, Jazz Jam Sessions, night jazz
cruise, and Jazz Brunch which often turns
into a jam, all featuring some of the "nation's top traditional jazz bands" playing in
the clubs of Beale Street. FOODS SERVED:
"Southern cookin'." ADMISSION: tickets
available per event or as a patron package.
ACCOMMODATIONS: motels and hotels,
B&B's, campgrounds. RESTAURANTS: fast
foods, family, elegant. CONTACT: Davis E.
Tillman, 203 Beale St., Suite 303, Memphis, TN 38103, (901) 522-9260. 1,200

HERITAGE DAYS *second weekend in October,* Rogersville, Hawkins Co., to celebrate "the people and heritage of the area." More than 150 arts and crafts booths and demonstrations of local crafts, games; lots of music such as bluegrass and gospel, high school bands, dancing, clogging. FOODS SERVED: local. ADMISSION: free. ACCOMMODATIONS: motels and hotels, B&B's, campgrounds, RV parks. RESTAURANTS: family, elegant. CONTACT: Heritage Days, c/o Heritage Association, Rogersville, TN 37857, (615) 272-2186. 40,000

OKTOBERFEST *October 13–17,* Memphis, Shelby Co., at the Civic Center Plaza, to celebrate fall. Arts and crafts, 15k Run at Mud Island, Memphis music with "everything from oompah to country, blues, jazz, and rock." FOODS SERVED: German, Greek, Italian, Russian, barbecue including knockwurst with sauerkraut, toasted tamales, Polish sausage, gyros, French pastries. ADMISSION: free. ACCOMMODATIONS: motels and hotels, B&B's, campgrounds. RESTAURANTS: fast foods, family, elegant. CONTACT: Center City Commission, 147 Jefferson Ave., Suite 1001, Memphis, TN 38103, (901) 526-6840. 40,000

MOUNTAIN MAKINS FESTIVAL *last full weekend in October,* Morristown, Hamblen Co., at the Rose Center, to celebrate the crafts and arts traditions of the area. Crafts sales and demonstrations including baskets, handwoven wearables, jewelry, tole and decorative painting, waterfowl carving, folk art, stenciling, stained glass, musical instruments, wooden crafts, beeswax candles, ships in bottles, folk dolls, dollhouses and furnishings, raffiatying, smocking, quilts, pottery, cross stitching, dulcimers, corn husk dolls, pine-needle baskets; country store, Tsoyia Indian Dancers, cloggers, bluegrass bands, square dancers, gospel music, medicine show, children's activities including petting zoo, pumpkin decorating, face-painting, Children's Touch Museum, balloons, mimes, and games. FOODS SERVED: "traditional Appalachian." ADMISSION: adults $2.00, children 10 and under free. ACCOMMODATIONS: motels and hotels, campgrounds. RESTAURANTS: fast foods, family. CONTACT: Rose Center, 442 W. Second North St., Morristown, TN 37815, (615) 581-4330. 10,000

MONROE COUNTY TOBACCO AND HARVEST FESTIVAL *fourth weekend in October,* Sweetwater, Monroe Co., at the Tobacco Warehouse, to honor the tobacco farmer. More than 100 arts, crafts, and commercial booths, parade, clogging competition, gospel singing all-day Sunday, well known country-western singers, bluegrass, fiddling, and guitar contests, dance party. FOODS SERVED: local concessions. ADMISSION: free. ACCOMMODATIONS: motels and hotels, campgrounds, RV parks. RESTAURANTS: fast foods, family, elegant. CONTACT: Tobacco Warehouse, N. Main St., Sweetwater, TN 37874, (615) 337-7234.

GATLINBURG'S CHRISTMAS FESTIVAL *Thanksgiving weekend (late November) through week before Christmas,* Gatlinburg, Sevier Co., to celebrate Christmas in the Smokies and the "customs and traditions of an old-fashioned yuletide combined with contemporary events." City of Gatlinburg is decorated with "millions of white lights," lighted parade, Christmas Tree Display with more than fifty trees decorated in regional, national, and international themes and mostly hand-crafted ornaments. Smoky Mountain Living Christmas Tree which stands more than twenty-six feet tall and holds seventy singers from the Gatlinburg Community Chorale who perform three times each Christmas; Candlelight Ball, Festival of Christmas Past, Madrigal Feast, Bavarian Christmas, and an outdoor Living Musical Nativity. ADMISSION: free, charge for dances. ACCOMMODATIONS: motels and hotels, campgrounds, RV parks. RESTAURANTS: fast foods, family, elegant ("come as you are"). CONTACT: Gatlinburg Chamber of Commerce, P.O. Box 527, Gatlinburg, TN 37738,

(800) 251-9868 outside Tennessee or (800) 824-4766 inside Tennessee. 75,000

NASHVILLE'S COUNTRY HOLI-DAYS *Thanksgiving (late November) through New Year's Day,* Nashville, Davidson Co. More than forty events including the Opryland Hotel's "Ceremony of the Yule Log," Christmas storytelling sessions with country music greats; "Christmas at Twitty City," Conway Twitty's nine-acre fantasy world featuring more than 250,000 twinkling lights; Barbara Mandrell welcomes visitors to bring an ornament from home to place on her tree at Barbara Mandrell Country, and Minnie Pearl often greets fans at Grinder's Switch; candlelight tours of historic homes, "Trees of Christmas" display of trees from around the world, holiday-craft fairs throughout Nashville; southern, Victorian, traditional, and international music. FOODS SERVED: concessions. ADMISSION: free to some events, charges for others.

ACCOMMODATIONS: motels and hotels, B&B's, campgrounds, RV parks. RESTAURANTS: fast foods, family, elegant. CONTACT: Nashville Area Chamber of Commerce, 161 Fourth Avenue North, Nashville, TN 37219, (615) 259-3900.

FESTIVAL OF LESSONS AND CAROLS *first weekend in December,* Sewannee, Franklin Co., at the University of the South, to celebrate Advent and the birth of Christ. The reading of lessons from the Bible, interspersed with Christmas carols and hymns sung by choirs and soloists and played by musicians ranging from the brass of the Nashville Symphony Orchestra to organist Robbe Delcamp. ADMISSION: free. ACCOMMODATIONS: motels and hotels. RESTAURANTS: fast foods, family. CONTACT: Latham W. Davis, The University of the South, Office of Public Relations, Sewanee, TN 37375, (615) 598-5931. 3,500

WEST VIRGINIA

DOGWOOD ARTS AND CRAFTS FESTIVAL *fourth weekend in April,* Huntington, Cabell Co., to celebrate the blooming of local dogwood trees. Arts and crafts sales and demonstrations, continuous entertainment. FOODS SERVED: variety. ADMISSION: $1.50. ACCOMMODATIONS: motels and hotels, B&B's, campgrounds, RV parks. RESTAURANTS: fast foods, family, elegant, Chinese, Polynesian, Italian, Mexican, Cajun. CONTACT: Loretta Covington at (304) 696-5940 or the Huntington Area Chamber of Commerce, 522 Ninth St., Huntington, WV 25716, (304) 525-5131. 20,000

WEBSTER COUNTY WOODCHOPPING FESTIVAL *third week in May through Memorial Day (late May),* Webster

Springs, Webster Co. Contestants from all over the world converge on Webster Springs to compete in the World Championship Woodchopping Contest, West Virginia State Championship Turkey Calling Contest, axe shaving, Jack and Jill crosscut sawing, nail driving, parades, square dancing. FOODS SERVED: concessions. ADMISSION: free. ACCOMMODATIONS: motels and hotels, campgrounds, RV parks. RESTAURANTS: fast foods, family. CONTACT: Randy Underwood, P.O. Box 227, Webster Springs, WV 26288, (304) 847-7666.

THREE RIVERS COAL FESTIVAL *third or fourth weekend in May,* Fairmont, Marion Co., to celebrate coal and its role in local heritage. Arts and crafts show and sale, the Mock Coal Mine, industrial and commercial exhibits, continuous entertainment which has included the Scott Brothers, The Hollanders, Just Another Band, Marionette Star Theatre, and local groups. FOODS SERVED: "variety." ADMISSION: free until 3:00 P.M., from 3:00–10:00 P.M. $4.00. ACCOMMODATIONS: motels and hotels. RESTAURANTS: fast foods, family, elegant. CONTACT: Three Rivers Coal Festival, P.O. Box 1604, Fairmont, WV 26554, (304) 363-2625, or the Marion Co. Chamber of Commerce, P.O. Box 208, Fairmont, WV 26555, (304) 363-0442. 20,000

WEST VIRGINIA DANDELION FESTIVAL *third or fourth weekend in May,* White Sulphur Springs, Greenbrier Co., to celebrate dandelions and spring. Arts and crafts, carnival, 10k Run, wine tasting, live entertainment such as magician Glen Gary, the Populaires from Greenbrier and Sunshine Express from Columbus, Ohio. FOODS SERVED: "good food." ADMISSION: free. ACCOMMODATIONS: motels and hotels, B&B's, campgrounds, RV parks. RESTAURANTS: family, elegant. CONTACT: White Sulphur Springs Chamber of Commerce, P.O. Drawer A, White Sulphur Springs, WV 24986, (304) 536-3842. 4,000

MOUNTAIN FESTIVAL *Memorial Day (late May),* Bluefield, Mercer Co. More than 100 events including arts and crafts, bicycle races, foot races, mountain climbing, tennis and bowling tournaments, parachute jumps, Mr. and Mrs. Body Building Contest, plays, square dancing, fireworks. FOODS SERVED: mountain and concessions. ADMISSION: free. ACCOMMODATIONS: motels and hotels, campgrounds. RESTAURANTS: fast foods, family. CONTACT: Greater Bluefield Chamber of Commerce, P.O. Box 4098, Bluefield, WV 24701, (304) 327-7184.

VANDALIA GATHERING *Memorial Day weekend (late May),* Charleston, Kanawha Co., on the Capitol lawn and in the Cultural Center, to highlight West Virginia's ethnic and traditional music. Craft exhibits and demonstrations, quilt exhibit, Liar's Contest, banjo and fiddle contests, loads of bluegrass and West Virginia traditional music. FOODS SERVED: concessions. ADMISSION: free. ACCOMMODATIONS: motels and hotels, campgrounds, RV parks. RESTAURANTS: fast foods, family, elegant. CONTACT: Department of Culture and History, Cultural Center, Capitol Complex, Charleston, WV 25305, (304) 348-0220.

WEST VIRGINIA STRAWBERRY FESTIVAL *last weekend in May,* Buckhannon, Upshur Co., to celebrate the strawberry season. Crafts, Strawberry Auction, strawberry recipes, antique car parade, quilt judging, Fireman's Parade, Grand Feature Parade, barbecues, concerts by the U. S. Navy Band and high school bands from throughout the United States. FOODS SERVED: barbecue, and variety of others. ADMISSION: free. ACCOMMODATIONS: motels and hotels, campgrounds, RV parks. RESTAURANTS: fast foods, family, elegant. CONTACT: Buckhannon Upshur Chamber of Commerce, P.O. Box 442, Buckhannon, WV 26201, (304) 472-1722.

MOUNTAIN HERITAGE ARTS AND CRAFTS FESTIVAL *second weekend in June,* between Harpers Ferry and Charles Town, Jefferson Co. Juried arts and crafts show, bluegrass music. FOODS SERVED: wide variety. ADMISSION: adults $4.00, children 6–12 $2.00, under 6 free. ACCOMMODATIONS: motels and hotels, B&B's, campgrounds. RESTAURANTS: fast foods, family, elegant nearby, Italian, German, Chinese. CONTACT: Jefferson Co. Chamber of Commerce, Inc., P.O. Box 426, Charles Town, WV 25414, (304) 725-2055. 25,000

TRI-STATE FAIR AND REGATTA *June 13 through August 1,* Ashland, Huntington, and Ironton, as a celebration of the area's interdependence. Arts and crafts festival, custom-classic car show, Sternwheel Regatta, Sailboat Regatta, canoe races, Bass Boat Races, water ski show, Industrial Fun-O-Limp-ics, queen pageant, Budweiser Cup Races, kite flying competition, antique show, Alpha Charity Horse Show, All-American Soap Box Derby; live entertainment including Fox Wagon, McGuffy Lane, Dick Hawkins and the All Stars, Willis Family Puppets, Lucky Jazz Band, Kenny Yahn's Country Nights, and square dancing, Hank Hallers' Bavarians, the Musik Elite, Stark Raven, Midway Cloggers. FOODS SERVED: concessions. ADMISSION: free. ACCOMMODATIONS: motels and hotels, B&B's, campgrounds. RESTAURANTS: fast foods, family, elegant, international. CONTACT: Huntington Area Chamber of Commerce, 522 Ninth St., Huntington, WV 25716, (304) 525-5131.

WEST VIRGINIA STATE FOLK FESTIVAL *third weekend in June*, Glenville, Gilmer Co., downtown. Authentic folk music and square dancing, parade, fiddle and banjo contests, traditional music concerts, country store with handmade crafts. FOODS SERVED: traditional and concessions. ADMISSION: free. ACCOMMODATIONS: motels and hotels. RESTAURANTS: family. CONTACT: Diane Bach, P.O. Box 362, Glenville, WV 26351, (304) 462-7361, ext. 224.

MOUNTAIN STATE ART AND CRAFT FAIR *July 4th "plus one weekend,"* Ripley, Jackson Co., at the Cedar Lakes Conference Center to celebrate "Appalachian Heritage." Mountain and traditional crafts exhibits and demonstrations, children's activities, door prizes, art show, mountain-heritage music such as dulcimers, fiddles, banjos, storytelling, clogging, Kathy Mattea, Tom T. Hall, Billy Ed Wheeler and Mountain Edge, West Virginia Public Radio Performers. FOODS SERVED: Appalachian and other foods. ADMISSION: free. ACCOMMODATIONS: motels and hotels, campgrounds, RV parks. RESTAURANTS: fast foods, family, elegant. CONTACT: Mountain State Art and Craft Fair, P.O. Box 389, Ripley, WV 25271, (304) 372-3247. 33,000

JAMBOREE-IN-THE-HILLS *third weekend in July*, St. Clairsville, Ohio Co., at Brush Run Park, 15 miles west of Wheeling, WV. "A full array of major country-music stars participate in this premier outdoor country-music extravangaza featuring nineteen hours of continuous music." FOODS SERVED: concessions. ADMISSION: charges. ACCOMMODATIONS: motels and hotels, campgrounds. RESTAURANTS: fast foods, family. CONTACT: Kathy Oliver, 1015 Main St., Wheeling, WV 26003, (304) 232-1108 or (800) 624-5456 from outside West Virginia. 60,000

UPPER OHIO VALLEY ITALIAN FESTIVAL *third weekend in July*, Wheeling, Ohio Co., a "six-county celebration (that) pays homage to the local Italian population, their ancestors and heritage." More than 100 food and arts and crafts booths, sporting events, continuous entertainment including Italian music and singing. FOODS SERVED: lots of Italian specialties. ADMISSION: free. ACCOMMODATIONS: motels and hotels, campground, RV parks. RESTAURANTS: fast foods, family, elegant. CONTACT: Central Union Building, 14th and Market St., Wheeling, WV 26003, (304) 233-1090 or the Wheeling Area Chamber of Commerce, 1012 Main St., Wheeling, WV 26003, (304) 233-2575.

WEST VIRGINIA WATER FESTIVAL *second week in August*, Hinton, Summers Co. National Power Boat races on Bluestone Lake, parades, Queen Mermaid coronation, Firemen's Parade, flower show, arts and crafts, dog show, bingo and other games, bluegrass music. FOODS SERVED: barbecue, concessions. ADMISSION: free. ACCOMMODATIONS: motels and hotels, B&B's, campgrounds, RV parks. RESTAURANTS: fast foods, family, elegant. CONTACT: Summers Co. Chamber of Commerce, P.O. Box 309, Hinton, WV 25951, (304) 466-5332. 100,000

APPALACHIAN ARTS AND CRAFTS FESTIVAL *last weekend in Au-*

gust, Beckley, Raleigh Co., at the Armory–Civic Center. Crafts displays and demonstrations, live entertainment including gospel, country, bluegrass, cloggers, square dancers. FOODS SERVED: homemade ice cream, funnel cakes, apple cider, baked goods, sandwiches. ADMISSION: adults $2.00, senior citizens $1.50, students $1.00. ACCOMMODATIONS: motels and hotels, campgrounds. RESTAURANTS: fast foods, family, elegant, Italian, Chinese. CONTACT: Beckley–Raleigh Co. Chamber of Commerce, P.O. Box 1798, Beckley, WV 25802, (304) 252-7328. 15,000

CHARLESTON STERNWHEEL REGATTA FESTIVAL *last week in August through Labor Day (early September),* Charleston, Kanawha Co., "the largest river festival east of the Mississippi." Arts and crafts fair, sternwheel and tow-boat races, hot air balloon race, 15mi. distance run, "New Orleans-style funeral parade," fireworks. FOODS SERVED: concessions. ADMISSION: free. ACCOMMODATIONS: motels and hotels, campgrounds, RV parks. RESTAURANTS: fast foods, family, elegant. CONTACT: Charleston Sternwheel Regatta Festival, Box 2749, Charleston, WV 25330, (304) 348-6419 or the Charleston Regional Chamber of Commerce, 818 Virginia St., E., Charleston, WV 25301, (304) 345-0770.

WEST VIRGINIA ITALIAN HERITAGE FESTIVAL *Labor Day weekend (early September),* Clarksburg, Harrison Co., to celebrate the Italian heritage of many residents. Man- and Woman-of-the-Year coronations, Italian singing and dancing, wine making and bocci contests, parade, big-name entertainers have included Al Martino, Jerry Vale, Dick Contino, Anna Maria Alberghetti, Mary Lou Retton, Joe DiMaggio, and Frankie Avalon in addition to Rocco del Sud, Christine Corelli, Damian, I Campagnoti, U. S. Air Force Band, River City Brass Band, Pinocchio's Mini Circus; wine and cheese receptions, sidewalk cafes, Italian films, poetry readings. FOODS SERVED: Italian.

ADMISSION: free. ACCOMMODATIONS: motels. RESTAURANTS: fast foods, family, elegant, Italian. CONTACT: West Virginia Italian Heritage Festival, Inc., P.O. Box 1632, Clarksburg, WV 26301, (304) 624-8694. 110,000

STONEWALL JACKSON ARTS AND CRAFTS JUBILEE *Labor Day weekend (early September),* near Weston, Lewis Co., at Jackson's Mill State 4-H Camp, to celebrate local heritage. Arts and more than 100 craftspeople display and demonstrate their skills including glassblowing, woodchopping and needle arts, quilt show and contest, photography show and judging, West Virginia State Fruit Pie Baking Contest, Civil War Reenactment Unit, West Virginia State Horseshoe Pitching Tournament, petting zoo, wildlife display, tours of historic Jackson's Mill, clown face painting, heritage music. FOODS SERVED: "mouth watering" heritage foods such as cornbread and beans, pancakes and sausage, chicken and beef barbecues. ADMISSION: adults $3.00, senior citizens $2.00, children $1.00. ACCOMMODATIONS: motels and hotels, campgrounds. RESTAURANTS: fast foods, family. CONTACT: Stonewall Jackson Arts and Crafts Jubilee, P.O. Box 956, Weston, WV 26452, (304) 269-1863. 30,000

WEST VIRGINIA RAILROAD HERITAGE FESTIVAL *second weekend in September,* Grafton, Taylor Co. Railroad memorabilia, art and quilt exhibits, street fair, live entertainment, rail excursions. FOODS SERVED: local specialties, concessions. ADMISSION: free. ACCOMMODATIONS: motels and hotels, campgrounds. RESTAURANTS: fast foods, family. CONTACT: West Virginia Railroad Heritage Festival, P.O. Box 66, Grafton, WV 26534, (304) 265-2529 October–June, (304) 265-1957 July–October 1.

KING COAL FESTIVAL *third week in September,* Williamson, Mingo Co., in the Tug Valley, to celebrate the coal industry. Track meet, apple butter making, pet

show, beauty contests, gospel meet, horseshoe pitching, all-day outdoor market, bluegrass festival, crowning of King Coal, hot air balloon rides, parade, country and bluegrass bands. FOODS SERVED: apple products, concessions. ADMISSION: free. ACCOMMODATIONS: motels and hotels. RESTAURANTS: fast foods. CONTACT: Mae Stallard, President, Action in Mingo, 28 Oak St., Williamson, WV 25661, (304) 235-1510. 15,000

PRESTON COUNTY BUCKWHEAT FESTIVAL *last full weekend in September,* Kingwood, Preston Co., to celebrate the grain harvest. Arts and crafts fair, antique car show, cattle, hog, and sheep exhibits and judging, coronation of Queen Ceres and King Buckwheat, Firemen's Gigantic Parade including more than 100 Tri-State bands and fire departments; School Day Parade, Lamb Dressing Contest, Bicycle Decorating Contest, Most Congenial Award, Turkey Calling Contest, pet show, Farmers' Day Parade, Band Spectacular, arm wrestling, Banjo and Fiddlers' Contests, youth livestock-sale, Western Square Dance; major entertainers have included Barbara Mandrell and Sisters, Atlanta, and the Louise Mandrell Show. FOODS SERVED: buckwheat dinners including buckwheat cakes, sausage, and syrup. ADMISSION: free, buckwheat dinner $4.00 for all-you-can-eat. ACCOMMODATIONS: motels and hotels, campgrounds, RV parks. RESTAURANTS: fast foods, family, elegant. CONTACT: Kingwood Volunteer Fire Department, P.O. Box 336, Kingwood, WV 26537, (304) 329-0101, or the Kingwood Area Chamber of Commerce, P.O. Box 67, Kingwood, WV 26537, (304) 324-0466. 100,000

FALL MOUNTAIN HERITAGE ARTS AND CRAFTS FESTIVAL *last weekend in September,* between Harpers Ferry and Charles Town, Jefferson Co. Juried arts and crafts show, bluegrass music. FOODS SERVED: wide variety. ADMISSION: charge. ACCOMMODATIONS: motels and hotels, B&B's, campgrounds. RESTAURANTS: fast foods, family, elegant nearby, Italian,

German, Chinese. CONTACT: Jefferson Co. Chamber of Commerce, Inc., P.O. Box 426, Charles Town, WV 25414, (304) 725-2055. 25,000

WEST VIRGINIA HONEY FESTIVAL *last weekend in September,* Parkersburg, Wood Co., at City Park, as a salute to the honey industry. Arts and crafts, Baking Contest, 3mi. Honey Run, man with a live bee-beard, live entertainment, "educational and cultural experiences," honey products. FOODS SERVED: baked goods and other foods featuring honey, concessions. ADMISSION: free. ACCOMMODATIONS: motels and hotels, campgrounds, RV parks. RESTAURANTS: fast foods, family, elegant. CONTACT: Sarah Jalbert, P.O. Box 2149, Parkersburg, WV 26102, (304) 485-7068.

MOUNTAIN STATE FOREST FESTIVAL *last weekend in September through first weekend in October,* Elkins, Randolph Co., to celebrate fall and mountain glory. Arts and crafts shows, coronations, parades, cabarets, carnivals, contests, big-name entertainment such as Ronnie Milsap and Kathy Mattea, "several well-known gospel groups." FOODS SERVED: concessions. ADMISSION: free, charges for concerts. ACCOMMODATIONS: motels and hotels, B&B, campgrounds, RV parks. RESTAURANTS: fast foods, family, elegant. CONTACT: Elkins Area Chamber of Commerce, P.O. Box 1169, Elkins, WV 26241, (304) 636-2717. 90,000

WEST VIRGINIA BLACK WALNUT FESTIVAL *early October,* Spencer, Roane Co., to salute the black walnut. Four-day festival includes arts and crafts show, auto show, canoe races, majorette and band festival, sale of hulled walnuts. ADMISSION: free. ACCOMMODATIONS: motels and hotels. RESTAURANTS: fast foods, family. CONTACT: Jeff Boyles, 207 Church St., Spencer, WV 25276, (304) 927-5957, or the Roane Co. Chamber of Commerce, P.O. Box 1, Spencer, WV 25276, (304) 927-1780.

BRIDGE WALK FESTIVAL *second Saturday in October,* New River Gorge Bridge on U. S. Route 19, near Oak Hill, Fayette Co., to celebrate the New River Gorge Bridge itself on the only day of the year when people can legally walk on the bridge "and take in the excellent view of the gorge that it offers." More than 250 arts and crafts vendors, continuous entertainment on stage such as the Michael James Gang, The Sparkling Highsteppers, and dancers. FOODS SERVED: Greek, American such as cornbread and beans, concessions. ADMISSION: free. ACCOMMODATIONS: motels and hotels, campgrounds, RV parks. RESTAURANTS: fast foods, family, elegant, Chinese, French. CONTACT: Fayette–Plateau Chamber of Commerce, 214 Main St., Fayetteville, WV 25901, (304) 465-5617. 200,000

MOUNTAIN STATE APPLE HARVEST FESTIVAL *third weekend in October,* Martinsburg, Berkeley Co., to celebrate the apple harvest. Arts and crafts, tours of experimental farms and the farmers' market, Mountain State Apple-Pie Baking Contest, coronation of Apple Harvest Queen, Celebrity Sports Breakfast, Opening of the Hunt including Blessing of the Hounds, Apple Pie Auction, 10k Apple Trample, Grand Feature Parade, Apple Bowl of Little League Football, Panhandlers Square Dance, Big Apple Tournament of Bands, antique car show, Grand Ball, appearance of Ronald McDonald and friends, drawing for the championship Mountain State Quilt. FOODS SERVED: pancake breakfasts, apple pies and other apple products, concessions. ADMISSION: free. ACCOMMODATIONS: motels and hotels, B&B's, campgrounds. RESTAURANTS: fast foods, family, elegant, Chinese. CONTACT: Mountain State Apple Harvest Festival, P.O. Box 1362, Martinsburg, WV 25401, (304) 253-2500, or the Martinsburg–Berkeley Co. Chamber of Commerce, 110 W. Burke St., Martinsburg, WV 25401, (304) 267-4841. 6,000

Deep South

Alabama / 83

Arkansas / 87

Florida / 90

Georgia / 102

Louisiana / 105

Mississippi / 108

South Carolina / 110

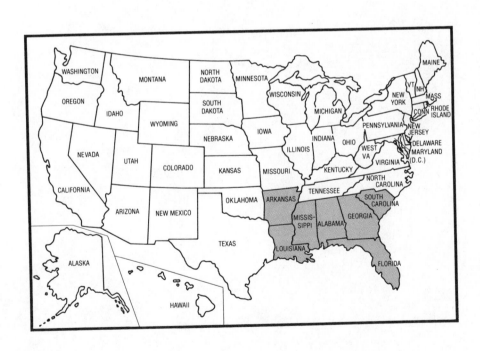

ALABAMA

MARDI GRAS *week prior to Lent,* Mobile, Mobile Co. Pre-Lenten celebration featuring street parades put on by mystic societies, masked balls nightly, coronation of King and Queen the Saturday of Mardi Gras week; Family Day activities at Fort Conde, Joe Cain Parade on Sunday, in which the public is invited to participate, big-name entertainers at masked balls, local hotels feature special entertainment indoors and outdoors during the week. ADMISSION: free, charges to balls. ACCOMMODATIONS: motels and hotels, B&B's. RESTAURANTS: fast foods, family, elegant, international. CONTACT: Mobile Area Chamber of Commerce, P.O. Box 2187, Mobile, AL 36652, (205) 433-6951. 500,000

HISTORIC SELMA PILGRIMAGE AND ANTIQUE SHOW *last weekend in March,* Selma, Dallas Co. Tours of historic buildings and homes, antique show and sale, country crafts, barbecue Friday night, presentation of the Pilgrimage Court featuring young ladies in antebellum gowns escorted by cadets from Marion Military Institute, walking tours, tours of Heritage Village composed of five relocated historic structures, Pilgrimage 10K and 2 mi. runs, art exhibit and sale. FOODS SERVED: Tea Room, barbecue Friday only. ADMISSION: Pilgrimage Package "includes day tour, antique show, country crafts, Friday evening tour, Pilgrimage Pluses," $15.00, day tour adults $10.00, students $6.00, single house $4.00, Friday evening tour $5.00. ACCOMMODATIONS: motels and hotels, B&B's, campgrounds, RV parks. RESTAURANTS: fast foods, family. CONTACT: Selma–Dallas Co. Historic Preservation Society, P.O. Box 586, Selma, AL 36702, (205) 872-8265, or the Selma Area Chamber of Commerce, P.O. Drawer D, Selma, AL 35701, (205) 875-7241. 25,000

MOBILE INTERNATIONAL FESTIVAL *second Sunday in April,* Mobile, Mobile Co., in the City Auditorium. More than forty countries participate, offering their own cultural dancing and singing, cultural booths, authentic costumes. FOODS SERVED: ethnic foods from countries exhibiting. ADMISSION: charge. ACCOMMODATIONS: motels and hotels, B&B's, RV parks. RESTAURANTS: fast foods, family, elegant. CONTACT: Sydney de Gervais, 1413 Polaris Drive, Mobile, AL 36609, (205) 666-5969.

BIRMINGHAM FESTIVAL OF ARTS *third week in April,* Birmingham, Jefferson Co., throughout the city, each year honoring and featuring the culture of a different country. Events include artisans, acrobats, zoo animals, music and dance, parade, theatrical and operatic presentations, dinner honoring the ambassador of the country, book and author luncheon and a 10-day international fair featuring many countries and highlighting the year's honored country. FOODS SERVED: foods of the honored country and others. ADMISSION: $2.00 to international fair, charges for some events. ACCOMMODATIONS: motels and hotels, B&B's, campgrounds. RESTAURANTS: fast foods, family, elegant. CONTACT: Sara Crowder at (205) 323-5461 or the Greater Birmingham Convention and Visitors Bureau, 2027 First Ave., N., Birmingham, AL 35203-4167, (205) 252-9825. 100,000

GREEK FOOD FESTIVAL *last weekend in April,* Birmingham, Jefferson Co., at the Greek Orthodox Cathedral on the Southside, to celebrate Greek culture and foods. Greek folk dancers and musicians. FOODS SERVED: loads of Greek food specialties including lunch and dinner. ADMISSION: free. ACCOMMODATIONS: motels and hotels, B&B's, campgrounds. RESTAURANTS: fast foods, family, elegant. CON-

TACT: Greek Orthodox Cathedral, 307 19th St., So., Birmingham, AL 35233, (205) 252-5195 or the Greater Birmingham Convention and Visitors Bureau, 2027 First Ave., N., Birmingham, AL 35203-4167, (205) 252-9825. 8,000

CAHAWBA FESTIVAL *fourth Saturday in May,* Old Cahawba, located twelve miles from Selma, Dallas Co., in celebration of Cahawba's status as Alabama's first state capital. Frog jumping, greased-pole climbing, strumming, pickin' and cloggin', bluegrass music, Prettiest Possum Contest. FOODS SERVED: barbecue and Brunswick stew. ADMISSION: $2.00 per car. ACCOMMODATIONS: motels and hotels, B&B's, campgrounds, RV parks. RESTAURANTS: fast foods, family, elegant. CONTACT: Selma Area Chamber of Commerce, P.O. Drawer D, Selma, AL 35701, (205) 875-7241. 10,000

ALABAMA JUBILEE HOT-AIR BALLOON CLASSIC *Memorial Day weekend (May),* Point Mallard Park, Decatur, Morgan Co. Races include fifty hot-air balloons, softball, raquetball, and tennis tournaments, arts and crafts, parachutists, antique car show. FOODS SERVED: "regional cuisine." ADMISSION: free. ACCOMMODATIONS: motels and hotels, B&B's, campgrounds, RV parks. RESTAURANTS: fast foods, family, elegant. CONTACT: Decatur Convention and Visitors Bureau, P.O. Box 2003, Decatur, AL 35602, (205) 350-2028. 15,000

ALABAMA JUNE JAM *second Saturday in June,* Fort Payne High School grounds, Fort Payne, DeKalb Co., an annual event sponsored by country music band Alabama, featuring country-music stars such as Alabama, Willie Nelson, Charlie Daniels, John Schneider, Gary Morris, Mel Tillis, and the Forester Sisters; sky-diving show, fireworks. FOODS SERVED: all-American hot dogs, hamburgers, ice cream, cokes. ADMISSION: before May 31, $15.95; June 1 to Jam, $18.00. Charities benefit. ACCOMMODATIONS: mo-

tels, B&B's, campgrounds, RV parks, others available in Chattanooga, TN. RESTAURANTS: fast foods, family. CONTACT: Alabama Fan Club, P.O. Box 529, Fort Payne, AL 35967, (205) 845-1646. 60,000 Note: Bring lawn chairs or blankets, picnic baskets allowed; no glass, no alcoholic beverages.

ALABAMA BLUEBERRY FESTIVAL *third Saturday in June,* Jefferson Davis, Jr. College, Brewton, Escambia Co., and dedicated to Dr. W. T. Brightwell, whose improved varieties of the Rabbiteye blueberry were introduced December, 1961, in the Brewton area, now the only town in Alabama shipping blueberries commercially. Arts and crafts, antique cars, street rods, Blueberry Baking Contest, tasting party, local cloggers perform, cookbooks sold. FOODS SERVED: homemade blueberry foods including blueberry cobbler, blueberry ice cream and snow cones, blueberry waffles, layered desserts. ADMISSION: free. ACCOMMODATIONS: motels. RESTAURANTS: fast foods, family. CONTACT: Greater Brewton Chamber of Commerce, Box 19, Brewton, AL 36427, (205) 867-3224. 18,000

BLESSING OF THE FLEET *third weekend in June,* Bayou La Batre, Mobile Co., near Mobile, in recognition of Bayou La Batre's importance as a seafood and boat-building area. Procession of decorated shrimp boats, captains invite visitors aboard to participate in the boat parade. Arts and crafts sales and exhibits, Blessing of the Fleet, mass, Land Parade. FOODS SERVED: seafood lunches. ADMISSION: free. ACCOMMODATIONS: small motels in area, others in nearby Mobile. RESTAURANTS: family, seafood. CONTACT: St. Margaret's Church, P.O. Box 365, Bayou La Batre, AL 36509, (205) 824-2415.

SUMMER MUSIC FESTIVAL *third weekend in June,* DeSoto Caverns, Childersburg, Talladega Co. A showcase of Alabama musical and artistic talent including visual arts and bluegrass, jazz, folk and country music, choral and barbershop singing in the unusual setting of the De-Soto Caverns' Onyx Draperies and 2,000-year-old Indian burial ground discovered by Spanish explorer Hernando DeSoto in 1540. European-style outdoor market featuring arts and crafts, antiques, collectibles. A benefit for The King's Ranch, a home for abandoned, abused, or neglected children. FOODS SERVED: fresh-food mart and fun-foods fair. ADMISSION: charge, children under four free. ACCOMMODATIONS: motels. RESTAURANTS: fast foods, family, seafood. CONTACT: Caryl Lynn Mathis, 93 Ivy Trail, N. E., Atlanta, GA 30352, (404) 261-6179.

MENTONE CRAFTS FESTIVAL *first weekend after July 4,* Mentone, DeKalb Co., in Brow Park. 100 artists and craftspeople exhibit and sell their work, plus demonstrations of shingle splitting, quilting, beekeeping, clogging, and other mountain skills. FOODS SERVED: local concessions. ADMISSION: free. ACCOMMODATIONS: motels, B&B, campgrounds, and RV parks in Fort Payne, AL. RESTAURANTS: fast foods, family. CONTACT: Fort Payne Area Chamber of Commerce, P.O. Box 125, Fort Payne, AL 35967, (205) 845-2741.

ALABAMA SHAKESPEARE FESTIVAL *mid-July and August,* Montgomery, Montgomery Co., at the Alabama Shakespeare Complex. Professional performances Tuesday through Saturday and weekend matinees. Pre-show and After-theatre Discussions plus "Meet the Cast" parties for all theatregoers. Elizabethan church service at two "Shakespeare Sundays" during the season, weekly chamber-music concerts on Saturdays in the historic Church of Saint Michael and All Angels, student conservatory performs workshop productions during August. ADMISSION: $10.00–$15.00, group rates available. ACCOMMODATIONS: motels and hotels, B&B's, campgrounds, RV parks. RESTAURANTS: fast foods, family, ethnic,

southern specialties. CONTACT: Alabama Shakespeare Festival, P.O. Box 20350, Montgomery, AL 36120-0350, (205) 272-1640.

W. C. HANDY MUSIC FESTIVAL *first full weekend in August,* Florence, Muscle Shoals, Sheffield, and Tuscumbia, Lauderdale Co., in recognition of local musical heritage and the contribution of Florence-native W. C. Handy, "father of the blues." Riverside jazz, ABC's of Jazz for children, spiritual music at the church where Handy's father and grandfather were pastors, Century Bike Ride, DaDooFunRun, sidewalk cafe, Street Strut, major concert has featured stars such as Dizzy Gillespie, the late Count Basie, Manhattan Transfer, Roberta Flack, Carrie Smith, Emil Orth and the River City Six, and the Dukes of Dixieland, plus "scores of musicians who record at Muscle Shoals studios. FOODS SERVED: barbecue, southern foods. ADMISSION: many events are free, some up to $10.00. ACCOMMODATIONS: motels and hotels, campgrounds, RV parks. RESTAURANTS: fast foods, family, elegant, Greek. CONTACT: Music Preservation Society, Inc., 217 E. Tuscaloosa St., Florence, AL 35630, (205) 766-7642 or (205) 766-9719. 30,000

OCTOBERFEST *fourth weekend in September,* Birmingham, Jefferson Co., at the Jefferson Civic Center Exhibition Hall, downtown Birmingham. Three "well-known" German bands provide music for listening and folk dancing. FOODS SERVED: lots of German food specialties and beers. ADMISSION: charge. ACCOMMODATIONS: motels and hotels, B&B's, campgrounds. RESTAURANTS: fast foods, family, elegant. CONTACT: Mina Keasler at (205) 923-6564 or the Greater Birmingham Convention and Visitors Bureau, 2027 First Ave., N., Birmingham, AL 35203-4167, (205) 252-9825. 20,000

OUTDOOR ARTS AND CRAFTS SHOW *last weekend in September,* Fine Arts Museum of the South, Langan Park,

Mobile, Mobile Co. More than 300 artists from several states exhibit their work; music, fun and games for children. FOODS SERVED: local food booths. ADMISSION: free. ACCOMMODATIONS: motels and hotels, B&B's, RV parks. RESTAURANTS: fast foods, family, elegant. CONTACT: Fine Arts Museum of the South, P.O. Box 8404, Mobile, AL 36608, (205) 343-2667.

HARVEST FESTIVAL *first Friday and Saturday in October,* Boaz, Marshall Co., in the Sand Mountain area, celebrating the harvest of soybeans and corn. Sidewalk sale, arts and crafts, Snead State Jr. College Jazz Band, fashion show, Miss Harvest Festival Pageant, Gizmo the Clown, Cowboy's Pistol Shootout, antique car show. FOODS SERVED: home-baked and canned goods. ADMISSION: free. ACCOMMODATIONS: one motel. RESTAURANTS: fast foods, family. CONTACT: Boaz Chamber of Commerce, P.O. Box 563, Boaz, AL 35957, (205) 593-8154. 75,000

KENTUCK FESTIVAL *first weekend in October,* Kentuck Park, Northport, Tuscaloosa Co., to celebrate southern heritage and the arts. 150 juried exhibitors from throughout U. S., with demonstrations by southern folk artists including weavers, basket makers, carvers, blacksmiths, painters, country and bluegrass music, square dancing, clogging, dulcimers. FOODS SERVED: "traditional southern" such as sausage and biscuits cooked on wood-burning stoves, barbecue, fried chicken. ADMISSION: adults $2.50, children and seniors $1.50. ACCOMMODATIONS: motels and hotels, campgrounds. RESTAURANTS: fast foods, family, elegant, Chinese, Mexican, Italian. CONTACT: Kentuck Museum Association, P.O. Box 127, Northport, AL 35476, (205) 333-1252. 23,000

RIVERFRONT MARKET *second Saturday in October,* Selma, Dallas Co., on historic Water Avenue. More than 250 arts and crafts booths line both sides of the "only antebellum river-front business district intact in the United States." Dixieland music. FOODS SERVED: regional food specialties are one of the main attractions of this event. ADMISSION: free. ACCOMMODATIONS: motels and hotels, B&B's, campgrounds, RV parks. RESTAURANTS: fast foods, family. CONTACT: Selma Area Chamber of Commerce, P.O. Drawer D, Selma, AL 35701, (205) 875-7241.

ALABAMA TALE TELLIN' FESTIVAL *second weekend in October,* National Guard Armory on Dallas Ave., Selma, Dallas Co. Telling of ancient legends, folklore, ghostly and ghastly tales of the supernatural, humorous tales of natural and unnatural happenings of the south, bonfire Saturday night. Performers might include David Holt, Syd Lieberman, Loralee Cooley, and Kathryn Tucker Windham. FOODS SERVED: catfish supper at 5:00 P.M. ADMISSION: advance family, $10.00, adults $3.00, children under 12 $2.00. ACCOMMODATIONS: motels and hotels, B&B's, campgrounds, RV parks. RESTAURANTS: fast foods, family. CONTACT: Public Library of Selma and Dallas Co., 1103 Selma Ave., Selma, AL 36701, (205) 875-3535, or Selma Area Chamber of Commerce, P.O. Drawer D, Selma, AL 35701, (205) 875-7241. 2,000

NATIONAL SHRIMP FESTIVAL *second full weekend in October,* Gulf Shores, Baldwin Co., on the public beach area of Pleasure Island, in honor of the shrimping industry. Arts and crafts, musical entertainment including bluegrass, jazz, country-western, and Top 40 music, plus the United States Air Force Reserve Band; children's entertainment, Sand Sculpture Contest, parade, dance, gymnastic and karate exhibitions. FOODS SERVED: many seafood booths, especially local shrimp dishes. ADMISSION: free. ACCOMMODATIONS: motels and hotels, campgrounds, RV parks, condominiums. RESTAURANTS: fast foods, family, elegant, seafood specialties. CONTACT: Alabama Gulf Coast Area Chamber of Commerce, P.O. Drawer 457, Gulf Shores, AL 36542, (205) 968-7511. 150,000

NATIONAL PEANUT FESTIVAL *two weeks in mid-October,* Dothan, Houston Co., in the Wiregrass area to honor the peanut farmer and peanut industry. National Peanut Festival Recipe Contest, selection of Peanut Farmer-of-the-Year, arts and crafts shows, theatre productions, antique auto show, bowling, racquetball, golf, and tennis tournaments, Southern Regional Open Karate Tournament, circus big tent, hog shows, Coca-Cola professional Frisbee and Footbag Team Show, greased-pig contest, Goober Gamboleers Square Dance, coloring contest, Black Man- and Woman-of-the-Year Banquet, BMX Freestyle Exhibition, Halloween Costume Contest, entertainment such as Louise Mandrell, El DeBarge, Hank Williams, Jr., Chubby Checker, gospel groups, and Little Jimmy Dickens. FOODS SERVED: southern specialties and many peanut products and concoctions. ADMISSION: adults $4.00, children $3.00. ACCOMMODATIONS: motels and hotels, B&B's, campgrounds, RV parks. RESTAURANTS: fast foods, family, elegant. CONTACT: National Peanut Festival, 1691 Ross Clark Circle, S.E., Dothan, AL 36301, (205) 793-4323. 100,000

ARKANSAS

ARKANSAS FOLK FESTIVAL *third weekend in April,* Mountain View, Stone Co., at the Ozark Folk Center and in Court Square. Folk musicals, craft show and demonstrations, parade, Southern Regional Mountain Dulcimer and Hammered Dulcimer Contest, rodeo, impromptu musicals. FOODS SERVED: home-cooked and concessions. ADMISSION: from $4.25 up, varies by show. ACCOMMODATIONS: motels and hotels, B&B's, campgrounds, RV parks. RESTAURANTS: fast foods, family. CONTACT: Mountain View Area Chamber of Commerce, P.O. Box 133, Mountain View, AR 72560, (501) 269-8068. 50,000

DOGWOOD FESTIVAL *fourth weekend in April,* Siloam Springs, Benton Co., at the Downtown Park, to celebrate the blooming of dogwood trees and spring. 180 arts and crafts booths, daily entertainment, beauty pageant, tiny tots pageant, dogwood tree giveaway. FOODS SERVED: country. ADMISSION: free. ACCOMMODATIONS: motels and hotels, B&B's, campgrounds, RV park. RESTAURANTS: fast foods, family, elegant, Mexican. CONTACT: Chamber of Commerce, P.O. Box 476, Siloam Springs, AR 72761, (501) 524-6466. 35,000

FESTIVAL OF TWO RIVERS *first weekend in May,* Arkadelphia, Clark Co., on the lawn of the County Courthouse. Arts and crafts booths, judged art show, Clothesline Art Show, "tobacco spittin', cow-chip throwin', horseshoe pitchin', egg tossin'," theatrical events, musical entertainment including the Stateline Band, golf and tennis tournaments, U. S. Cycling Federation Bike Race, beauty pageant. FOODS SERVED: concessions. ADMISSION: free. ACCOMMODATIONS: motels and hotels, campgrounds. RESTAURANTS: fast foods, family. CONTACT: Festival of Two Rivers, Inc., P.O. Box 38, Arkadelphia, AR 71923, (501) 246-5542. 7,000

TOAD SUCK DAZE *first weekend in May,* Conway, Faulkner Co. Toad jumping, arts and crafts, King and Queen Toads, diaper dash, buggy race, softball and horseshoe-pitching tournaments, cow-chip throw, puppet show, old-fashioned melodrama, sack races, banjo picking, Mass Band Concert, fireworks display, tug-o-war, children's center, street dance, all to benefit Toad Suck Scholarships. FOODS SERVED: sausage-on-a-stick, funnel cakes, pie supper. ADMISSION: free. ACCOMMODATIONS: motels and hotels, campgrounds, RV parks. RESTAURANTS: fast foods, family. CONTACT: Chamber of Commerce, P.O. Box 1492, Conway, AR 72032, (501) 327-7788. 60,000

ARKANSAS FUN FESTIVAL *first weekend in June for four days,* centered in Hot Springs, Garland Co., in Diamond Lakes Country. National Rock Skipping Contest, Bath Tub Parade down Bath House Row, Speakeasy Talent Show, raft races on Lake Hamilton, concert, All-Arkansas Talent Show, arts and crafts, 5k Foot Race, Street Rod Fun Run, Small Fry Fishing Derby. FOODS SERVED: Taste Hot Springs features samplings of ethnic and gourmet foods from local restaurants. ADMISSION: free with charges to some events. ACCOMMODATIONS: motels and hotels, campgrounds. RESTAURANTS: fast foods, family, elegant. CONTACT: Hot Springs Chamber of Commerce, P.O. Box 1500, Hot Springs, AR 71901, instate: (800) 272-2081; out of state: (800) 643-1570. 45,000

WYNNE FUNFEST *second weekend in June,* near Wynne, Cross Co., at Village Creek State Park in the Crowley's Ridge area. Arts and crafts display and sales, country music by "Crossroads," rock music by R. T. Scott band, Air Force Band, local gospel groups, games for all ages, barbecue contest, 5k Run. FOODS SERVED: local specialties including barbecue. ADMISSION: free. ACCOMMODATIONS: motel, campground, RV park. RESTAURANTS: fast foods, family, elegant. CONTACT: Wynne Chamber of Commerce, P.O. Box 234, Wynne, AR 72396, (501) 238-2601. 12,000

PINK TOMATO FESTIVAL *second full weekend in June,* Warren, Bradley Co., in the Piney Bayou country of Southeast Arkansas, to honor the tomato harvest. Music jamboree, arts and crafts, beauty pageant, parade, street dance, puppet show, tomato bobbing, greased-pole climb, coon hunt and show, tobacco-spitting contests for men and women, mechanical bull ride, square dance, beard-growing contest, prayer breakfast, library book sale, children's art contest, tomato-eating contest, tour of tomato fields, arm wrestling, Ugliest Dog Contest. FOODS SERVED: All-Tomato Luncheon, concessions. ADMISSION: free. ACCOMMODATIONS: motels and hotels. RESTAURANTS: fast foods, family. CONTACT: Warren–Bradley Co. Chamber of Commerce, 206 N. Myrtle, Warren, AR 71671, (501) 226-5225. 10,000

HOPE WATERMELON FESTIVAL *third week in August,* Hope, Hempstead Co., at Hope Fair Park, in celebration of the harvest of "huge watermelons" in "The Home of the World's Largest—200 lbs." Watermelon-eating and seed-spitting contests, arts and crafts show, country-western music and dance, log burling, cow-chip tossing, wrestling, motorcycle rally, swim meet, barrel race, egg tossing, bingo, arm wrestling, early-days gas-engine show, antique car show, historic photography display, 4mi Run, chess and tennis tournaments, parade, dog show, Lip Sync Contest, gospel singing. FOODS SERVED: fish fry, watermelon, concessions, hand-dipped ice cream, Homemade Ice Cream Supper. ADMISSION: free to most events, charges to some special events. ACCOMMODATIONS: motels and hotels, campgrounds, RV park. RESTAURANTS: fast foods, family, Cantonese. CONTACT: Hope–Hempstead Co. Chamber of Commerce, P.O. Box 250, Hope, AR 71801, (501) 777-3640. 40,000

BEAVER LAKE WATER FESTIVAL *weekend before Labor Day weekend (early September),* Rogers, Benton Co., at the Horseshow Bend Recreation area on Beaver Lake. Fishing tournament, beauty pageant, water ski and water-related exhibitions, arts and crafts, boat parade, boat show, bass boat races. FOODS SERVED: local concessions. ADMISSION: free. ACCOMMODATIONS: motels and hotels, campgrounds, RV parks. RESTAURANTS: fast foods. CONTACT: Rogers Chamber of Commerce, Box 428, Rogers, AR 72757, (501) 636-1240. 20,000

TEXARKANA QUADRANGLE ARTS AND CRAFTS FESTIVAL *last Saturday in September,* Texarkana in the Ark–La–Tex area. Large arts and crafts exhibition and sale, 5k and 10k races, traditional music such as fiddling, blue-grass, country-western, cloggers and square dancers, Caddo Indian Dance Exhibition, pet show, children's art tent, antique automobile show, prizes. FOODS SERVED: fast foods including Mexican, soul food, Cajun. ADMISSION: free. ACCOMMODATIONS: motels and hotels, campgrounds, RV parks. RESTAURANTS: fast foods, family, elegant, Asian, Mexican, Italian. CONTACT: Texarkana Quadrangle Arts and Crafts Festival Committee, P.O. Box 2343, Texarkana, TX 75504 or Texarkana Chamber of Commerce, P.O. Box 1468, Texarkana, AR 75504, (214) 792-7191. 35,000

BELLA VISTA ARTS AND CRAFTS FESTIVAL *third weekend in October,* Bella Vista Village, at the Town Center in Blowing Springs Park. More than 450 exhibitors from twenty states exhibit, demonstrate, and sell their wares ranging from hand-crafted porcelain dolls, oil paintings, silver jewelry to tatted snowflakes, tin animals, and hand puppets, glue-in for children to create from precut wood, in a lovely setting and ambiance. FOODS SERVED: baked potatoes, candies, pork skins, funnel cakes, hamburgers, chili, pizza, barbecue, picnics encouraged. ADMISSION: free. ACCOMMODATIONS: motels and hotels, furnished houses and townhouses. RESTAURANTS: fast foods, family, elegant, Italian, Mexican, Chinese. CONTACT: Bella Vista Arts and Crafts Festival, 303 Towncenter, Bella Vista, AR 72714, (501) 855-3741. 100,000

OKTOBERFEST *third weekend in October,* Hot Springs, Garland Co., in Diamond Lakes Country. Polka and polka-costume contests, arts and crafts, German dog show, softball tournament, oompah music. FOODS SERVED: German food and "Northeast Arkansas wine in the Bavarian tradition." ADMISSION: charges for some contests. ACCOMMODATIONS: motels and hotels, campgrounds. RESTAURANTS: fast foods, family, elegant. CONTACT: Hot Springs Chamber of Commerce, P.O. Box 1500, Hot Springs, AR 71901, instate: (800) 272-2081; out of state: (800) 643-1570. 35,000

OZARKS ARTS AND CRAFTS FAIR ("The War Eagle Fair") *third full weekend in October,* War Eagle, Benton Co., at the War Eagle Mills Farm. Local Ozark artists and craftspeople working with native materials; demonstrations and sales. FOODS SERVED: "homestyle food and snacks," picnics encouraged. ADMISSION: free. ACCOMMODATIONS: (in nearby towns) motels and hotels, B&B's, campgrounds, RV parks. RESTAURANTS: (in nearby towns) fast foods, family, elegant, Italian, Chinese. CONTACT: Ozark Arts and Crafts Fair Association, Inc., Rt. 1, Box 157, War Eagle Farm, Hindsville, AR 72738, (501) 789-5398. 100,000

ORIGINAL OZARK FESTIVAL *last weekend in October and first weekend in November,* Eureka Springs, Carroll Co., to celebrate Ozark heritage. "Seventy-five professional musicians play only traditional Ozark music and songs that must be at least 75-years-old on non-electrified instruments" such as guitars, banjos, fiddles, harmonicas, dulcimers, Elizabethan music and songs, square dancing, jig and clogging. Native crafts including pottery, woodcraft, leather craft and painting. FOODS SERVED: traditional Ozark. ADMISSION: adults $5.00, children $3.00; admission free to arts and crafts show. ACCOMMODATIONS: motels and hotels, B&B's, campgrounds, RV parks. RESTAURANTS: fast foods, family, elegant, continental,

Asian, Cajun. CONTACT: Eureka Springs Chamber of Commerce, P.O. Box 551, Eureka Springs, AR 72632, (501) 253-8737. 10,000

WORLD'S CHAMPIONSHIP DUCK CALLING CONTEST AND WINGS OVER THE PRAIRIE FESTIVAL *week of Thanksgiving (November),* Stuttgart, Arkansas Co., downtown and at the Auditorium. Duck Calling Contest, Queen Mallard Beauty Pageant, Duck Gumbo Cook-off, carnival, Great 10k Duck Race, arts and crafts fair, Sportsman's Dinner and Dance, trap shoot. Celebrities such as Wally Schirra, Whitey Herzog, Jim Ed Brown, Jerry Clower have appeared. FOODS SERVED: duck gumbo, barbecue. ADMISSION: free except $3.00 to Queen Mallard Beauty Pageant and Duck Gumbo Cook-off. ACCOMMODATIONS: motels and hotels. RESTAURANTS: fast foods, family. CONTACT: Stuttgart Chamber of Commerce, P.O. Box 932, Stuttgart, AR 72160, (501) 673-1602. 75,000

FLORIDA

OLD ISLAND DAYS *January through March,* Key West, Monroe Co. At least forty-six events in three months, including a craft show in late January, historic house and garden tours led by ladies in red shawls on weekends during February and mid-March, a sidewalk art festival sponsored by the Key West Art Center and Key West Players on the third weekend in February, the Island Food Festival featuring Cuban and Bahamian foods, as well as local seafood on the third weekend in February, the fabulous orchid show the third weekend in March, and the Conch Shell Blowing Contest on the third Saturday in March, featuring "the finest in conch shell music!" This is a real community-wide festival and worthy of spending time in old Key West. FOODS SERVED: wide variety including Cuban sandwiches and lots of seafood. ADMISSION: free to many events, charges for others. ACCOMMODATIONS: motels and hotels, B&B's, campgrounds, RV parks. RESTAURANTS: fast foods, family, elegant. CONTACT: Old Island Restoration Foundation, Inc., P.O. Box 689, Key West, FL 33041, (305) 294-9501.

FLORIDA KEYS RENAISSANCE FAIRE *third weekend in January,* Marathon, Monroe Co., in the Florida Keys in recognition of the 16th century. Jousting knights on horseback, heroes and villains fighting out a human chess game, battle-ax toss, kings and queens, lords and ladies, and "a fair pleasing wench or two," jousters, New Riders of the Golden Age, Sticks and Stones Puppet Theatre, SAK Theatre from Epcot Center, The Royal Chessmen, 100 arts, crafts and food booths. FOODS SERVED: "kingly feasts of turkey legs, pig roasts, etc." ADMISSION: adults $3.00, children under 10 free. ACCOMMODATIONS: motels and hotels, B&B's, campgrounds, RV parks. RESTAURANTS: fast foods, family, elegant, Asian, Cuban, Italian, Mexican. CONTACT: Florida Keys Renaissance Faire, 427 89th St., Marathon, Florida Keys, FL 33050, (305) 743-4386. 10,000

ORLANDO SCOTTISH HIGHLAND GAMES *third weekend in January,* Orlando, Orange Co., at the Central Florida Fairgrounds. "Competitions in nine heavy Scottish athletic events," Highland dancing, pipebands such as Stirling and Rosie O'Grady's, drumming, abundance of Scottish souvenirs for sale. FOODS SERVED: Scottish and Celtic. ADMISSION: $6.00. ACCOMMODATIONS: motels and hotels, campgrounds, RV parks. RESTAURANTS: fast foods, family, elegant. CONTACT: Orlando Scottish Highland Games, Scottish-American Society of Central Florida, Inc., P.O. Box 2149, Orlando, FL 32802, or The Greater Orlando Chamber of Commerce, P.O. Box 1234, Orlando, FL 32802, (305) 425-1234. 8,000

PIRATE FEST AND GASPARILLA INVASION *February 9,* Tampa, Hillsborough Co., to celebrate the Gasparilla Invasion and Tampa's buccaneer history. Annual entrance of Tampa's Pirates-for-a-Day businessmen aboard the "Jose Gaspar" into Tampa Bay, pirate invasion onto Bayshore Boulevard amidst a flotilla of Tampa's watercraft, surrendering ceremony, parade; at the Franklin Street Mall there's live entertainment for children and adults including magicians, puppets, mimes, fireworks, and musical showcase featuring stars such as the Crystals, the Shirelles, and Little Anthony. FOODS SERVED: concessions. ADMISSION: free. ACCOMMODATIONS: motels and hotels, campgrounds, RV parks. RESTAURANTS: fast foods, family, elegant, international. CONTACT: Tampa–Hillsborough Convention and Visitors Association, Inc., P.O. Box 519, Tampa, FL 33601, (813) 223-1111 or (800) 826-8358. 650,000

FIESTA DAY *second Saturday in February,* Tampa, Hillsborough Co., in the Ybor City area to celebrate "Gasparilla events." Ybor City blocks reflect the music, culture, and ceremonial performances of Italy, Cuba, and Spain, including artists' exhibits and demonstrations, strolling musicians, puppeteers, traditional Latin children's games, farmers' market, hot air balloons, annual costume contest. FOODS SERVED: Spanish bean soup, Cuban bread, and cafe con leche. ADMISSION: free. ACCOMMODATIONS: motels and hotels, campgrounds, RV parks. RESTAURANTS: fast foods, family, elegant, international. CONTACT: Susan McVicker, 1800 E. 9th Ave., Tampa, FL 33605, (814) 248-3712 or the Tampa–Hillsborough Convention and Visitors Association, Inc., P.O. Box 519,

Tampa, FL 33601, (813) 223-1111 or (800) 826-8358. 30,000

MIAMI BEACH OUTDOOR FESTIVAL OF THE ARTS *second weekend in February,* Miami Beach, Dade Co., at the Outside Miami Beach Convention Center. Arts and crafts from fine arts to cottage crafts, musical and theatrical events, children's corner, children's art display, "artists in all media from all over the country." Awards include $1,750 Purchase Awards for Best of Show, $4,350 in cash prizes, and $25,000 in Advance Patron Purchases. FOODS SERVED: international. ADMISSION: free. ACCOMMODATIONS: motels and hotels. RESTAURANTS: fast foods, family, elegant. CONTACT: Miami Beach Fine Arts Board, P.O. Bin "O", Miami Beach, FL 33119 or the Miami Beach Chamber of Commerce, 1920 Meridian Ave., Miami Beach, FL 33139, (305) 672-1270. 250,000

FLORIDA CITRUS FESTIVAL *second weekend and third week in February,* Winter Haven, Polk Co., in celebration of the citrus harvest. Orange pie-eating contest, cow-chip throwing and greased-pig contests, fine arts, language arts, homemaking and artistic fruit displays, parade, Citrus Queen Pageant, golf tournament, Citrus Classic Road Race, carnival, cloggers, Billy "Crash" Craddock, Paul Lennon, The Platters, Sawyer Brown, Exile, Bonnie Nelson, Jeannie C. Riley, The Stalneckevs. FOODS SERVED: "all kinds from hot dogs to elephant ears." ADMISSION: General $3.00, charges for specific events. ACCOMMODATIONS: motels and hotels, B&B's, campgrounds, RV parks. RESTAURANTS: fast foods, family, elegant, seafood. CONTACT: Florida Citrus Showcase, P.O. Box 9229, Winter Haven, FL 33880, (813) 293-3175. 146,000

GRANT SEAFOOD FESTIVAL *third weekend in February,* Grant, Brevard Co., to celebrate local seafood and promote conservation and environmental awareness. Arts and crafts, many seafood booths, continuous entertainment includ-

ing bluegrass, country, big band, dixieland; educational and informational booths. FOODS SERVED: seafood such as oysters, clams, crab, scallops, frog legs. ADMISSION: free. ACCOMMODATIONS: motels and hotels, RV parks. RESTAURANTS: fast foods, family. CONTACT: Grant Community Club, Inc., P.O. Box 44, Grant, FL 32949. 50,000

SWAMP CABBAGE FESTIVAL *third weekend in February*, LaBelle, Mendry Co., to recognize Florida's state tree, the Sabal Palm, known locally as "cabbage palms." The Sabal Palm served settlers as both food and building material, and is known today in food circles as "hearts of palm." Local and Indian arts and crafts, quilt show, Bass Tournament, Swamp Stomp 5,000m Run for men and women, Baby Contest, golf tournament, beauty pageant, Coronation Ball, mini-parade, rodeo, dance, country-western dance, continuous entertainment featuring dancers and bands such as Dillon Thomas, Dixie Star, and The South. FOODS SERVED: chicken and dumplings dinner, park dinners include steak, roast beef, ribs, chicken, hamburgers, sloppy joes, breads, fruits. ADMISSION: free. ACCOMMODATIONS: motels and hotels, campgrounds, RV parks. RESTAURANTS: fast foods, family. CONTACT: Greater LaBelle Chamber of Commerce, P.O. Box 456, LaBelle, FL 33935, (813) 675-0125. 25,000

COCONUT GROVE ARTS FESTIVAL *third weekend in February*, Miami, Dade Co., in the village atmosphere of Coconut Grove, to celebrate the arts. More than 320 visual artists present their work, fifty culinary artists offer every edible from ethnic and one-of-a-kind Greek salad, Tex/Mex fajitas, Israeli falafel, Japanese tempura, Italian sausage to banana-rum fritters, stone crabs, conch chowder. Art Watch demonstrators show their skills of printmaking, watercolor, sculpture, papermaking, weaving, ceramics, basketry, and painting. Performing arts program includes artists such as Dizzy Gillespie, Jeff

Palmer and Randy Bernsen and the Ocean Sound Band, The Turtles featuring Flo and Eddie, Peter Graves' Atlantean Driftwood Band, The Shirelles, Herbie Mann and The Family of Mann, Stanley Tarrentine. FOODS SERVED: see above "Culinary Artists." ADMISSION: free. ACCOMMODATIONS: motels and hotels, B&B's, campgrounds, RV parks. RESTAURANTS: fast foods, family, elegant. CONTACT: The Coconut Grove Association, P.O. Box 330757, Coconut Grove, FL 33133, (305) 447-0401. 1,000,000

HATSUME FAIR *last weekend in February*, Delray Beach, Palm Beach Co., celebrating the "First bud of the year." Japanese performing arts, demonstrations, bonsai, plants, Sushi-eating Contest, children's corner, Soh Daiko Drum Group, Deems Tsutakawa (jazz), Chitose Fujima Kabuki dance, bonsai demonstrations, martial arts. FOODS SERVED: Japanese and American. ADMISSION: adults $2.00, children under 12 free. ACCOMMODATIONS: motels and hotels. RESTAURANTS: fast foods, family. CONTACT: The Morikami, Inc., 4000 Morikami Park Rd., Delray Beach, FL 33445, (305) 495-0233. 20,000

GASPARILLA SIDEWALK ARTS FESTIVAL *last weekend in February or first weekend in March*, Tampa, Hillsborough Co. Largest art festival in Tampa with $20,000 in prizes to be awarded in thirteen fine-arts categories, with more than 300 of "the nation's top artists" participating. FOODS SERVED: concessions. ADMISSION: free. ACCOMMODATIONS: motels and hotels, campgrounds, RV parks. RESTAURANTS: fast foods, family, elegant, international. CONTACT: Bill Grey, P.O. Box 10591, Tampa, FL 33679, (813) 221-5333 or the Tampa-Hillsborough Convention and Visitors Association, Inc., P.O. Box 519, Tampa, FL 33601, (813) 223-1111 or (800) 826-8358. 150,000

CHALO NITKA *first full weekend in March*, Moore Haven, Glades Co. Country music, Indian and local arts and crafts,

Chalo Nitka (Big Bass in Miccasukie language) Queen Contest. FOODS SERVED: Seminole including pumpkin bread and fry bread. ADMISSION: donation. ACCOMMODATIONS: motels and hotels, campgrounds, RV parks. RESTAURANTS: family. CONTACT: Glades Co. Chamber, P.O. Box 490, Moore Haven, FL 33471, (813) 946-0440.

RIVER FESTIVAL *March,* Jacksonville, Duval Co., at the Florida National Pavillion in Metropolitan Park, to celebrate "our clean St. John's River." Music, river activities includes sailboarding race, cigarette boat race, para-sailers, kite contest, swim contest, 9.1mi River Run. FOODS SERVED: seafood and international. ADMISSION: free. ACCOMMODATIONS: motels and hotels, B&B's, campgrounds, RV parks. RESTAURANTS: fast foods, family, elegant, Asian, Mexican, Greek, Italian, German. CONTACT: Dale Eldridge or Lisa Braren, City of Jacksonville, 220 E. Bay St., Rm. 107, Jacksonville, FL 32203, (904) 633-2890. 50,000

FLORIDA STRAWBERRY FESTIVAL AND HILLSBOROUGH COUNTY FAIR *first 11 days in March,* Plant City, Hillsborough Co., to celebrate the strawberry harvest. Strawberry production field, Youth, Baby, and Grand Feature parades, festival gift shop, Coronation Ceremony; Strawberry Stemming, Strawberry-Shortcake Eating, Milking, Rooster Crowing, Meadow Muffin Toss contests; country-music star shows, Pioneer Post Office, fine arts shows, horticulture, livestock. FOODS SERVED: strawberries in every form and concoction possible, strawberry food products available to take home. ADMISSION: $2.50 advance, $3.50 at the gate. ACCOMMODATIONS: motels and hotels, campgrounds, RV parks. RESTAURANTS: fast foods, family. CONTACT: Florida Strawberry Festival and Hillsborough Co. Fair, P.O. Drawer 1869, Plant City, FL 34289-2869, (813) 752-9194. 691,000

BACH FESTIVAL AT WINTER PARK *first week in March,* Winter Park, Orange Co., at Rollins College's Knowles Memorial Chapel. Five concerts and lectures focusing on a theme of Bach's compositions and featuring the Bach Festival Choir, the Florida Symphony Orchestra, Concert Royal Baroque Orchestra, and various artists such as Juliana Gondek, Marianna Busching, Steven Rickards, John Aler, Douglas Lawrence, Alexander Anderson, and the Orlando Deanery Boys Choir. ADMISSION: $15.00 individual concert, $50.00 for five concerts. ACCOMMODATIONS: motels and hotels, campgrounds. RESTAURANTS: fast foods, family, elegant, international. CONTACT: The Bach Festival Society of Winter Park, Rollins College, Box 2763, Winter Park, FL 32789, (305) 646-2182. 2,000

STRAWBERRY FESTIVAL *first weekend through second weekend in March,* Tampa, Hillsborough Co., at Plant City, to celebrate its strawberry crop. Strawberry Queen competition, Strawberry Parade, midway with rides, Strawberry Shortcake Contest, country-music entertainment with stars such as Crystal Gayle, Mel Tillis, Conway Twitty, Pat Boone, Crysty Lane, Roy Clark, Reba McEntire, Golden Boys of Bandstand, George Strait, John Conlee. FOODS SERVED: lots of strawberry shortcake and other strawberry products, concessions. ADMISSION: $3.50. ACCOMMODATIONS: motels and hotels, campgrounds, RV parks. RESTAURANTS: fast foods, family, elegant, international. CONTACT: Patsy Brooks, P.O. Box 1869, Plant City, FL 33566, (813) 752-9194 or the Tampa-Hillsborough Convention and Visitors Association, Inc., P.O. Box 519, Tampa, FL 33601, (813) 223-1111 or (800) 826-8358. 400,000

DELIUS FESTIVAL *first weekend in March,* Jacksonville, Duval Co., to celebrate the music of English composer Frederick Delius and his contemporaries. Festival date coincides with Delius' arrival in Florida. Events take place at Jacksonville University and other musical and educational institutions in Jacksonville. Musical and historial events such as recitals, concerts, lectures, exhibits of "Deliana" at local libraries, performances of the works of Delius, composition contest for young composers, presentations by officers of the Delius Trust in London. ADMISSION: free. ACCOMMODATIONS: motels and hotels, B&B's. RESTAURANTS: fast foods, family, elegant. CONTACT: Thomas H. Gunn, Delius Association of Florida, P.O. Box 5621, Jacksonville, FL 32247-5621 or the Jacksonville Chamber of Commerce, P.O. Box 329, Jacksonville, FL 32202, (904) 353-0300.

KISSIMMEE BLUEGRASS FESTIVAL *first weekend in March,* Kissimmee, Osceola Co., in the Kissimmee–St. Cloud resort area. Lots of bluegrass music including performers such as Bill Monroe, Lewis Family, Johnson Mountain Boys, Foster Family, Ralph Stanley. FOODS SERVED: fast foods, barbecue. ADMISSION: adults $10.00 per day. ACCOMMODATIONS: motels and hotels, campgrounds, RV parks. RESTAURANTS: fast foods, family, Mexican, Chinese, Italian. CONTACT: Lee P. Eldridge, First Federal Osceola, P.O. Box 98, St. Cloud, FL 32769, (305) 892-1200. 10,000

PIONEER PARK DAYS *first weekend in March,* Zolfo Springs, Hardee Co., in Pioneer Park, to further appreciation of steam and gas engines. Model steam and gas engines, antique gas and steam engines, oil-pull tractors, Old Fashioned Parade, antique cars, giant flea market, Civil War reenactment, live entertainment including local country and gospel singers. FOODS SERVED: "American, Spanish, and Mexican." ADMISSION: free. ACCOMMODATIONS: campgrounds. RESTAURANTS: fast foods, family, Spanish, Mexican. CONTACT: Hardee Co. Chamber of Commerce, P.O. Box 683, Wauchula, FL 33873, (813) 773-6967. 300,000

CARNAVAL MIAMI *second week in March through the day before Lent,* Little Havana, Miami, Dade Co. Carnaval Miami is the "umbrella" name for nine days of joyous pre-Lenten celebration including *Calle Ocho,* "the largest street festival in the United States," and features several stages on which salsa, cha cha cha, mambo, merengue, flamenco, jazz country-western, bluegrass are performed; Carnival Night includes an all-star variety show, "televised throughout the Americas," huge fiesta, fireworks; *Paseo* is a "traditional parade of floats, decorated trucks, cars and street dancers, streamers and confetti along the street; Miami Cup International Soccer at the Orange Bowl features teams from Argentina, Brazil, Colombia and "Team U.S.A."; the *Calle Ocho* 8k Run followed by a "lively celebration," Carnival Miami Bike Dash, which is a bicycle race throughout the main streets of Little Havana; Carnaval Miami Dance at Flagler Greyhound Track includes a Battle of the Bands featuring top Latin bands and dancing until the wee hours, Miami Spice Cooking Contest, poster and photo contests, carnival disco for teenagers at the Dinner Key Auditorium. During the *Calle Ocho* "the entire Hispanic community throws a block party (twenty-three blocks) for everyone." FOODS SERVED: pan con lechon, rice and beans, tacos, shish-ke-bobs, American and Latin foods. ADMISSION: free, charges for few events. ACCOMMODATIONS: motels and hotels, B&B's, condominiums. RESTAURANTS: fast foods, family, elegant, international. CONTACT: Kiwanis Club of Little Havana, 900 S. W. First St., Suite 202, Miami, FL 33130, (305) 324-7349. 1,000,000

DOWN HOME DAYS *second week in March,* Madison, Madison Co., as a salute to farmers. Parade, crafts, live entertainment, competitive sports, fashion shows, beauty pageant, stock shows. FOODS SERVED: "traditionally southern." ADMISSION: free. ACCOMMODATIONS: motels and hotels, campgrounds, RV parks. RESTAURANTS: fast foods, family. CONTACT: Madison Co. Chamber of Commerce, 105 N. Range St., Madison, FL 32340, (904) 973-2788. 10,000

ORANGE BLOSSOM FESTIVAL *second weekend through third weekend in March*, Davie, Broward Co. Three art shows, carnival, hot air balloon race, Fitness Fair, 5mi. and 1mi. runs, raft race, sock hop, Orange Juice Squeeze, country fair, tea, library book sale, rodeo; youth, Queen and 50 Plus pageants; gospel concerts, Gold Coast Cloggers and performances by local dance studios. FOODS SERVED: Seminole Indian, orange juice, pancake breakfast, barbecue, Greek, Italian, Spanish, Chinese. ADMISSION: free. ACCOMMODATIONS: motels and hotels, campgrounds, RV parks. RESTAURANTS: fast foods, family, elegant. CONTACT: Davie–Cooper City Chamber of Commerce, 4185 S. W. 64th Ave., Davie, FL 33314, (305) 581-0790. 80,000

SPECKLED PERCH FESTIVAL *third weekend in March*, Okeechobee, Okeechobee Co., the "Speckled Perch Capital of the World." Arts and crafts, game booths, parade, continuous live music including country-western and bluegrass, parade, fish fry. FOODS SERVED: speckled perch, Seminole Indian specialties. ADMISSION: free. ACCOMMODATIONS: motels and hotels, campgrounds, RV parks. RESTAURANTS: fast foods, family. CONTACT: Okeechobee Co. Chamber of Commerce, Okeechobee, FL 33472, (813) 763-6464. 15,000

WINTER PARK SIDEWALK ART FESTIVAL *third weekend in March*, Winter Park, Orange Co., in Central Park. Exhibits by more than 250 artists in oils, acrylics, watercolor, photography, metal, glass, clay, and fiber compete for over $20,000 in prize money. Children's exhibit, children's art workshop, live performances by artists such as Herbie Mann, Dave Brubeck, Florida Symphony Orchestra, and the Southern Ballet Co. FOODS SERVED: gyros, fruit, salads, all-American. ADMISSION: free. ACCOMMODATIONS: motels and hotels, campgrounds, RV parks. RESTAURANTS: fast foods, family, elegant, French. CONTACT: Winter Park Sidewalk Art Festival, P.O. Box 597, Winter Park, FL 32790 or the Winter Park Chamber of Commerce, P.O. Box 280, Winter Park, FL 32790, (305) 644-8281. 300,000

ST. PETERSBURG FESTIVAL OF STATES *last week in March through first week in April*, St. Petersburg, Pinellas Co., in the Tampa Bay area. Nearly 200 events including three major parades, hydroplane races, jetski, and windsurfing contests, foot races, antique auto show, fireworks, concerts including jazz and high school marching bands competition. FOODS SERVED: concessions. ADMISSION: free except field show of bands, $4.00–$9.00. ACCOMMODATIONS: motels and hotels, B&B's, campgrounds, RV parks. RESTAURANTS: fast foods, family, elegant, international. CONTACT: Festival of States, P.O. Box 1731, St. Petersburg, FL 33731, (813) 821-4069. 750,000

COUNTRY MUSIC FESTIVAL *April*, Jacksonville, Duval Co., at the Florida National Pavillion in Metropolitan Park. Country-western music featuring stars such as Ronnie Milsap, Sylvia, Earl Thomas Conley, Billy "Crash" Craddock, and the Whiskey River Band. FOODS SERVED: seafood and international. ADMISSION: free. ACCOMMODATIONS: motels and hotels, B&B's, campgrounds, RV parks. RESTAURANTS: fast foods, family, elegant, Asian, Mexican, Greek, Italian, German. CONTACT: Dale Eldridge or Lisa Braren, City of Jacksonville, 220 E. Bay St., Rm. 107, Jacksonville, FL 32203, (904) 633-2890. 50,000

CATFISH FESTIVAL *first Saturday in April*, Crescent City, Putnam Co. World's Catfish Skinning Contest, more than 100 artists and craftspeople from throughout Florida, King Catfish Parade, Catfish Run, free bluegrass concert, Gospel Jubilee, Tot Ribbon Run. FOODS SERVED: fried catfish dinners featuring fingerling-size blues and channel cats, steamed blue crabs, swamp cabbage, catfish chowder, alligator tail, chicken dinners, hot dogs, strawberry shortcake. (Serving begins at 9:00 A.M.)

ADMISSION: $5.00. ACCOMMODATIONS: motels, B&B's, campgrounds, RV parks. RESTAURANTS: family. CONTACT: Putnam Co. Chamber of Commerce, P.O. Box 550, Palatka, FL 32078, (904) 328-1503. 40,000

SPRING ARTS FESTIVAL *first weekend in April*, Gainesville, Alachua Co., in Gainesville historic district to celebrate the beginning of spring. More than 300 artists and craftspeople displaying two and three-dimensional arts, youth art area featuring hands-on opportunities, youth art displays, Children's Emporium with works by festival artists in the $1.00–$10.00 range for those 12 and under, continuous entertainment by groups such as the Gainesville Civic Ballet/Dance Alive! Youth Ensemble, Crosscreek Cloggers, Theatre for the Deaf, and Sante Fe Community College Theatre for Young People; concessions. FOODS SERVED: kosher, Greek, Italian, American, natural/health, Hispanic/Latin. ADMISSION: free. ACCOMMODATIONS: motels and hotels, campgrounds, RV parks. RESTAURANTS: fast foods, family, elegant, continental, Indian. CONTACT: Spring Arts Festival, P.O. Box 1530, Gainesville, FL 32602, (904) 372-1976. 100,000

DE SOTO CELEBRATION *second week in April*, Bradenton, Manatee Co., in the Tampa Bay area, to celebrate Spanish explorer Hernando De Soto's landing at the mouth of the Manatee River in 1539. Landing reenactment, seafood fest, 10k Run, Plastic Bottle Boat Regatta, children's parade, Coronation Ball, Grande Parade, Stadium Country Music Show, Celebrity All-Star Softball Game with the Tampa Bay Bucaneers. FOODS SERVED: seafood, Spanish, American. ADMISSION: free with charges to some events. ACCOMMODATIONS: motels and hotels, campgrounds, RV parks. RESTAURANTS: fast foods, family, elegant. CONTACT: The De Soto Celebration, 4301 32nd St., W., Suite C-3, Bradenton, FL 33505, (813) 755-0338. 30,000

COCOA BEACH EASTER SURFING FESTIVAL *Easter weekend (April)*, Cocoa Beach, Brevard Co., on Canaveral Pier, to begin the surfing season. Bikini Contest, jet-ski races, professional and amateur surfing contests, wind-surfing competition, sand sculpture contests, mimes, jugglers, entertainment including groups such as No Dice, Mint Condition, John Sebastian, local groups, and Indian dances. FOODS SERVED: Cherokee Indian. ADMISSION: free. ACCOMMODATIONS: motels and hotels, B&B's, campgrounds, RV parks. RESTAURANTS: fast foods, family, elegant. CONTACT: American Professional Surfers, P.O. Box 1370, Cocoa Beach, FL 32931, (305) 783-5813. 80,000

APOPKA ART AND FOLIAGE FESTIVAL *fourth weekend in April*, Apopka, Orange Co. Juried art show, school art displays, bus tour of rose farms and greenhouses, exotic foliage and plants from area growers for sale, horticultural consultations, entertainment from local schools and churches. FOODS SERVED: concessions. ADMISSION: free, $2.00 for bus tours. ACCOMMODATIONS: motels and hotels, campgrounds, RV parks. RESTAURANTS: fast foods, family. CONTACT: Apopka Woman's Club, P.O. Box 336, Apopka, FL 32703, (305) 889-2872. 20,000

WEEK OF THE OCEAN FESTIVAL *last week in April through first week in May*, Fort Lauderdale, Broward Co., to celebrate "the influence of the ocean on our lives." Sea turtle release, art show, sea chantey concerts, Mother Ocean Day, Fort Lauderdale Billfish Tournament, Sierra Club beach walk, scuba demonstrations, sundown serenade on the waterway, school marine fair. FOODS SERVED: seafood, "sometimes under-utilized species" such as eel or squid. ADMISSION: mostly free, park entrance fees from $1.00–$25.00. ACCOMMODATIONS: motels and hotels, B&B's, campgrounds, RV parks. RESTAURANTS: fast foods, family, elegant, international. CONTACT: Cynthia

Hancock, 516 Bontona Ave., Fort Lauderdale, FL 33301, (305) 462-5573. 40,000

CHAUTAUQUA FESTIVAL *April through third Saturday in May*, DeFuniak Springs, Walton Co., on the Emerald Coast, to recognize the educational history of the Florida Chautauqua from 1885–1920. Okaloosa Symphony in concern in March, one-week residence by the Gainesville Civic Ballet's Dance Alive! in April, lunchtime concerts in April by brass quintet Top Brass, Chautauqua Day entertainment by Fantasy Theatre Factory and a gospel concert by The Kingsmen; performances by Little Theatre and the community choir, and dance and dramatic presentations for the public and in schools. FOODS SERVED: variety. ADMISSION: free. ACCOMMODATIONS: motels and hotels, campgrounds. RESTAURANTS: fast foods, family, elegant (on the beach). CONTACT: Chautauqua Festival, Inc., P.O. Box 29, DeFuniak Springs, FL 32433, (904) 892-3191. 5,000

INTERNATIONAL FESTIVAL *May*, Jacksonville, Duval Co., at the Southbank Riverwalk. "Food from all over the world served at booths set up along 1.9 mile-long Riverfront Boardwalk" with entertainers from singers and musicians to clowns, mimes, and dancers. FOODS SERVED: international and seafood. ADMISSION: free. ACCOMMODATIONS: motels and hotels, B&B's, campgrounds, RV parks. RESTAURANTS: fast foods, family, elegant, Asian, Mexican, Greek, Italian, German. CONTACT: Dale Eldridge or Lisa Braren, City of Jacksonville, 220 E. Bay St., Rm. 107, Jacksonville, FL 32203, (904) 633-2890. 40,000

SPRING MUSIC FESTIVAL *May*, Jacksonville, Duval Co., at the Florida National Pavillion in Metropolitan Park. Two days of nostalgic music, singing, and entertainment featuring artists such as The Four Tops, The Platters, The Spinners, and The Beach Boys. FOODS SERVED: seafood and international. ADMISSION: free. AC-

COMMODATIONS: motels and hotels, B&B's, campgrounds, RV parks. RESTAURANTS: fast foods, family, elegant, Asian, Mexican, Greek, Italian, German. CONTACT: Dale Eldridge or Lisa Braren, City of Jacksonville, 220 E. Bay St., Rm. 107, Jacksonville, FL 32203, (904) 633-2890. 100,000

PALM HARBOR DAY ARTS CRAFTS AND MUSIC FESTIVAL *first Saturday in May*, Palm Harbor, Pinellas Co., to celebrate the founding of Palm Harbor. Arts and crafts show, continuous entertainment including cloggers, country and bluegrass music, children's games. FOODS SERVED: barbecue, concessions, beer garden. ADMISSION: free. ACCOMMODATIONS: motels and hotels, campgrounds, RV parks. RESTAURANTS: fast foods, family, elegant. CONTACT: Greater Palm Harbor Area Chamber of Commerce, 100 U. S. 19 North, Suite 300, Palm Harbor, FL 33563, (813) 787-1776. 7,000

ISLE OF EIGHT FLAGS SHRIMP FESTIVAL *first weekend in May*, Fernandina Beach, Nassau Co., at Amelia Island, in recognition of Florida's shrimp industry. Arts and crafts exhibits, antiques, continuous entertainment. FOODS SERVED: "lots of shrimp" and American. ADMISSION: free. ACCOMMODATIONS: motels and hotels, B&B's, campgrounds, RV parks. RESTAURANTS: fast foods, family, elegant, seafood. CONTACT: Amelia Island–Fernandina Beach Chamber of Commerce, P.O. Box 472, Fernandina Beach, FL 32034, (904) 261-3248. 130,000

FLORIDA FOLK FESTIVAL *Memorial Day weekend (late May)*, White Springs, Hamilton Co., in the Suwannee Valley at Stephen Foster State Folk Culture Center to encourage folk arts within the cultural groups in which they survive. Many arts and crafts demonstrations and sales, hundreds of performers including traditional singers, tale tellers, musicians, and dancers, workshop performances include puppets, folk music, fiddles, banjos, gui-

tars, tsabounas, and dulcimers. FOODS SERVED: regional and ethnic foods such as chicken and dumplings, egg rolls, tabouli salad, fish and hush puppies, barbecue pork and beef, hoppin' john, okra and tomatoes, boiled and parched peanuts, Seminole fry bread, cakes and pies. ADMISSION: adults $7.00, children $1.50, group rates available. ACCOMMODATIONS: nearby motels, campgrounds, RV parks. RESTAURANTS: fast foods, family. CONTACT: Florida Department of State, Division of Historical Resources, Bureau of Florida Folklife Programs, P.O. Box 265, White Springs, FL 32096, (904) 396-2192. 10,000

ZELLWOOD SWEET CORN FESTIVAL *Memorial Day weekend (late May)*, Zellwood, Orange Co., to celebrate the sweet corn harvest. Arts and crafts show, carnival rides for children, continuous entertainment including country and bluegrass music, cloggers. FOODS SERVED: "all the corn you can eat," southern ham and trimmings, plus one nationality featured each year. ADMISSION: adults $5.00 advance, $7.00 at the gate. ACCOMMODATIONS: motels and hotels, B&B's, campgrounds, RV parks. RESTAURANTS: fast foods, family, elegant, Italian, Chinese. CONTACT: Zellwood Sweet Corn Festival, P.O. Box 628, Zellwood, FL 32798, (305) 886-0014. 25,000

MUSIC FESTIVAL OF FLORIDA *first three weeks in June*, Sarasota, Sarasota Co., on Florida's West Coast. "A learning experience with emphasis upon instrumental techniques and musical approaches as they apply to chamber music repertoire." Master classes in strings, woodwinds, brass, and piano, seminars and workshops. Three weekends of concerts by faculty artists and participant orchestras; Ensemble-in-Residence: Florida String Quartet. Students rehearse and perform major literature for chamber ensembles including string quartets, woodwind quintets, brass quintets. ADMISSION: charges for concerts from $8.00–$15.00 single concert, $30.00–$70.00 for six con-

certs. ACCOMMODATIONS: motels and hotels, campgrounds, RV parks. RESTAURANTS: fast foods, family, elegant. CONTACT: Florida West Coast Music, Inc., Music Festival of Florida, 709 N. Tamiami Trail, Sarasota, FL 33577, (813) 952-9634. 9,000

BILLY BOWLEGS FESTIVAL *second week in June*, Fort Walton Beach, Okaloosa Co., in Northwest Florida, to remember when pirates took over the city. "Captain Billy Bowlegs, a real pirate who ruled the area in the late 1700s, storms the city on his pirate ship 'Blackhawk' and takes over the city for a week of pageantry and fun." Parades, arts and crafts show, international food fair, ballet and concerts in the park, fireworks, sailboat regattas, Midnight Run, golf and softball tournaments, Krewe coronation, big bands, jazz, country-western music. FOODS SERVED: international. ADMISSION: free. ACCOMMODATIONS: motels and hotels, B&B's, campgrounds, RV parks. RESTAURANTS: fast foods, family, elegant, Asian, Greek, French, Mexican. CONTACT: Greater Fort Walton Beach Chamber of Commerce, P.O. Box 640, Fort Walton Beach, FL 32549, (904) 244-8191. 100,000

FLORIDA PRO *Labor Day weekend (early September)*, Sebastian Inlet State Park, Brevard Co., benefiting kidney dialysis research and treatment. Professional surfers compete for $10,000 purse, bikini contests, lots of water events, entertainers such as Juice Newton, Piece by Piece, and Dick Jones. FOODS SERVED: international, fast foods. ADMISSION: $1.50 per day. ACCOMMODATIONS: motels and hotels, campgrounds, RV parks. RESTAURANTS: family. CONTACT: American Professional Surfers, P.O. Box 1370, Cocoa Beach, FL 32931, (305) 783-5813. 80,000

DESTIN SEAFOOD FESTIVAL *first weekend in October*, Destin, Okaloosa Co., at the Kelly Docks. Entertainment, arts and crafts, 10k races, lots of food booths. FOODS SERVED: locally caught and prepared seafood, ethnic foods. ADMISSION: free. ACCOMMODATIONS: motels and hotels, campgrounds, RV parks. RESTAURANTS: fast foods, family, elegant, seafood. CONTACT: Destin Chamber of Commerce, P.O. Box 8, Destin, FL 32541, (904) 837-6241. 25,000

FALL FESTIVAL *second Saturday in October,* Lakeland, Polk Co., in Munn Park in Lakeland's historic district. Sidewalk art show featuring work of more than 150 artists, belly dancers, cloggers, singers, and guitarists. FOODS SERVED: regional specialties. ADMISSION: free. ACCOMMODATIONS: motels and hotels, campgrounds, RV parks. RESTAURANTS: fast foods, family, elegant, international. CONTACT: Arts on the Park, 115 N. Kentucky Ave., Lakeland, FL 33801, (813) 680-2787, or the Lakeland Chamber of Commerce, Box 3538, Lakeland, FL 33802, (813) 688-8551. 7,000

JACKSONSONVILLE JAZZ FESTIVAL *second weekend in October,* Jacksonville, Duval Co., at the Florida National Pavillion in Metropolitan Park. Three-day event including piano competition, two days of jazz and food. Guest artists may include Miles Davis, Special EFX, Rare Silk, Branford Marsalis, Spyro Gyra, Tito Puente, Ella Fitzgerald, Ray Charles, Della Reese, Dizzie Gillespie, and Excelsior Brass Band. FOODS SERVED: seafood, Mexican, Italian, Greek. ADMISSION: free, patron tickets $100.00 including parking, dinner, entertainment. ACCOMMODATIONS: motels and hotels, B&B's, campgrounds, RV parks. RESTAURANTS: fast foods, family, elegant, Asian, Mexican, Greek, Italian, German. CONTACT: City of Jacksonville, 220 E. Bay St., Rm. 107, Jacksonville, FL 32203, (904) 633-2890 or Dan Kossof at WJCT Radio, (904) 353-7770. 100,000

INDIAN SUMMER SEAFOOD FESTIVAL *second weekend in October,* Panama City Beach, Bay Co. Arts and crafts, fireworks, children's rides, Ober Gatlin-burg Ski Show, Florida State University Flying Circus, entertainment such as Kris Kristopherson, George Jones, Spyro Gyra, Bertie Higgins, and area cloggers and bands, jazzercise. FOODS SERVED: seafood such as shrimp, crab, oysters, fish, funnel cakes, elephant ears, veg-ka-bobs, hot dogs, ices. ADMISSION: $1.00. ACCOMMODATIONS: motels and hotels, B&B's, campgrounds, RV parks. RESTAURANTS: fast foods, family, elegant, Asian, Italian, Mexican. CONTACT: Panama City Beach Resort Council, P.O. Box 9473, Panama City Beach, FL 32407, (904) 234-0292. 30,000

WINTER PARK AUTUMN ART FESTIVAL *second weekend in October,* Winter Park, Orange Co., on the campus of Rollins College. More than seventy-five juried artists exhibit and sell their work, awards made, music and dance including local country, jazz, folk, rock'n'roll, children's art workshops. FOODS SERVED: all-American snacks. ADMISSION: free. ACCOMMODATIONS: motels and hotels, B&B's, campgrounds, RV parks. RESTAURANTS: fast foods, family, elegant. CONTACT: Crealde Arts, 600 St. Andrews Blvd., Winter Park, FL 32792, (305) 671-1886, or the Winter Park Chamber of Commerce, P.O. Box 280, Winter Park, FL 32790, (305) 644-8281. 25,000

BOGGY BAYOU MULLET FESTIVAL *third weekend in October,* Niceville, Okaloosa Co., "to glorify the mullet, an underdog among seafoods." Large arts and crafts show featuring artists and craftspeople from southeastern states, continuous professional entertainment including country music, rock'n'roll, rhythm and blues, gospel, bluegrass, and jazz, comedy, clowns, and celebrities such as Red Holland. FOODS SERVED: mullet is the food focus, with an abundance of other seafoods such as shrimp, oysters, and gumbo, and specialties from Europe, Latin America, and Southeast Asia. ADMISSION: free. ACCOMMODATIONS: motels, campgrounds. RESTAURANTS: fast foods, family, seafood. CONTACT: Boggy Bayou Mullet Festival, P.O. Box 231, Niceville, FL 32578, (904) 678-2323. 200,000

BRANDON BALLOON FESTIVAL
fourth Saturday in October, Tampa, Hillsborough Co. Ballooning games and competition exhibits, carnival midway, Chili Cook-off; main stage and local entertainment has included the Nitty Gritty Dirt Band, Exile, and Cheap Trick. FOODS SERVED: international food pavilion and chili. ADMISSION: $3.50. ACCOMMODATIONS: motels and hotels, campgrounds, RV parks. RESTAURANTS: fast foods, family, elegant, international. CONTACT: Tampa–Hillsborough Convention and Visitors Association, Inc., P.O. Box 519, Tampa, FL 33601, (813) 223-1111 or (800) 826-8358. 50,000

JOHN'S PASS SEAFOOD FESTIVAL
fourth weekend in October, John's Pass Village, Pinellas Co., near Madeira Beach. Music, arts and crafts, entertainment, educational displays on ecology and preservation, abundance of seafood. FOODS SERVED: seafood in many forms. ADMISSION: free. ACCOMMODATIONS: motels and hotels, B&B's, campgrounds, RV parks. RESTAURANTS: fast foods, family, elegant, seafood. CONTACT: Madeira Beach Chamber of Commerce, 501 150th Ave., Madeira Beach, FL 33708, (813) 391-7373. 100,000

PIONEER DAYS FOLK FESTIVAL
fourth weekend in October, Orlando, Orange Co., at the Pine Castle Center for the Arts, in remembrance of the "Florida Pioneer Era." A step into the past and then into the present farm life of old central Florida, featuring folklife demonstrations of sugar-cane grinding and syrup making, rocking chairs, beekeeping, palm weaving, meat smoking and diddley-bow playing; farm exhibits; traditional crafts demonstrations of basketry, blacksmithing, broom making, chair caning, pottery, quilting, soap making, spinning and weaving; children's area includes storytelling, miniatures, children's art, games, tum-

bling, face painting, pony rides and moonwalk; Bass Fishing Contest, Turkey Shoot, other hunting and fishing contests, community parade; entertainment such as clogging groups, Foster Family, Ernie Maynard and Southland Express, Moses Williams on his diddley bow, and folksinger Russ Russell. FOODS SERVED: barbecued ribs, "cracker fixin's," biscuits and syrup, cakes and pies. ADMISSION: $3.00. ACCOMMODATIONS: motels and hotels, B&B's, campgrounds, RV parks. RESTAURANTS: fast foods, family, elegant, continental, Cuban, Mexican, Indian. CONTACT: Pine Castle Center of the Arts, 5903 Randolph St., Orlando, FL 32809, (305) 855-7461. 15,000

FLORIDA FOREST FESTIVAL
last weekend in October, Perry, Taylor Co. "World's Largest Free Fish Fry," King Tree Parade, antique auto show, arts and crafts show and sale, 10k Great Race, beauty pageants, fireworks, children's games, carnival, tennis tournament, state 4-H Ecology Contest, FFA Forestry Contest, banquet, local bands and entertainers, banquet features artists such as Jerry Clower, Paul Harvey, Grady Nutt. FOODS SERVED: fish and fish, southern specialties such as cheese grits and hush puppies. ADMISSION: free except to buffet and carnival. ACCOMMODATIONS: motels and hotels, campgrounds. RESTAURANTS: fast foods, family, elegant, Chinese. CONTACT: Florida Forest Festival, P.O. Box 892, Perry, FL 32347, (904) 584-5366. 50,000

GUAVA-WEEN HALLOWEEN EXTRAVAGANZA
October 31, Tampa, Hillsborough Co., in the Ybor City area of Tampa, as a "spoof of V. M. Ybor's attempt to grow guavas vs. cigars in Ybor City," a largely Cuban-American neighborhood. Parade down Ybor City's 7th Avenue, major name bands, costume balls, street dancing, and the Johnny G. Lyons Band. FOODS SERVED: "the Great Ybor City Cuban Sandwich Extravaganza— World's Largest Cuban." ADMISSION: free. ACCOMMODATIONS: motels and hotels,

campgrounds, RV parks. RESTAURANTS: fast foods, family, elegant, international. CONTACT: Michael Shea, P.O. Box 384, Tampa, FL 33601, (813) 247-4497 or the Tampa–Hillsborough Convention and Visitors Association, Inc., P.O. Box 519, Tampa, FL 33601, (813) 223-1111 or (800) 826-8358. 30,000

FLORIDA SEAFOOD FESTIVAL *first Saturday in November,* Apalachicola, Franklin Co., in the Apalachicola Bay Area, in "thanksgiving to the sea for its gifts." Arts and crafts, Florida State Oyster Shucking Championship, oyster-eating contest, Blue Crab Race, Blessing of the Fleet, Redfish Run 5k Road Race, King Retsyo Ball, street dance, antique car show, parade, live entertainment such as country-western and rock bands, gospel singing, clogging and modern dancers, sky-diving exhibitions and Air Force and Army bands. FOODS SERVED: "seafood of all kinds," barbecue, concession foods. ADMISSION: adults $1.00, children under 12 free. ACCOMMODATIONS: motels and hotels, B&B's, campgrounds, RV parks. RESTAURANTS: family, elegant. CONTACT: Florida Seafood Festival, 45 Market Street, Apalachicola, FL 32320, (904) 653-8051. 25,000

FESTIVAL OF THE ARTS *first Saturday in November,* Innverness, Citrus Co., in Central Florida. Display of arts and crafts, including traditional local crafts, performances by local dance studios, bagpipers and school bands. FOODS SERVED: concessions. ADMISSION: free. ACCOMMODATIONS: motels and hotels, campgrounds, RV parks. RESTAURANTS: fast foods, family, elegant. CONTACT: Citrus Co. Chamber of Commerce, 208 W. Main St., Innverness, Fl 32650, (904) 726-2801 or the Citrus Co. Art League, Inc., P.O. Box 32, Lecanto, FL 32661, (904) 726-1600. 8,000

HIGHLANDS ART LEAGUE SIDEWALK ART FESTIVAL *first Saturday in November,* Sebring, Highlands Co. Arts and crafts exhibits and demonstrations, street entertainment, high school band, middle school band, purchase awards. FOODS SERVED: baked goods, concessions. ADMISSION: free. ACCOMMODATIONS: motels and hotels, campgrounds, RV parks. RESTAURANTS: fast foods, family, elegant. CONTACT: Highlands Art League, P.O. Box 468, Sebring, FL 33870, (813) 385-5312. 15,000

YBOR CITY FOLK FESTIVAL *second weekend in November,* Tampa, Hillsborough Co., in Ybor City, to celebrate its ethnic history. Hispanic crafts, authentic costuming from the diverse ethnic groups of Ybor City, Santeria, old-time vendors, street singers and musicians, folklore, including more than 100 performers during the three days of festivities. FOODS SERVED: Hispanic from Spain and Cuba, Italian. ADMISSION: free. ACCOMMODATIONS: motels and hotels, campgrounds, RV parks. RESTAURANTS: fast foods, family, elegant, international. CONTACT: Joan Jennewein, P.O. Box 5421, Tampa, FL 33675, (813) 247-1434 or the Tampa–Hillsborough Convention and Visitors Association, Inc., P.O. Box 519, Tampa, FL 33601, (813) 223-1111 or (800) 826-8358. 20,000

COLLARD FESTIVAL *fourth Saturday in November,* Ponce de Leon, Holmes Co., in the Northwest Florida Panhandle to recognize "the lowly collard greens." Arts and crafts show, fine arts show, gopher race, horseshoe-throwing contest, cloggers, country-western bands, clowns, timber-industry display. FOODS SERVED: collard greens along with "typical southern dinner." ADMISSION: free, charge for the dinner. ACCOMMODATIONS: motels and hotels, campgrounds, RV parks. RESTAURANTS: fast foods, family, elegant. CONTACT: Delbert Young or LaVerral Fox, R & L Fox Realty, Inc., P.O. Box 247, Ponce de Leon, FL 32455, (904) 836-4747. 1,500

ST. CLOUD ART FESTIVAL *first weekend in December,* St. Cloud, Osceola Co., in Central Florida to benefit local charities. Juried art show and demonstrations of arts and crafts including oils and acrylics, watercolors, graphics, pastels, sculpture, photography, country crafts; cloggers, school bands and choruses, magician, Indians. FOODS SERVED: concessions and salt water taffy. ADMISSION: free. ACCOMMODATIONS: motels and hotels, campgrounds, RV parks. RESTAURANTS: fast foods, family. CONTACT: St. Cloud Junior Woman's Club, Inc., P.O. Box 522, St. Cloud, FL 32769, (305) 892-8200. 10,000

PALM HARBOR ARTS, CRAFTS, AND MUSIC FESTIVAL *first weekend in December,* Palm Harbor, Pinellas Co. Arts and crafts show featuring artists from all over the United States, continuous musical entertainment including folk, bluegrass, and contemporary music. FOODS SERVED: "20–25 food vendors from meals to snacks." ADMISSION: free. ACCOMMODATIONS: motels and hotels, campgrounds, RV parks. RESTAURANTS: fast foods, family, elegant. CONTACT: Greater Palm Harbor Area Chamber of Commerce, 1000 U. S. 19 North, Suite 300, Palm Harbor, FL 33563, (813) 787-1776. 30,000

GEORGIA

ST. PATRICK'S FESTIVAL *March 7– March 22,* Dublin, Laurens Co., in the Magnolia Midlands, to celebrate St. Patrick's Day. "The largest Dublin outside the Emerald Isle celebrates St. Patrick's Day longer and harder than any city in America or Ireland." Leprechaun Contest, Miss Emerald City Pageant, contemporary crafts and folk art, theatrical presentation, softball, tennis, and golf tournaments, Irish feast and fashions, Teenage Skater's Ball, St. Patrick's Ball, parade, jazz festival, Mini-Leprechaun 2mi. Race, Leprechaun 10k Race, Masquerade Ball and Bash, Irish Invitational Speed Meet, appearances by runners such as Bill Rogers, entertainment by the Air Lingus Airline group from Dublin, Ireland, and Dr. Billy Dodd and his jazz friends. FOODS SERVED: Irish beefstew luncheon, pancake supper, lots of Irish food. ADMISSION: free, charge for some events up to $7.50. ACCOMMODATIONS: motels and hotels, campgrounds, RV parks. RESTAURANTS: fast foods, family, elegant, Chinese, Mexican. CONTACT: Dublin–Laurens Co. Chamber of Commerce, P.O. Box 818, Dublin, GA 31040, (912) 272-5546. 50,000

OLD SOUTH CELEBRATION *first three weekends in April,* Stone Mountain Park, DeKalb Co., in recognition of antebellum plantations. Nineteenth-century arts, crafts, music, storytelling, cooking, exhibits, and Civil War reenactments. FOODS SERVED: "southern and simple, open-hearth cooking and sampling." ADMISSION: adults $2.50, children 6–11 $1.50, $4.00 per car entry fee to park. ACCOMMODATIONS: motels and hotels, campgrounds. RESTAURANTS: fast foods, family, Chinese. CONTACT: Public Relations Dept., Stone Mountain Park, P.O. Box 778, Stone Mountain, GA 30086, (404) 498-5637. 30,000

LINDBERGH DAYS: A FESTIVAL OF LIGHT *April 25,* Americus, Sumter Co., at Southern Field outside Americus in recognition of the solo flight made by Charles Lindbergh originating from Southern Field and as a salute to all aviators. Static air display of vintage planes, aviation pioneers speak, display of Lindbergh memorabilia, Army and other military band concerts, high school "show choir," Georgia Southwestern College band and music students perform, other high school bands. FOODS SERVED: southern. ADMISSION: $2.00. ACCOMMODATIONS: motels and hotels, B&B's, campgrounds, RV parks. RESTAURANTS: fast foods, family, elegant, Chinese. CONTACT: Americus–Sumter Co. Chamber of Commerce, 400 W. Lamar St., Americus, GA 31709-3473, (912) 924-2646. 8,000

SPRINGFEST AND BBQ PORK COOK-OFF *first weekend in May,* Stone Mountain Park, DeKalb Co., near Atlanta. More than 150 artists, BBQ Pork Cook-off, clogging festival, crafts sale, country-music festival. FOODS SERVED: "strictly southern" featuring barbecued pork. ADMISSION: free except $4.00 entry per car to park. ACCOMMODATIONS: motels and hotels, campgrounds. RESTAURANTS: fast foods, family, Chinese. CONTACT: Public Relations Dept., Stone Mountain Park, P.O. Box 778, Stone Mountain, GA 30086, (404) 498-5637. 50,000

PRATER'S MILL COUNTRY FAIR *Mother's Day (early May) and second weekend in October,* Dalton, Whitfield Co., at Prater's Mill, in the foothills of the Appalachian Mountains. Arts and crafts including the works of recognized artists, new talents, and craftspeople producing traditional crafts such as blacksmithing, spinning, weaving, and "Dalton's famous hand-tufted bedspread-making." Entire festival reflects life at the turn-of-the-century including an operational 1855 grist mill, corn grinding, 1800s music such as fiddlers, gospel singers, and square dancers, juggler, magician, cloggers, country bands, and singers, pony rides, canoe rides, and cartoon animals wander around the grounds. FOODS SERVED: country cooking and southern such as greens, cornbread, deep-pit barbecue, fried pork rinds, soup, churned ice cream, baked breads, fried pies, funnel cakes. ADMISSION: adults $3.00, children 12 and under free. ACCOMMODATIONS: motels and hotels, B&B's, campgrounds, RV parks. RESTAURANTS: fast foods, family, elegant, Asian, Mexi-

can, Greek, Italian. CONTACT: The Prater's Mill Foundation, 216 Riderwood Dr., Dalton, GA 30722 or the Dalton–Whitfield Chamber of Commerce, P.O. Box 99, Dalton, GA 30722, (404) 278-7373. 40,000

VIDALIA ONION FESTIVAL *third weekend in May,* Vidalia, Toombs Co., to celebrate the sweet onion harvest. Arts and crafts, Onion Festival Cooking School, Sweet Onion Cook-off, Vidalia Onion Eating Contest, Onion Fun Run (2mi.), Onion Run (10,000m), beauty pageant, street dance, rodeo; tennis, golf, and volleyball tournaments, Sweet Onion Century Ride Bike Race, prayer breakfast, Nashville country band, jazz, gospel singers. FOODS SERVED: Vidalia sweet onion concoctions, other southern specialties. ADMISSION: free, arts and crafts $2.00–$3.00. ACCOMMODATIONS: motels and hotels, campgrounds, RV parks nearby. RESTAURANTS: fast foods, family, elegant, Chinese, Greek. CONTACT: Vidalia Onion Festival, P.O. Box 1213, Vidalia, GA 30474, (912) 537-4466, or the Vidalia Chamber of Commerce, P.O. Box 306, Vidalia, GA 30474, (912) 537-4466. 70,000

GEORGIA FOLK FESTIVAL *Memorial Day weekend (late May),* Eatonton, Putnam Co., to recognize Georgia's folk history. Arts and crafts, demonstrations of blacksmithing, soap making, storytelling, sheep-shearing, yarn spinning, painting, cooking, folk singing, dancing, all using old-fashioned instruments. FOODS SERVED: "old southern foods." ADMISSION: adults $3.00, youth $1.00. ACCOMMODATIONS: motels and hotels, B&B's, campgrounds. RESTAURANTS: fast foods, family. CONTACT: Rock Eagle 4–H Center, Eatonton, GA 31024, (404) 485-2831, or the Eatonton–Putnam Chamber of Commerce, P.O. Box 656, Eatonton, GA 31024, (404) 485-7701. 6,000

PUTNAM CO. DAIRY FESTIVAL *first Saturday in June,* Eatonton, Putnam Co., in Courthouse Square, in recognition of the local dairy industry. Road races, 10k

and 1 mi Fun Run, arts and crafts, live entertainment including cloggers, gospel singers, country music, puppet shows, beauty contest, parade. FOODS SERVED: barbecue; free milk, cheese, and ice cream; concessions. ADMISSION: free. ACCOMMODATIONS: motels and hotels, B&B's, campgrounds. RESTAURANTS: fast foods, family. CONTACT: Eatonton–Putnam Chamber of Commerce, P.O. Box 656, Eatonton, GA 31024, (404) 485-7701. 15,000

WINTERVILLE MARIGOLD FESTIVAL *weekend after Father's Day (late June)*, Winterville, Clarke Co., in the Athens area to salute locally grown marigolds, "the friendship flower." Arts and crafts, parade, clogging, beauty pageant, crafts demonstrations, gospel singing in the park, bluegrass, dances, entertainers such as Kenny Rogers and Marianne Gordon. FOODS SERVED: "all kinds." ADMISSION: free. ACCOMMODATIONS: (in Athens) motels and hotels, B&B's, campgrounds. RESTAURANTS: fast foods, family, elegant, Asian, Mexican, Greek. CONTACT: Winterville Marigold Festival, City Hall, P.O. Box 306, Winterville, GA 30683 or the Athens Area Chamber of Commerce, P.O. Box 948, Athens, GA 30603, (404) 549-6800. 15,000

POWERS' CROSSROADS COUNTRY FAIR & ART FESTIVAL *Labor Day weekend (early September)*, Powers' Crossroads, 12 miles west of Newnan, Coweta Co. More than 300 artists and craftspeople display and demonstrate, authentic syrup mill and grist mill, marching and military bands, bluegrass music by the Bullsboro Bluegrass Band, U. S. Marine Drum and Bugle Corps, square dancing, and the Sugar Cane Cloggers. FOODS SERVED: home-cooked southern foods including barbecued pork and chicken. ADMISSION: adults $3.00, children 5–12 $1.00, children 4 and under free. ACCOMMODATIONS: (in area) motels and hotels, B&B's, campgrounds. RESTAURANTS: fast foods, family, elegant, Mexican, Chinese. CONTACT: Coweta Festivals, Inc., P.O.

Box 899, Newnan, GA 30264, (404) 253-6361. 60,000

YELLOW DAISY FESTIVAL *first weekend after Labor Day (mid-September)*, Stone Mountain Park, DeKalb Co., to recognize the "rare Confederate Daisy growing only around Stone Mountain." More than 450 artists and craftspeople, bluegrass music and fiddle competitions, bluegrass jam sessions, mandolin and guitar competition, flower show, cloggers, square dancers, lots of bands, Curb Market featuring fresh produce, cloggers, hog calling contest, Bojangles, Showcase of Stars, big-name entertainment in the coliseum. FOODS SERVED: southern specialties such as barbecued ribs, beef, and pork, baked beans, Brunswick stew, salad bar and fruit. ADMISSION: free, charges for BBQ Buffet, $4.00 per car entry-fee to park. ACCOMMODATIONS: motels and hotels, campgrounds. RESTAURANTS: fast foods, family, Chinese. CONTACT: Public Relations Dept., Stone Mountain Park, P.O. Box 778, Stone Mountain, GA 30086, (404) 498-5637. 150,000

BARNESVILLE BUGGY DAYS *third weekend in October*, Barnesville, Lamar Co., in recognition of Barnesville as the 1800s "Buggy Capital of the South." Arts and crafts festival, parade, street dance, beauty pageant, tours of homes, steam engine train, greased-pig chase, local bands, cloggers, square dancing, magicians, gospel singing. FOODS SERVED: barbecued pork and chicken, funnel cakes, concessions. ADMISSION: free. ACCOMMODATIONS: motel, B&B, campgrounds. RESTAURANTS: fast foods, family, elegant. CONTACT: Chamber of Commerce, City Hall, 109 Forsyth St., Barnesville, GA 30204, (404) 358-2732. 40,000

HERITAGE HOLIDAYS *third week and weekend in October*, Rome, Floyd Co., in the Coosa Valley area. Riverboat rides, wagon train and trail ride, parade, arts and crafts fair, clogging, rock dances, historical tours, performances by chorus groups, local theatrical groups, country and rock groups, and regional television personalities. FOODS SERVED: southern. ADMISSION: free, arts and crafts fair— adults $2.00, children $1.00. ACCOMMODATIONS: motels and hotels, campgrounds, RV parks. RESTAURANTS: fast foods, family, elegant, Greek, Italian, Mexican, Chinese. CONTACT: Heritage Holidays, Inc., P.O. Drawer H, Rome, GA 30163, (404) 291-3819. 15,000

GEORGIA SWEET POTATO FESTIVAL *last Saturday in October,* Ocilla, Irwin Co., to celebrate the sweet potato harvest. Arts and crafts, beauty pageant, cooking contests featuring sweet potatoes and other southern specialties, parade, "twenty-one stars from the West Coast" including Robert Fuller and Joseph Mascola. FOODS SERVED: sweet potatoes and lots of others. ADMISSION: free. ACCOMMODATIONS: motel, RV park. RESTAURANTS: fast foods, family, elegant. CONTACT: Ocilla Business Association, Irwin Co. Chamber of Commerce, P.O. Box 104, Ocilla, GA 31774, (912) 468-9114. 15,000

LOUISIANA

RIVER CITY BLUES FESTIVAL *first weekend in April (rain date second weekend in April),* Baton Rouge, East Baton Rouge Parish, downtown. Legendary bluesmen from Baton Rouge and the surrounding areas perform blues music all day long. FOODS SERVED: lots of food and drink. ADMISSION: free. ACCOMMODATIONS: motels and hotels, B&B's, campgrounds, RV parks. RESTAURANTS: fast foods, family, elegant, international, Cajun. CONTACT: Baton Rouge Convention and Visitors Bureau, P.O. Drawer 4149, Baton Rouge, LA 70821, (504) 383-1825.

FESTFORALL *Memorial Day weekend (late May),* Baton Rouge, East Baton Rouge Parish. Juried arts and crafts show and sale, craftspeople's demonstrations such as wicker, wood carving, weaving and quilting, children's village, video expo, face painting, mimes, clowns, performances by the Baton Rouge Ballet Theatre, the Bell Ringers, blues and rock groups, zydeco groups, gospel and folk singers, classical musicians, Children's Theatre, mid-eastern dancers. FOODS SERVED: Cajun, Asian, sausage and crawfish breads, funnel cakes, concessions. ADMISSION: free. ACCOMMODATIONS: motels and hotels, RV parks nearby. RESTAURANTS: fast foods, family, elegant, many ethnic selections. CONTACT: River City Festivals Association, 427 Laurel St., Baton Rouge, LA 70801, (504) 344-3328, or the Greater Baton Rouge Chamber of Commerce, P.O. Box 3217, Baton Rouge, LA 70821, (504) 381-7125. 250,000

LOUISIANA BALLOON FESTIVAL AND AIRSHOW *fourth weekend in May,* Hammond, Tangipahoa Parish, at the Municipal Airport. Balloon races, military display, carnival, fireworks, air show, and live entertainment. FOODS SERVED: southern. ADMISSION: charge. ACCOMMODATIONS: motels and hotels, campgrounds, RV parks. RESTAURANTS: fast foods, family, Cajun, seafood. CONTACT: Hammond Chamber of Commerce, P.O. Box 1458, Hammond, LA 70404, (504) 345-4457.

MUDBUG MADNESS *last weekend in May,* Shreveport, Caddo Parish, in the Ark–La–Tex area, to recognize the crawfish. Mudbug (crawfish) Eating Contest, street dance; local and regional entertainers includes Cajun and country music. FOODS SERVED: Cajun, crawfish. ADMIS-

SION: free. ACCOMMODATIONS: motels and hotels, B&B's, campgrounds, RV parks. RESTAURANTS: fast foods, family, elegant, international, Cajun. CONTACT: Shreveport Chamber of Commerce, P.O. Box 20074, Shreveport, LA 71120, (318) 226-8521. 15,000

JAMBALAYA FESTIVAL AND ART SHOW *second weekend in June,* Gonzales, Ascension Parish, on Burnside Street. Crafts, bicycle races, art show, carnival, live entertainment. FOODS SERVED: lots of southern food and seafood, beverages. ADMISSION: free. ACCOMMODATIONS: motels and hotels, campgrounds. RESTAURANTS: fast foods, family, southern. CONTACT: Greater Gonzales Chamber of Commerce, P.O. Box 1204, Gonzales, LA 70737, (504) 647-7487.

BLACK ARTS FESTIVAL *mid-June,* Shreveport, Caddo Parish, in the Ark–La–Tex area, to celebrate Black culture and artistic talents of Black residents of the area. Arts, crafts, and entertainment including local and regional Cajun and Black music bands. FOODS SERVED: "southern style." ADMISSION: free. ACCOMMODATIONS: motels and hotels, B&B's, campgrounds, RV parks. RESTAURANTS: fast foods, family, elegant, international, Cajun. CONTACT: Gloria Gipaon at (318) 221-7964 or the Shreveport Chamber of Commerce, P.O. Box 20074, Shreveport, LA 71120, (318) 226-8521. 5,000

GOSPEL MUSIC FESTIVAL *third Saturday in June,* Baton Rouge, East Baton Rouge Parish, at Catfish Town Marketplace. Gospel groups, solo artists, a capella choirs, gospel puppet shows, clowns, and contemporary Christian music groups perform all day. ADMISSION: free. ACCOMMODATIONS: motels and hotels, B&B's, campgrounds, RV parks. RESTAURANTS: fast foods, family, elegant, international, Cajun. CONTACT: Baton Rouge Convention and Visitors Bureau, P.O. Drawer 4149, Baton Rouge, LA 70821, (504) 383-1825.

CAJUN BASTILLE DAY *second weekend in July,* Baton Rouge, East Baton Rouge Parish, at Catfish Town Marketplace. Three-day showcase of Cajun music, dance, cultural exhibits, films, children's activities, all emphasizing Louisiana's French heritage. ADMISSION: free. ACCOMMODATIONS: motels and hotels, B&B's, campgrounds, RV parks. RESTAURANTS: fast foods, family, elegant, international, Cajun. CONTACT: Baton Rouge Convention and Visitors Bureau, P.O. Drawer 4149, Baton Rouge, LA 70821, (504) 383-1825.

NATCHITOCHES–NORTHWEST-ERN FOLK FESTIVAL *third weekend in July,* Natchitoches, Natchitoches Co., at Prather Coliseum on the Northwestern State University of Louisiana campus, to celebrate Louisiana folk art. Forty crafts booths, many displays, three music stages featuring local and regional artists in twenty-five musical groups performing Cajun, blues, bluegrass, and traditional Anglo-American music, big-name stars, crafts workshops, "talking sessions on feature exhibit," films, videos. FOODS SERVED: fifteen food booths offer Cajun, Creole, Afro-American, Anglo-American, Indian, Spanish foods. ADMISSION: Friday and Saturday daytime concerts, adults $5.00, children $3.00; Friday and Saturday night concerts, adults $4.00, children free. ACCOMMODATIONS: motels and hotels, B&B's, campgrounds, RV parks. RESTAURANTS: fast foods, family, elegant, Chinese, Cajun, Creole. CONTACT: Donald W. Hatley, Director, Louisiana Folklife Center, Box 3663 NSU, Natchitoches, LA 71497-0014, (318) 357-4332. 20,000

LOUISIANA SHRIMP AND PETROLEUM FESTIVAL *Labor Day weekend (early September),* Morgan City, St. Mary Parish, to celebrate the shrimp and petroleum industries' significance to the area. Historic Blessing of the Fleet ceremony, water parade, fireworks display, arts and crafts show, outdoor Catholic mass, children's day activities, street fair, corona-

tion court and pageant, street parade, food fest, music in the park by performers such as Pierre Descant, Impulse, Lagniappe on the Bayou Festival Singers, U.S. Air Force Band, Red Alert, and Bah-Humbug. FOODS SERVED: "famous Cajun cuisine." ADMISSION: free. ACCOMMODATIONS: motels and hotels, campgrounds. RESTAURANTS: fast foods, family, elegant, Chinese, Mexican, Cajun, Creole. CONTACT: Benny Villa, P.O. Box 103, Morgan City, LA 70381, (504) 385-0703 or the Atchafalaya Delta Tourist Commission, P.O. Box 2332, Morgan City, LA 70381, (504) 395-4905. 75,000

FESTIVALS ACADIENS *third weekend in September,* Lafayette, Lafayette Parish, in Acadiana, to celebrate the Cajun culture and its development since the first Acadiens settled in Louisiana after leaving a French colony in eastern Canada. Lafayette is known as "the capital of French Louisiana." Cajun Music Festival features the sounds of centuries-old folk music sung in French and intended to inspire dancing. The Bayou Food Festival offers Cajun cooking from crawfish gumbo to alligator sausage and corn maque-chou, combining the flavors of France, Spain, Africa, Germany, and the Gulf Coast. The Louisiana native crafts festival features handmade Cajun crafts and demonstrations of works such as blacksmiths, duck decoy carvers to storytellers and alligator skinners. Businessmen and tradesmen display products of modern Acadiana, a midway with rides, games, and petting zoo. The University Art Museum hosts the Louisiana Film/Video Festival and the Louisiana contemporary crafts festival showcases "the best craftsmen and women working in clay, wood, fiber, glass, leather, quilting, and metal." The University of Southwestern Louisiana hosts its annual Deep South Writers' Conference highlighted by lectures and workshops featuring published authors from throughout the country, storytelling, and preservation of the Acadian language and history. The RSVP Senior Fair and Craft Show offers for sale a variety of arts and crafts created by the senior citizens of Acadiana. FOODS SERVED: Cajun! ADMISSION: most events free, charges for Writers' Conference, native crafts festival, and the Jaycees' Acadiana Fair and Trade Show. ACCOMMODATIONS: motels and hotels, B&B's, campgrounds, RV parks. RESTAURANTS: fast foods, family, elegant, Cajun (French-Acadien), international. CONTACT: Lafayette Convention & Visitors Commission, P.O. Box 52066, Lafayette, LA 70505, (318) 232-3808. 130,000

RAYNE FROG FESTIVAL *third weekend in September,* Rayne, Acadia Parish, to herald the frog in the "Frog Capital of the World." Opening "Fais-do-do" features Cajun music, Frog Eating Contest in which contestants are judged both on speed and table manners, Frog Festival Run, Diaper Derby, Little Mr. and Miss Tadpole, golf and tennis tournaments, frog racing and jumping contests, Catholic mass, cooking contest. FOODS SERVED: frogs and Cajun, concessions. ADMISSION: free. ACCOMMODATIONS: motels and hotels, campgrounds. RESTAURANTS: fast foods, family, Cajun. CONTACT: Frog Festival, Rayne Chamber of Commerce and Agriculture, P.O. Box 383, Rayne, LA 70578, (318) 334-2332. 70,000

RED RIVER REVEL *first week in October,* Shreveport, Gaddo Parish, in Ark–La–Tex area, to celebrate the arts. Arts and crafts displays and sales, demonstrations, children's workshops, film festival, live performances by stars such as Irma Thomas, Neville Brothers, A-Train, a Tribute to Leadbelly. FOODS SERVED: Cajun, Italian, Greek, Mexican, and American. ADMISSION: free. ACCOMMODATIONS: motels and hotels, B&B's, campgrounds, RV parks. CONTACT: Director of Red River Revel, City of Shreveport Parks and Recreation, 800 Snow St., Shreveport, LA 71101, (318) 424-4000. 400,000

INTERNATIONAL ALLIGATOR FESTIVAL *third weekend in October,* Franklin,

St. Mary Parish, in Acadiana, to celebrate the end of alligator-harvest season. Alligator Cooking Contest, Alligator Eating Contest, giant auction, pre-festival dance, crafts booths, game and fun booths, music by the Fa-Tras Cajun Band, Atchafalaya, and other local artists and musicians. Pre-festival tours by local alligator trappers can be arranged, as can slide and film presentations for groups. FOODS SERVED: alligator sauce piquant, fried alligator, alligator boudin, Acadien and concession foods. ADMISSION: free, pre-festival dance $15.00. ACCOMMODATIONS: motels and hotels, B&B's, campgrounds, RV parks. RESTAURANTS: fast foods, family, elegant, Chinese, Cajun. CONTACT: International Alligator Festival, St. John and Hanson Schools, 903 Anderson St., Franklin, LA 70538, (318) 828-3487. 8,000

NATCHITOCHES CHRISTMAS FESTIVAL OF LIGHTS *first Saturday in December,* Natchitoches, Natchitoches Parish, downtown. Festival Run, all-day entertainment on the riverbank stage, Junior Parade, Main Parade, fireworks, Christmas lights turned on after fireworks, parade's grand marshalls have included George Peppard, Lorne Green, Deidre Hall, Vanna White, and Ron Hale. FOODS SERVED: Natchitoches meat pie and its variations, concessions. ADMISSION: $2.00 per car. ACCOMMODATIONS: motels and hotels, B&B's, campgrounds, RV parks. RESTAURANTS: fast foods, family, elegant, Chinese. CONTACT: Natchitoches Chamber of Commerce, P.O. Box 3, Natchitoches, LA 71458-0003, (318) 352-4411. 150,000

MISSISSIPPI

WORLD CATFISH FESTIVAL *first Saturday in April,* Belzoni, Humphreys Co., on the Courthouse lawn and surrounding area, to celebrate the "Catfish Capital of the World." Arts and crafts show, Catfish Eating Contest, tours of catfish ponds, operetta for children, coronation of Catfish Queen, 10k Race, tours of Wister Garden, fiddling contest, live bands including the "Young-at-Heart Washboard Band," the Neshoba County Senior Citizens Group, and Chris Quevas on the Courthouse steps. FOODS SERVED: catfish, catfish and hush puppy lunch, Chinese, Italian, American. ADMISSION: free. ACCOMMODATIONS: campgrounds and RV parks. RESTAURANTS: fast foods, family. CONTACT: Mr. Tommy Taylor, Box 239, Belzoni, MS 39038, (601) 247-3743, or the Humphreys Co. Chamber of Commerce, P.O. Box 268, Belzoni, MS 39038, (601) 247-2616. 30,000

AMORY RAILROAD FESTIVAL *fourth weekend in April,* Amory, Monroe Co., to celebrate Amory's railroad heritage. Arts and crafts, train rides, mini-train, Hobo Parade, antique car show, fishing rodeo, 10k Run, Fun Run, Boat Show, Remote-Control Airplane Show, helicopter rides, continuous entertainment including local television personalities, bluegrass, rock, country, contemporary, and gospel music; hobo "Steam-train" Maury Graham judges the Hobo Parade. FOODS SERVED: concessions including barbecue. ADMISSION: free. ACCOMMODATIONS: motels and hotels, campground, RV parking on school campus. RESTAURANTS: fast foods, family. CONTACT: Amory–North Monroe Chamber of Commerce, P.O. Box 128, Amory, MS 38821, (601) 256-7194. 50,000

GUM TREE FESTIVAL *second weekend in May,* Tupelo, Lee Co. Art show on Courthouse Square lawn, largest 10k Run in Mississippi with 2,000 runners, 6.2mi. Run, street dance every night, super sales at all businesses, Tupelo Community Theatre presents a special production such as "Showboat" each year. ADMISSION: free, $6.00 to enter 10k Run. ACCOMMODATIONS: motels and hotels, B&B's, campgrounds, RV park. RESTAURANTS: fast foods, family, elegant, Chinese, Italian, Mexican, Greek. CONTACT: Community Development Foundation, P.O. Drawer A, Tupelo, MS 38801, (601) 842-4521. 15,000

GREAT RIVER DAYS *second or third week in May,* Aberdeen, Monroe Co. Arts and crafts show, bands, concessions, fireworks, sternwheelers, concerts and candlelight walking tour of the Aberdeen Lock and Dam. FOODS SERVED: concessions. ADMISSION: free. ACCOMMODATIONS: motels and hotels, campgrounds, RV parks. RESTAURANTS: fast foods, family. CONTACT: Aberdeen–South Monroe Chamber of Commerce, P.O. Box 727, Aberdeen, MS 39730, (601) 369-6488.

GREENWOOD ARTS FESTIVAL *fourth weekend and following two days in May,* Greenwood, Leflore Co., in the Delta area, to celebrate the arts. Art and literary contests, race and Fun Run, Jazz in the Park, Patrons Party, Sun Fest, children's activities, literary seminar, Little Theater production, parades, Cottonlandia Collectors Exhibit, in the past entertainment has included Shirley Jones, the Jackson Symphony Orchestra, Ballet Mississippi, and The Fifth Dimension. FOODS SERVED: "southern Delta hospitality" including catfish, barbecue, crawfish. ADMISSION: free to most events, charges to Patrons' Party from $17.50 to $100.00. ACCOMMODATIONS: motels and hotels. RESTAURANTS: fast foods, family, elegant, "Delta atmosphere." CONTACT: Chamber of Commerce, P.O. Box 848, Greenwood, MS 38930, (601) 453-4152. 5,000

JIMMIE RODGERS MEMORIAL FESTIVAL *last full week of May (subject to change),* Meridian, Lauderdale Co., to honor and celebrate the memory of Jimmie Rodgers, the "Father of Country Mu-

sic." "Five nights of the best country music anywhere," which has included stars such as Janie Fricke, Mel Tillis and his band, Tammy Wynette, Steve Wariner, Keith Stegall, The Kendalls, and many more, "old-time" country music and gospel singing in the park, talent contest, kickoff dance, the Bluegrass Jamboree at the Ralph Morgan Rodeo Arena, beauty pageant, commemoration services and wreath-laying ceremony, Jimmie Rodgers Memorial Run, flea market, antique car show. FOODS SERVED: barbecue and lots of other food. ADMISSION: General Admission $6.00, Reserved Seats $10.00. ACCOMMODATIONS: motels and hotels, campground, RV parks. RESTAURANTS: fast foods, family. CONTACT: Jimmie Rodgers Foundation, Inc., P.O. Drawer 2170, Meridian, MS 39302, (601) 483-JRMF. 20,000

RED HILLS FESTIVAL *Memorial Day weekend (late May),* Louisville, Winston Co., on South Columbus Avenue. Arts and crafts exhibits, 10k Race, 1mi. Fun Run, live entertainment by local and Mississippi groups. FOODS SERVED: homemade ice cream, pork skins, Polish sausage, homemade donuts, fried chicken, hamburgers. ADMISSION: free. ACCOMMODATIONS: motels and hotels, B&B's, RV parks. RESTAURANTS: fast foods, family, elegant. CONTACT: Louisville–Winston Co. Chamber of Commerce, P.O. Box 551, Louisville, MS 39339, (601) 773-3921. 5,000

MISSISSIPPI DEEP SEA FISHING RODEO *July 4th weekend,* Gulfport, Harrison Co., on the Mississippi Gulf Coast. The "World's Largest Fishing Rodeo," and Mississippi's Official Sport Fishing Classic. Fishing contests, "fun and games," rides, concessions, fish and fishing-related displays, live entertainment by several local bands on stage. FOODS SERVED: seafood galore, hamburgers, hot dogs, pizza, general concessions.. ADMISSION: free. ACCOMMODATIONS: motels and hotels, B&B's, campgrounds, RV parks. RESTAURANTS: fast foods, family, elegant. CON-

TACT: Mississippi Deep Sea Fishing Rodeo, P.O. Box 1289, Gulfport, MS 39502-1289, (601) 863-2713. 150,000

CHOCTAW INDIAN FAIR *second week in July*, Philadelphia, Neshoba Co., at the Mississippi Band of Choctaw Indians Reservation 8 miles west of Philadelphia on Highway 16. Non-Indians are welcome at this four-day celebration featuring cultural programs such as demonstrations of native arts, crafts, and dances, blowgun, rabbit-stick and dance competitions; World Stickball Series, midway, Princess Pageant, film festival, museum; grandstand entertainment includes Choctaw Social Dancers, Fancy Feather Dancers, Hoop Dancers, local and native bands and singing groups, stars recently featured include Iron Eyes Cody, Nuchie Nashoba, Nikki Watson, Paul Ott, Billy Joe Royal, Tom T. Hall, Billy Thunderkloud, John Anderson, Dottie West, Klaudt Indian Family, Jerry Reed, Gary Morris, Jim Glaser, and Steve Wariner. FOODS SERVED: Choctaw native foods, fast foods. ADMISSION: daily, adults $6.00, student $4.00; season, adult $12.00, student $10.00. ACCOMMODATIONS: motels and hotels, campgrounds, RV parks. RESTAURANTS: fast foods, family. CONTACT: Bob Ferguson or Ann Kibitlewski, The Mississippi Band of Choctaw Indians, Rt. 7, Box 21, Philadelphia, MS 39350, (601) 656-5251. 16,000

C.R.O.P. DAY (Cotton Row on Parade Day) *first Saturday in August*, Greenwood, Leflore Co., in the Delta area, to salute King Cotton. Arts and crafts, flea market, Cotton Seed Pulling Contest, mud wrestling, air show, Cotton Bale Give-Away, Historic Cotton Row office open for tours, river raft races, pony rides, summer clearance sales, live entertainment including the Parchman State Band, local rock 'n' roll groups, bluegrass bands, jazz, and cloggers. FOODS SERVED: catfish, barbecue, ice cream, watermelons. ADMISSION: free. ACCOMMODATIONS: motels and hotels. RESTAURANTS: fast foods, family, elegant "Delta Atmosphere." CONTACT: Chamber of Commerce, P.O. Box 848, Greenwood, MS 38930, (601) 453-4152. 15,000

SOUTH CAROLINA

LOWCOUNTRY OYSTER FESTIVAL *third Sunday in January*, Charleston, Charleston Co., at Boone Hall Plantation, to celebrate the abundance of Lowcountry oysters and seafood, "The Largest Oyster Festival in South Carolina." Best Dressed Oyster Contest in which public is invited to enter, regional bands and other live entertainment. FOODS SERVED: "all the steamed oysters you can eat, along with home-cooked chili and hot dogs." ADMISSION: adults $10.00 advance and $12.00 at the gate, children under 10 free. ACCOMMODATIONS: motels and hotels, B&B's, resorts. RESTAURANTS: family, elegant, seafood. ("January is Visitor Appreciation Month . . . area hotels/motels and restaurants offer discount rates.") CONTACT: Joe Sliker, Owner, 83 Queen Restaurant, Corner of King and Queen, Charleston, SC 29401, (803) 723-7591 or the Charleston Trident Chamber of Commerce, P.O. Box 975, Charleston, SC 29402, (803) 577-2510. 6,500

FLOWERTOWN FESTIVAL *first weekend in April*, Summerville, Dorchester Co., at Azalea Park, to celebrate the azaleas and "provide cultural enjoyment." More than 100 artists and craftspeople present their works; puppet shows, tours of homes in the historic district, carriage rides, balloon rides, golf tournament,

Azalea 100 Stock Car Racing, live entertainment and bands "from all over South Carolina and even some neighboring states." FOODS SERVED: Lowcountry specialties, Greek, Italian. ADMISSION: free, charges for horse-carriage ride and house tour. ACCOMMODATIONS: motels and hotels, B&B's, campgrounds, RV park. RESTAURANTS: fast foods, family, Greek, Lowcountry seafood. CONTACT: Mr. Tommy Tucker, Summerville Family YMCA, 900 Cross Creek Dr., Summerville, SC 29483, (803) 871-9622. 200,000

BETHUNE CHICKEN STRUT *second weekend in April,* Bethune, Kershaw Co., to honor the chicken. Talent show, parade, street dance, beauty contest. FOODS SERVED: "plenty of chicken" barbecued, fried, and in several other forms. ADMISSION: free. ACCOMMODATIONS: motels and hotels, B&B's. RESTAURANTS: fast foods, family. CONTACT: Kershaw Co. Chamber of Commerce, P.O. Box 605, Camden, SC 29020, (803) 432-2525. 10,000

PALMETTO BALLOON CLASSIC *second weekend in April,* Camden, Kershaw Co., in historic Camden. Arts and crafts and other exhibitors, hot air balloon races, Mass Balloon Ascension, parade, live entertainment including regional beach music groups. FOODS SERVED: concessions. ADMISSION: $4.00 per day or $7.00 for whole festival. ACCOMMODATIONS: motels and hotels, B&B's. RESTAURANTS: fast foods, family, elegant. CONTACT: Kershaw Co. Chamber of Commerce, P.O. Box 605, Camden, SC 29020, (803) 432-2525. 10,000

COME-SEE-ME *second weekend through third weekend in April,* Rock Hill, York Co., near Charlotte to celebrate the arrival of spring and the blooming of Glencairn Gardens. Art exhibits, garden tours, home tours, Gourmet Gardens, road race, bicycle race, softball and golf tournaments, children's activities, dances, live performances by Winthrop Theater Productions, Gootman Sauerkraut Band, Fantastic Shakers Band, Piedmont Highlanders Bagpipe Band, and a concert by the Winthrop College School of Music. FOODS SERVED: Greek, Oriental, Mexican, Spanish, French, American. ADMISSION: free, charges for some events. ACCOMMODATIONS: motels and hotels, campgrounds, RV parks. RESTAURANTS: fast foods, family, elegant, Chinese, Mexican. CONTACT: Rock Hill Area Chamber of Commerce, P.O. Box 590, Rock Hill, SC 29731-6590, (803) 324-7500. 50,000

ABBEVILLE SPRING FESTIVAL *first weekend in May,* Abbeville, Abbeville Co., in the Savannah River Valley, to open the summer tourist season. Crafts, flower show, photography contest, tours of historic homes, search for Confederate gold, stage play in historic Opera House, parades, live entertainment including clogging, street dance, guest stars like Stephen (Patch) Nichols of "Days of Our Lives." FOODS SERVED: variety. ADMISSION: free, home tours $8.00, charges for some events. ACCOMMODATIONS: motels and hotels, B&B's, campgrounds, RV parks. RESTAURANTS: fast foods, family, elegant, French. CONTACT: Abbeville Co. Festival Association, c/o Greater Abbeville Chamber of Commerce, 104 Pickens St., Abbeville, SC 29620, (803) 459-4600. 20,000

SOUTH CAROLINA FESTIVAL OF ROSES *first weekend in May,* Orangeburg, Orangeburg Co., to celebrate "roses blooming in the gardens" and as "a family festival for all." Large arts and crafts display in the Edisto Memorial Gardens, rose show, Basscatcher Tournament, Blackwater River Race (canoes), 10k and 2mi. Fun Runs, 10,000m Road Race, 2mi. walk, Pinewood Derby, beauty pageants, golf, tennis, and softball tournaments, Remote-Control Pattern Meet at Orangeburg, remote-control flying field, model display, model regatta and show featuring model boats, ships, airplanes, military, railroads, and other vehicles plus a miscellaneous category of animals, science fiction, doll houses, puppet shows, Bicycle Road Race; live entertainment including the Bennett Middle School Band, the Part Time Players, ventriloquist, magician, Claflin College and South Carolina State College choirs, country-western music, the Lowcountry Cloggers, and the Orangeburg Gospel Choral Union. FOODS SERVED: concessions. ADMISSION: free. ACCOMMODATIONS: motels and hotels, campgrounds. RESTAURANTS: fast foods, family, elegant, Greek, Chinese, Italian, southern barbecue. CONTACT: Orangeburg Co. Chamber of Commerce, P.O. Box 328, Orangeburg, SC 29116-0328, (803) 534-6821. 30,000

SPOLETO FESTIVAL U.S.A. *late May and early June,* Charleston, Charleston Co., to celebrate the performing and visual arts, in the spirit of Spoleto, Italy. Two–time Pulitzer Prize-winning Gian Carlo Menotti nears the end of his tenure as artistic director of the Spoleto Festival but still influences its outstanding programming and performance schedule. In the recent past operas performed include Richard Strauss' "Salome" featuring soprano Katharina Ikonomu, Jean-Philippe Rameau's "Platee," musical productions including a visiting major orchestra such as those of New York, Los Angeles, and Pittsburgh, a festival concert with The Spoleto Festival Orchestra and The Westminster Choir, thirty-two chamber music concerts, Spoleto's Finale Orchestral Concert and spectacular fireworks display; a Dance Gala, the Merce Cunningham Dance Company, Jelon Vieira Dance Brazil compete in the capoiera, a combination of dance form and martial art of the African slaves in Brazil, and the Jazz Tap Ensemble. Other artists who have performed at this festival include dancer Mikhail Baryshnikov, soprano Renata Scotto, cellist Yo-Yo Ma, and actress Colleen Dewhurst; art exhibitions and street performances. ADMISSION: $6.00–$36.00. ACCOMMODATIONS: motels and hotels, B&B's, campgrounds, RV parks. RESTAURANTS: fast foods, family, elegant, Asian, continental, Lowcountry, southern. CONTACT: Spoleto Festival, P.O. Box 157, Charleston, SC

29402, (803) 722-2764. (Note: subscription series and weekend packages available through January 31, single tickets and complete program available in February,) or the Charleston Trident Chamber of Commerce, P.O. Box 975, Charleston, SC 29402, (803) 577-2510. 75,000

APPLE FESTIVAL *first week in September,* Westminster and Long Creek, Oconee Co. Apple orchard tours, window display contest, local crafts, parade, golf tournament, Road Runners' Race, Apple Growers' Banquet, beauty pageant, square dance, clogging competition. FOODS SERVED: apple products and desserts, food booths. ADMISSION: free. ACCOMMODATIONS: campgrounds. RESTAURANTS: family. CONTACT: Oconee Co. Planning and Development Commission, P.O. Box 188, Walhalla, SC 29691, (803) 638-9585. 3,000

ATALAYA ARTS AND CRAFTS FESTIVAL *second weekend in September,* Murrells Inlet, Georgetown Co., as a salute to the visual and performing arts. Juried arts and crafts show, displays, dancing and music. FOODS SERVED: concessions. ADMISSION: free. ACCOMMODATIONS: motels and hotels, campgrounds, RV parks. RESTAURANTS: fast foods, family, elegant. CONTACT: Programs Section, State Parks Division, 1205 Pendleton St., Columbia, SC 29201, (803) 758-3622.

CATFISH FESTIVAL *third weekend in September,* Hardeeville, Jasper Co., to honor the catfish. Arts and crafts, parade, boat races, field events, country music. FOODS SERVED: catfish stew and other local delicacies. ADMISSION: free. ACCOMMODATIONS: motels and hotels, campgrounds, RV parks. RESTAURANTS: fast foods, family. CONTACT: Jasper Co. Chamber of Commerce, P.O. Box 1267, Ridgeland, SC 29936, (803) 726-8126.

THE TASTE OF CHARLESTON *third or fourth Sunday in September,* Charleston, Charleston Co., at Charles Towne

Landing, to celebrate Charleston Low-country Cooking. International food festival presents the foods and chefs of Charleston's fifty finest restaurants at one location and an opportunity to meet the chefs; waiter's race, Miss Taste of Charleston Beauty Pageant, live entertainment and "popular personalities." FOODS SERVED: international and regional cuisine. ADMISSION: $6.00. ACCOMMODATIONS: motels and hotels, B&B's, resorts. RESTAURANTS: family, elegant, seafood. CONTACT: Joe Sliker, Owner, 83 Queen Restaurant, Corner of King and Queen, Charleston, SC 29401, (803) 723-7591 or the Charleston Trident Chamber of Commerce, P.O. Box 975, Charleston, SC 29402, (803) 577-2510. 30,000

CAROLINA GOLDEN LEAF FESTIVAL *fourth week and weekend in September,* Mullins, Marion Co. Arts and crafts, home tours, beauty pageant, auctions, live entertainment. FOODS SERVED: local food booths. ACCOMMODATIONS: motels and hotels, campgrounds. RESTAURANTS: fast foods, family. CONTACT: Greater Mullins Chamber of Commerce, P.O. Box 595, Mullins, SC 29564, (803) 464-9330.

JUBILEE: FESTIVAL OF HERITAGE *fourth Sunday in September,* Columbia, Richland Co., to celebrate African-American heritage. Arts and crafts sales, storytelling, musical and dance performances, historical exhibits. FOODS SERVED: African-American and concessions. ADMISSION: free. ACOMMODATIONS: motels and hotels, campgrounds, RV parks. RESTAURANTS: fast foods, family, elegant. CONTACT: Marlena Hullum, Mann-Simons Cottage, 1493 Richland St., Columbia, SC 29201, (803) 252-1450.

MOJA ARTS FESTIVAL *first two weeks in October,* Charleston, Charleston Co., to celebrate the rich African-American culture in Charleston. Art exhibits, lectures, theatrical presentations, historic tours, jazz concerts, poetry readings.

FOODS SERVED: African-American, southern. ADMISSION: free, charges for some events. ACCOMMODATIONS: motels and hotels, campgrounds, RV parks. RESTAURANTS: fast foods, family, elegant. CONTACT: Office of Cultural Affairs, 133 Church St., Charleston, SC 29401, (803) 724-7305 or the Charleston Trident Chamber of Commerce, P.O. Box 975, Charleston, SC 29402, (803) 577-2510.

INTERNATIONAL ARTS FESTIVAL *first through second weekends in October,* Aiken, Aiken Co. Art shows, concerts, plays, dance performances, and food fairs representative of the cultures of France, China, Germany, Russia, Scotland, and Switzerland. FOODS SERVED: international. ADMISSION: charge to some events. ACCOMMODATIONS: motels and hotels, campgrounds, RV parks nearby. RESTAURANTS: fast foods, family, elegant. CONTACT: Charlotte N. Cassels, P.O. Box 2167, Aiken, SC 29802, (803) 648-3582 or the Greater Aiken Chamber of Commerce, P.O. Box 892, Aiken, SC 29802, (803) 648-0485.

AUTUMNFEST *Columbus Day weekend (near October 12),* Columbia, Richland Co., to welcome the fall season and the turning of leaves in Columbia. Crafts demonstrations, clowns, mimes, live entertainment and music. FOODS SERVED: local food booths. ADMISSION: free. ACCOMMODATIONS: motels and hotels, campgrounds, RV parks. RESTAURANTS: fast foods, family, elegant. CONTACT: Columbia Action Council, 1527 Senate St., Columbia, SC 29201, (803) 254-0253 or the Greater Columbia Chamber of Commerce, P.O. Box 1360, Columbia, SC 29202, (803) 733-1110.

SOUTH CAROLINA SWEET POTATO FESTIVAL *Columbus Day weekend (near October 12),* Darlington, Darlington Co., to salute the sweet potato crop. Arts and crafts, sweet potato recipe contest, sweet potato pie-eating contest, country-music concert. FOODS SERVED: lots of sweet potatoes. ADMISSION: free. ACCOM-MODATIONS: motels and hotels, camp-grounds nearby. RESTAURANTS: fast foods, family. CONTACT: Jimmy White, 305 Warley St., Darlington, SC 29532, (803) 662-3632 or the Darlington Chamber of Commerce, P.O. Box 274, Darlington, SC 29532, (803) 393-2641.

FALL FIESTA OF THE ARTS *third weekend in October,* Sumter, Sumter Co., at Swan Lake Gardens, to celebrate the performing and visual arts and crafts. Judged visual art and crafts show and sale with cash prizes awarded, juried young people's exhibit, live performances by local and professional talent including the Bits 'n' Pieces Puppet theatre, the South Carolina Philharmonic Orchestra, Bounce and Mademoiselle Ooo La La, and The Steel Bandits. ADMISSION: free. ACCOM-MODATIONS: motels and hotels, camp-grounds. RESTAURANTS: fast foods, family. CONTACT: Martha Greenway, County Courthouse, Sumter, SC 29150, (803) 773-1581. 15,000

OKTOBERFEST *third weekend in October,* Walhalla, Oconee Co., at Sertoma Field, to celebrate the German heritage of many Walhalla residents. Arts and crafts, carnival, sky divers, hot air balloons, live German music and dancers. FOODS SERVED: German and American. ADMISSION: adults $1.00, children, $.50. ACCOMMODATIONS: motels and hotels, campgrounds, RV parks. RESTAURANTS: fast foods, family. CONTACT: Greater Walhalla Chamber of Commerce, 203 E. Main St., Walhalla, SC 29691, (803) 638-2727. 20,000

CHRISTMAS IN CHARLESTON *November 28 through January 4,* Charleston, Charleston Co., to celebrate Christmas in the Lowcountry. Festival of Christmas Trees at the Omni Hotel, Grand Illumination on historic King Street and its Christmas decorations, parade of boats in the harbor, historic landmark walking tours, city-wide merchants' windows decorating contest, neighborhood Christmas doors competition, several theatrical presentations including the "Nutcracker," Annual Pops Christmas Concert by the Charleston Symphony Orchestra, caroling, traditional Negro spirituals, Hanukkah suppers and services, Christmas card (design) contest, holiday puppet show, holiday film festival, Concert of Champagne and Jazz at the Mills House Hotel, Christmas Parade, Charleston Renaissance Ensemble Christmas Concert, high tea at the Mills House Hotel, "Peter and the Wolf" Ballet. FOODS SERVED: Lowcountry cooking at some events, international cuisine at others. ADMISSION: free for some events, charges for others. ACCOMMODATIONS: motels and hotels, B&B's, resorts. RESTAURANTS: family, elegant, seafood. CONTACT: Charleston Trident Chamber of Commerce, P.O. Box 975, Charleston, SC 29402, (803) 577-2510. 125,000

ELGIN CATFISH STOMP *first weekend in December,* Elgin, Kershaw Co., to celebrate local catfish and its industry. Arts and crafts, parade, local and regional entertainers, live rock and country-western music. FOODS SERVED: catfish stew, fried catfish, southern fried chicken. ADMISSION: free. ACCOMMODATIONS: motels and hotels, B&B's. RESTAURANTS: fast foods, family. CONTACT: Kershaw Co. Chamber of Commerce, P.O. Box 605, Camden, SC 29020, (803) 432-2525. 10,000

MIDWEST

Illinois / 117

Indiana / 122

Iowa / 126

Kansas / 130

Michigan / 133

Minnesota / 138

Missouri / 143

Nebraska / 146

North Dakota / 148

Ohio / 149

Oklahoma / 155

South Dakota / 159

Wisconsin / 160

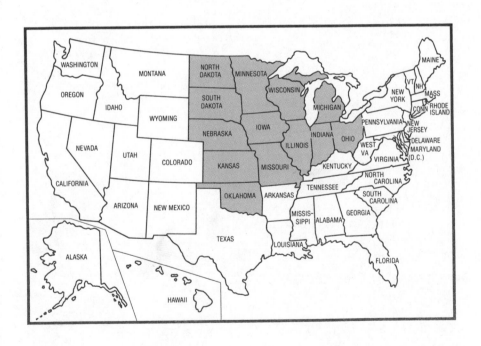

ILLINOIS

CELEBRATION: A FESTIVAL OF THE ARTS *last weekend in April,* Charleston, Coles Co., at Eastern Illinois University, to celebrate the arts. Arts and crafts exhibits and demonstrations, trumpet fanfare, 21st Century Steel Band, jazz bands, musical workshops, demonstrations of glassblowing, blacksmithing, folk art, storytellers, day-care center theatrical presentation, folk and traditional music concert, classical guitar, international students fair, Prairie Central Bluegrass, dance concert, new dance, baroque ensemble, special exhibits at the Tarble Arts Center, and a special evening performance by a big-name performer such as Burl Ives. FOODS SERVED: Dutch pastries, Polish sausage, tenderloins, baklava, turkey legs, and more. ADMISSION: free to $1.00. ACCOMODATIONS: motels and hotels, B&B's, campgrounds, RV parks. RESTAURANTS: fast foods, family, elegant. CONTACT: Dean, College of Fine Arts, Eastern Illinois University, Charleston, IL 61920, (217) 581-3110. 13,000

HERITAGE DAYS FESTIVAL *third weekend in May,* Streator, LaSalle Co., in City Park, to celebrate Streator's heritage. Open air concerts, arts and crafts, large flea market, jugglers, Civil War reenactments, Hot Cycle Race, children's rides, magicians. FOODS SERVED: ethnic foods from "German to Korean." ADMISSION: free. ACCOMODATIONS: motels and hotels, campgrounds. RESTAURANTS: fast foods, family. CONTACT: Kathy Morrison, Streatorland Historical Society, Inc., 205 W. 2nd, Streator, IL 61364, (815) 673-3186. 15,000

A TASTE OF THE ILLINOIS VALLEY *first weekend in June,* Peru, LaSalle Co., in the Illinois Valley, at the Illinois Valley YMCA. A "food festival celebrating the tremendous ethnic food specialties of the Illinois Valley in sample-sized proportions." Rides, games, crafts, auctions, live entertainment. FOODS SERVED: wide variety of ethnic foods. ADMISSION: charges for tastes, others free. ACCOMMODATIONS: motels and hotels, campgrounds, RV parks. RESTAURANTS: fast foods, family, elegant. CONTACT: Illinois Valley Area Chamber of Commerce, 300 Bucklin St., La Salle, IL 61301, (815) 223-0227.

HARVARD MILK DAY FESTIVAL *first weekend in June,* Harvard, McHenry Co., "Milk Center of the World," in the Stateline area at the border of Wisconsin and Illinois, to salute the dairy farmer. Cattle show, wee farm, Milk Day Roast, farm tours, queen contest, kiddie parade, big parade, carnival, food game, horse show, craft show, flea market, bed races, sock hop, talent show, Tractor and Truck Pull, entertainment such as Mickey Mouse, "vice-presidents' daughters, governors, senators." FOODS SERVED: southern, American, Italian, Mexican. ADMISSION: free, charges for some events. ACCOMMODATIONS: (nearby) motels and hotels. RESTAURANTS: fast foods, family, elegant, German. CONTACT: Harvard Milk Day, Inc., Municipal Building, 201 W. Front St., Harvard, IL 60033, (815) 943-4614. 77,000

DANCE OF THE NATIONS *second weekend in June,* Collinsville, Madison Co., in southwestern Illinois, to celebrate Native American Heritage. Competition dancing by nearly 600 Native American Indians, special Native American dancing and demonstrations, arts and crafts displays. FOODS SERVED: Native American. ADMISSION: free. ACCOMODATIONS: motels and hotels, B&B, campgrounds, RV parks. RESTAURANTS: fast foods, family, elegant, Chinese, Mexican. CONTACT: Southwestern Illinois Tourism and Convention Bureau, 2 Eastport Plaza Dr., Collinsville, IL 62234, (618) 344-2884. 60,000

OLD CANAL DAYS *third weekend in June,* Lockport, Will Co., in the Chicago area, to recognize the historic Illinois and Michigan Canal. Arts and crafts booths, photography, animal petting zoo, carnival rides, bingo, flea market, dunk tank, Civil War Camp, Indian Guide Encampment, mud volleyball games, parade, Pioneer Village, 10k Race, Soap Box Derby, Voyagers Landing, walking tours of the I and M Canal and Lockport Prairie, whippet (dog) races, musical entertainment such as roving musicians and stage performances at "one of the best-reserved canal towns in America." FOODS SERVED: concessions. ADMISSION: free except to Pioneer Village. ACCOMMODATIONS: motels and hotels, campgrounds, RV parks. RESTAURANTS: fast foods, family, elegant, French. CONTACT: Lockport Old Days, P. O. Box 31, Lockport, IL 60441, (815) 838-4744.

STEAMBOAT DAYS *Father's Day weekend (late June),* Peoria, Peoria Co., at Eckwood Park in the Tri-County area. Speedboat races, Homebuilt Paddlewheel Contest, water ski show, mud volleyball contest, Steamboat Classic Foot Race, arts and crafts, Miss Peoria Area Contest, baby crawl, parade of boats, bingo, live entertainment from jazz to rock. FOODS SERVED: brats, gyros, Belgian waffles, pork tenderloins, corn dogs, ice cream. ADMISSION: free. ACCOMMODATIONS: motels and hotesl, B&B's, campgrounds, RV parks. RESTAURANTS: fast foods, family, elegant, continental. CONTACT: Peoria Convention and Visitors Bureau, 331 Fulton, Suite 625, Peoria, IL 61602, (309) 676-0303. 200,000

SWEDISH DAYS *fourth week and weekend in June,* Geneva, Kane Co., to celebrate many residents' Swedish heritage. Arts and crafts including the Scandinavian art of rosemaking, entertainment on central stage, Kid's Day, parade, olympics, carnival, concessions, sidewalk sales, 10k Run, fireworks, Hot Air Balloon Rally. FOODS SERVED: Swedish buffet, American foods. ADMISSION: free. ACCOMMODA-TIONS: motels and hotels, B&B's. RESTAURANTS: fast foods, family, elegant. CONTACT: Geneva Chamber of Commerce, 5 N. Third, Geneva, IL 60134, (312) 232-6060. 100,000

OGLESBY CELEBRATION DAYS *fourth weekend in June,* Oglesby, La Salle Co. at Lehigh Park. "The famous Dannon-Oglesby 10k Road Race," 50's and 60's bands, polka bands, rock'n' roll, country music, arts and crafts show, square dancing, beer gardens, magic shows, flea market, carnival rides, fireworks. FOODS SERVED: local concessions, beer garden. ADMISSION: free. ACCOMMODATIONS: motels and hotels, campgrounds, RV parks. RESTAURANTS: fast foods, family, elegant. CONTACT: Illinois Valley Area Chamber of Commerce, 300 Bucklin St., La Salle, IL 61301, (815) 223-0227.

DIXON PETUNIA FESTIVAL *July 1–5,* Dixon, Lee Co., in the Rock River Valley, or Sauk Valley to celebrate the Fourth of July and the beautiful petunias in Page Park. Carnival, beer garden, raft race, 40's Dance, tennis tournament, flea market, art show, teen dance, big wheel race, Soap Box Derby, parade, fireworks, Taste of Sauk. FOODS SERVED: gourmet tastings from local restaurants; pancake and sausage breakfasts. ADMISSION: free. ACCOMMODATIONS: motels and hotels, B&B, campground, RV park. RESTAURANTS: fast foods, family. CONTACT: Dixon Petunia Festival Corporation, c/o Dixon Area Chamber of Commerce and Industry, 74 Galena Ave., Dixon, IL 61021, (815) 284-3361. 20,000

LINCOLNFEST *July 4,* Springfield, Sangamon Co. Parade, fireworks, nine stages with continous entertainment including stars such as Artie Shaw Orchestra, Nitty Gritty Dirt Band, Three Dog Night, Steve Wariner, Buckinghams, and Bobby Vee; special children's and junior's areas, arts and crafts, races, food booths. FOODS SERVED: Italian, Greek, German, Filipino, Spanish, American. ADMISSION: free. ACCOMMODATIONS: motels and hotels,

B&B's, campgrounds, RV parks. RESTAU-
RANTS: fast foods, family, elegant, Chinese, Thai, Greek. CONTACT: Lincolnfest,
624 E. Adams, Springfield, IL 62701,
(217) 789-2274. 250,000

TASTE CHICAGO *July 4th weekend,*
Chicago, Cook Co., at Grant Park. Forty
of Chicago's finest restaurants offer international and all-American epicurian delights, enhanced by continuous entertainment, including rock & roll, rhythm &
blues, polka, and country-western music;
concerts performed nightly by the Grant
Park Symphony Orchestra in the Petrillo
Music Shell; fireworks July 4th; Family
Oasis includes children's entertainment
such as clowns and magicians, and Parent-
Helper Tent. FOODS SERVED: see above.
ADMISSIONS: free, taste tickets six for
$5.00. ACCOMMODATIONS: hotels and mo-
tels. RESTAURANTS: fast foods, family, elegant, international. CONTACT: Mayor's
Office of Special Events, 121 N. LaSalle
St., Rm. 703, Chicago, IL 60602, (312)
744-3315. 2,400,000

WEST CHICAGO RAILROAD DAYS
second weekend in July, West Chicago,
DuPage Co., to highlight the railroad history of the community. Model railroad
show, arts and crafts, carnival, Rolling
Stock Exhibit, sidewalk sale, museum railroad exhibit, pie eating challenge, balloon
launch, slide programs on historic railroads, fireworks, 5k and 10k runs, Scheer
Brothers' Lumberjack Show of Champions, Soapbox Craze, big wheel race, baby
buggy race, 12"-softball tournament, live
entertainment by folk singer Peg Lehman,
Bruise Brothers, steel band, Wildwood
Pickers. FOODS SERVED: pig roast, corn
boil, breakfasts. ADMISSION: "most events
free." ACCOMMODATIONS: motels and hotels. RESTAURANTS: fast foods, family, elegant. CONTACT: Railroad Days Committee, P. O. Box 364, West Chicago, IL
60185, (312) 231-3004. 15,000

FIESTA DAYS *fourth week in July,* Mc-
Henry, McHenry Co. "Events for all ages

and interests," including Art in the Park,
antique car show, River Run, drum corps
show, parade, dances, banjo band, teen
nite, concert in the park, FOODS SERVED:
"variety." ADMISSION: free, charges for
some events. ACCOMMODATIONS: motels
and hotels, campgrounds, RV parks. RES-
TAURANTS: fast foods, family, elegant.
CONTACT: McHenry Area Chamber of
Commerce, 1257 N. Green St., Mc-
Henry, IL 60050, (815) 385-4300.
100,000

REDISCOVER CAHOKIA *first weekend
in August,* near Collinsville, Madison Co.,
at Cahokia Mounds State Historic Site, to
celebrate prehistoric Indian culture. Many
hands-on activities including pottery, flint-
knapping, face painting; atlatl contest, Ka-
hob and Choctaw dancing, Indian dancing,
displays of artifacts. ADMISSION: free. AC-
COMMODATIONS: motels and hotels, campgrounds. RESTAURANTS: fast foods, family, elegant. CONTACT: Cahokia Mounds
State Historic Site, Box 681, Collinsville,
IL 62234, (618) 344-5268. 13,000

**NATIONAL SWEET CORN FESTI-
VAL** *second weekend in August,* Mendota,
La Salle Co., in the Illinois Valley, as a
"Salute of the Golden Harvest" of sweet
corn. Arts and crafts fair, parades, queen
pageant, 10k Run, beer garden, tennis
tournament, water ski show, live musical
entertainment in the beer garden nightly,
and three bands on stage including "easy
listening" rock 'n' roll, 60's, drum and
bugle and marching bands, and a jazz concert. FOODS SERVED: "dozens of food concessions" including German, Bavarian,
Mexican, Japanese, Chinese, Polish, Italian, and Greek. ADMISSION: free. ACCOM-
MODATIONS: B&B, campgrounds. RES-
TAURANTS: fast foods, family, elegant,
Albanian, Chinese, Italian. CONTACT:
Mendota Area Chamber of Commerce,
Box 370 Mendota, IL 61342, (815) 539-
6507. 50,000

FRANKFORT FALL FESTIVAL *Labor
Day weekend (early September),* Frankfort,

Will Co., in the "downtown streets," to celebrate the fall harvest season in a "German town." More than 200 arts, crafts, and antiques exhibitors, carnival sponsored by volunteer fire department, street entertainment, parade, wagon tours of historic homes; lots of music including German in the beer tent, country, bluegrass, contemporary; clowns, strolling musicians, dog obedience show. FOODS SERVED: German in the beer tent, many organizations sponsor food and beverage booths along the streets. ADMISSION: free, "$2.50 to tent, redeemable for a sandwich inside." ACCOMODATIONS: motels and hotels, campgrounds and RV parks nearby. RESTAURANTS: fast foods, family, elegant, German, Italian. CONTACT: Frankfort Chamber of Commerce, P.O. Box 260, Frankfort, IL 60423, (815) 469-3356. 100,000

NATIONAL SWEETCORN FESTIVAL
Labor Day weekend (early September), Hoopeston, Vermillion Co., at McFerrin Park, to celebrate the "end of annual corn pack." National Sweetheart Pageant, talent show, children's games, antique auto show, flea market, Tractor Pull, demolition derby, 10k Race, parade. FOODS SERVED: free hot-buttered sweetcorn. ADMISSION: $1.00. ACCOMMODATIONS: motels and hotels, campgrounds, RV park. RESTAURANTS: fast foods, family. CONTACT: The National Sweetcorn Festival, c/o Hoopeston Jaycees, Box 28, Hoopeston, IL 60942, (217) 283-6057 or (217) 283-7873. 40,000

JUBILEE DAYS *Labor Day weekend (early September),* Zion, Lake Co. Queen contest, gospel rally, prayer breakfast, arts and crafts show, parade, "the best fireworks display in the county." FOODS SERVED: steer roast, sloppy joes, corn roast. ADMISSION: free. ACCOMMODATIONS: motels and hotels, campgrounds, RV parks. RESTAURANTS: fast foods, family, elegant, Greek. CONTACT: Rich Walker, Zion Park District, 2400 Dowie Memorial Dr., Zion, IL 60099, (312) 746-5500. 12,000

PEKIN MARIGOLD FESTIVAL *weekend after Labor Day (early September),* Pekin, Tazewell Co., downtown and at Mineral Springs Park, in memory of Senator Everett McKinley Dirksen and his efforts to make the marigold America's national flower. Flower show featuring marigolds, arts and crafts show, mud volleyball tournaments, big wheel races, Civil War reenactments, paddleboat racing, concerts, car show, flea market, dances, foot races, queen and princess contests. FOODS SERVED: "all kinds." ADMISSION: $6.00. ACCOMMODATIONS: motels and hotels, campgrounds, RV parks. RESTAURANTS: fast foods, family, elegant, Chinese, Italian. CONTACT: Pekin Area Chamber of Commerce, 116 S. Capitol St., Pekin, IL 61554, (309) 346-2106. 100,000

CEDARHURST CRAFT FAIR *first weekend after Labor Day (early September),* Mt. Vernon, Jefferson Co. National juried and invitational show featuring hand-crafted-work of more than 150 artists, supervised creative activities for children, performing artists such as St. Louis Levee Band, Patt Holt Singers, Stan Wagganer Show, Spatz. FOODS SERVED: "unusual" such as funnel cakes, shake-ups, tacos, meat ke-bobs, chicken strips, egg rolls. ADMISSION: free. ACCOMMODATIONS: motels and hotels, B&B's, campground, RV park. RESTAURANTS: fast foods, family, elegant, Greek, Chinese. CONTACT: Mitchell Museum Friends, P.O. Box 923, Mt. Vernon, IL 62864-0923, (618) 242-1236, or the Mt. Vernon Convention and Visitors Bureau, P.O. Box 2580, Mt. Vernon, IL 62864, (618) 242-3151. 40,000

FESTIVAL OF THE VINE *second weekend in September,* Geneva, Kane Co., in the Fox Valley, to celebrate autumn. Flavor Fare featuring "specialties of Geneva's fine restaurants" under one tent, biathalon including 10k run and 25mi. bike ride, Artists in Action, antique carriage rides, entertainment, street vendors, produce market. FOODS SERVED: see above. ADMISSION: free, charge for food tickets.

ACCOMMODATIONS: motels and hotels, B&B's. RESTAURANTS: fast foods, family, elegant. CONTACT: Geneva Chamber of Commerce, 5 N. Third, Geneva, IL 60134, (312) 232-6060. 35,000

OKTOBERFEST *second weekend in September,* Havana, Mason Co., the "Bridge to the Spoon River Country." Arts and crafts, lots of polka music, German food, beer, and wine. FOODS SERVED: see above. ADMISSION: free. ACCOMMODATIONS: motels and hotels, campground, RV parks. RESTAURANTS: fast foods, family. CONTACT: Havana Area Chamber of Commerce, P. O. Box 109, Havana, IL 62644, (309) 543-3528. 10,000

BUREAU COUNTY HOMESTEAD FESTIVAL AND PORK BBQ *second weekend in September,* Princeton, Bureau Co. Pioneer crafts, Civil War reenactment, flea market, 10,000m run, bed race, parade, car show, horse-drawn wagon rides, stage show, arts and crafts show, theatre production, street dance with orchestra, rock band in beer garden, hot air balloon rides. FOODS SERVED: pork barbecue, pancake breakfast, "all types of foods." ADMISSION: free. ACCOMMODATIONS: motels and hotels, campgrounds. RESTAURANTS: fast foods, family. CONTACT: Princeton Chamber of Commerce, 435 So. Main, Princeton, IL 61356, (815) 875-2616. 35,000

SWEETCORN AND WATERMELON FESTIVAL *third Saturday in September,* Mt. Vernon, Jefferson Co., to signal the "end of summer and beginning of fall" in what is known as the "King City." A week of activities culminates in this event featuring a two-block long flea market, parade, games, bike races, teen dances, greased-pole climb, rock and country-western music. FOODS SERVED: free sweetcorn and watermelon, barbecue, concessions. ADMISSION: "small charge." ACCOMMODATIONS: motels and hotels, B&B's, campground, RV park. RESTAURANTS: fast foods, family, elegant, Chi-

nese, Greek. CONTACT: Sweetcorn and Watermelon Festival, c/o American Savings, 12th and Broadway, Mt. Vernon, IL 62864, (618) 244-1400, or the Jefferson Co. Chamber of Commerce, P. O. Box 1047, Mt. Vernon, IL 62864, (618) 242-5725. 20,000

LITTLE VERMILLION FALL FESTIVAL *third weekend in September,* Danville, Vermillion Co., at Ellsworth Park. Arts and crafts exhibits and sales, contests, games, square dancers, ballet performances. FOODS SERVED: elephant ears, barbecue, tacos, Italian food. ADMISSION: free. ACCOMMODATIONS: motels and hotels. RESTAURANTS: fast foods, family, elegant. CONTACT: Danville Recreation Department, 100 W. Main, Danville, IL 61832, (217) 431-2272, 30,000

MORTON PUMPKIN FESTIVAL *third weekend in September,* Morton, Tazewell Co. "The Pumpkin Capital of the World!" in the Peoria area, to honor the pumpkin. "The largest, most colorful parade in Central Illinois" with 150 units and more than twenty-eight marching bands, Great Pumpkin Search, Giant Pumpkin Weigh-in, art show, auto show, Libby plant tours, Miss Morton Pageant, tennis tournament, carnival, children's art show, decorated pumpkins, flower and garden show, merchants' tent, food tent, Senior Citizens Day, kiddie parade, pumpkin cookery, Big Wheel Race, Ben Franklin Style Show, 10k and 2k Runs, pie eating contest, road rally. FOODS SERVED: pumpkin concoctions galore, pumpkin pancake breakfast, concessions. ADMISSION: free. ACCOMMODATIONS: motels and hotels, campgrounds, RV parks. RESTAURANTS: fast foods, family style. CONTACT: Morton Chamber of Commerce, 415 W. Jefferson, Morton, IL 61550, (309) 263-2491. 100,000

HONEY BEE FESTIVAL *first weekend in October,* Paris, Edgar Co. Honey exhibits throughout festival, high school homecoming, Homecoming and Honeybee Parade, Edgar County Historical Museum presents exhibits and demonstrations of early settler life including crafts such as pottery, weaving, log splitting, blacksmithing, wheat weaving, basketry, rope and soap making, quilting, lace and candle making. East Jasper Street Plaza features a flea market of crafts, food, beverages, and merchants' sales, arts and crafts galore, bluegrass music on the courthouse lawn; walking tours, 10k Run and Fun Run/Walk; vintage vehicles display on "Memory Lane," and "A Little Bit of Germany in Paris" in the Kiwanis Early Risers German Festival tent featuring German bands and groups, German food and beverages, coloring contest. FOODS SERVED: German, pancake breakfast, ham and beans, herbal concoctions, concession. ADMISSION: free. ACCOMMODATIONS: motels and hotels, campground, RV park. RESTAURANTS: fast foods, family. CONTACT: Paris Chamber of Commerce, P. O. Box 458, Paris, IL 61944, (217) 465-4179. 20,000

ETHNIC FEST FOR ALL *first weekend in November,* Peoria, Peoria Co., at the Exhibit Center of Peoria Civic Center, to recognize the "wide range of ethnic groups that live in Peoria." Ethnic arts and crafts, ethnic entertainment including dancing and singing and more than sixteen ethnic food booths. FOODS SERVED: Italian, German, French, Pakistani, Lebanese, Chinese, Jewish, Mexican, Latin American, Irish, Greek, Filipino, English, Korean, Vietnamese. ADMISSION: free, charges for food as fundraisers for each group. ACCOMMODATIONS: motels and hotels, B&B's, campgrounds, RV parks. RESTAURANTS: fast foods, family, elegant. CONTACT: Peoria Convention and Visitors Bureau, 331 Fulton, Suite 625, Peoria, IL 61602, (309) 676-0303. 25,000

INDIANA

RENAISSANCE FAIRE *fourth Saturday in April,* West Terre Haute, Vigo Co., at St. Mary-of-the-Woods College to recognize the "arts and crafts, fun and folly that dominated the Renaissance period." Juried art exhibition, full jousting tournament, several hundred actors, musicians, dancers, jesters, jugglers, knights, royalty, and village people in costume. Finale is the Jousting Tournament by Knights of Silver Sword of Chicago, musical and theatrical groups from Indianapolis and Bloomington. FOODS SERVED: Spanish, French and Italian. ADMISSION: adults $3.00, seniors and students $2.50. ACCOMMODATIONS: motels and hotels, B&B's, campgrounds, RV parks. RESTAURANTS: fast foods, family, elegant, German, Italian, Asian. CONTACT: Linda Cross Godfrey at (812) 535-5212, or the Terre Haute Convention and Visitors Bureau of Vigo Co., P. O. Box 500, Terre Haute, IN 47808, (812) 234-5555. 7,000

WABASH VALLEY FESTIVAL *last week in May,* Terre Haute, Vigo Co., at Fairbanks Park. Hydroplane races, carnival, with rides, flea market, local bands, religous music, Don Morris Band. FOODS SERVED: American and oriental. ADMISSION: free. ACCOMMODATIONS: motels and hotels, B&B's, campgrounds, RV parks. RESTAURANTS: fast foods, family, elegant, Italian, German, Asian. CONTACT: Pat Ralston at (812) 232-2727, or the Terre Haute Convention and Visitors Bureau of Vigo Co., P. O. Box 500, Terre Haute, IN 47808, (812) 234-5555. 150,000

HERITAGE DAYS FESTIVAL *third long weekend in June,* Huntington, huntington Co., to celebrate local heritage. Country marketplace, crafts and flea market, LaFontaine Art Festival, parade, 5 mi run, historic tours, bed race, all-day live entertainment. FOODS SERVED: "varied." AD-

MISSION: free, charges for some events. ACCOMMODATIONS: motels and hotels, B&B's, campgrounds, RV parks. RESTAURANTS: fast foods, family, German. CONTACT: Huntington Co. Chamber of Commerce, 12 W. Market St., Huntington, IN 46750, (219) 356-5300. 25,000

RIVERFRONT FESTIVAL *fourth Saturday in June,* Jeffersonville, Clark Co., on the Jeffersonville riverfront. Arts and crafts, fireworks, live musical entertainment, lots of food. ADMISSION: free. ACCOMMODATIONS: motels and hotels, B&B's, campgrounds, RV parks. RESTAURANTS: fast foods, family, elegant. CONTACT: Department of Redevelopment, 206 Eastern Blvd., Clarksville, IN 47130, (812) 283-7984. 18,000

THREE RIVERS FESTIVAL *Saturday after July 4,* running nine days, Fort Wayne, Allen Co. More than 250 events including arts and crafts, sports contests, celebrations of ethnic heritages, raft race, bed race, hot air balloon race, fireworks, lots of music (including concerts of rock, jazz, country, Big Band, folk, and classical), Children's Film Festival, folk art, aircraft display, boat rides, Juried Art Show, International Village, classic and current autos, farmers market, basketball, tennis, and racquetball tournaments, Jaguar Automobile Concourse, bicycle races and tour, edible wild plants hike, World's Longest Flea Market (1.2 miles), Philippine folk dancing, student paint-on, homemade wind machines, 10,000m run, Poker Rally, WQHK Bluegrass Blast/Fiddle and Banjo Contest, and much, much more! FOODS SERVED: sidewalk cafe, Hoo Sier Best Patio Chef gas grill competition, International Village featuring foods of China, Germany, Great Britain, Greece, India, Israel, Korea, Latin America, Pakistan, Philippines, Poland, Scandinavia, and the Third World. ADMISSION: most events free. ACCOMMODATIONS: motels and hotels. RESTAURANTS: fast foods, family, elegant, Indian, Chinese, Mexican, French. CONTACT: Three Rivers Festival, 2301

Fairfield Ave., Suite 107, Fort Wayne, IN 46807, (219) 745-5556. 1,300,000

IRON HORSE FESTIVAL *thrid weekend in July,* Logansport, Cass Co., to recognize railroading in Logansport. Model railroad exhibits, steam train excursions on former Pennsylvania Railroad lines, International Food Fair, arts and crafts, hot air balloon races, parade, farmers' market, Kiddies Korner, big name entertainment such as Johnny Cash, Louise Mandrell, Sylvia. FOODS SERVED: Italian, Greek, beef, and bread. ADMISSION: free. ACCOMMODATIONS: motels and hotels, campgrounds, RV parks. RESTAURANTS: fast foods, family, elegant, Chinese. CONTACT: Iron Horse Festival Association, P.O. Box 407, Logansport, IN 46947, or the Logansport/Cass Co. Chamber of Commerce, 300 E. Broadway, Suite 103, Logansport, IN 46947, (219) 753-6388. 100,00

SWISS DAYS *last Friday and Saturday in July,* Berne, Adams Co., to celebrate the Swiss heritage of many residents. Swiss folklore, Swiss travelog and films, Horse Pulling Contest, Maumee Valley Polka, Bonnet Singers, Swiss Style Show, Swiss puppeteers, gospel sing, handicapped races, Swiss Days Races, Swiss furniture making, yodeling contest, Kiddies Parade, concerts, Grand Parade, WMEE Record Hop; tours of First Mennonite Church, Swiss Village, Hitzer Stoves, softball, golf, bowling, tennis and Little League tournaments, Flower Show, pioneer crafts, German bands from Switzerland. FOODS SERVED: Swiss, German, and Amish. ADMISSION: free, charges for auditorium productions, from $4.50 to $7.50. ACCOMMODATIONS: motel, B&B, campgrounds, RV parks. RESTAURANTS: family style. CONTACT: Berne Chamber of Commerce, P. O. Box 85, Berne, IN 46711, (219) 589-2784. 35,000

BANKS OF THE WABASH DIXIELAND JAZZ FESTIVAL *weekend at the end of July and beginning of August,* Terre

Haute, Vigo Co. Dixieland jazz concerts at Fairbanks Park, farmers' market, after-hours jam session, Jazz Brunch. Performances by groups such as The Red Rose Ragtime Band, The Back Room Gang, New Reformation Jazz Band, Naptown Strutters, The Saints Dixieland Band, and Cakewalkin' Jazz Band. FOODS SERVED: New Orleans Jazz Brunch. ADMISSION: free, charges for some events. ACCOMODATIONS: motels and hotels, B&B's, campgrounds, RV parks, RESTAURANTS: fast foods, family, elegant, German, Italian, Asian. CONTACT: James Moore at (812) 299-1031, or the Terre Haute Convention and Visitors Bureau of Vigo Co., P. O. Box 500, Terre Haute, IN 47808, (812) 234-5555. 1,500

VAN BUREN POPCORN FESTIVAL *second weekend in August,* Van Buren, Grant Co., in the "Popcorn Capitol of the World." Small town fun includes big parade, crowning of the Popcorn Queen, helicopter rides, bed race, live music, arts and crafts booths and displays. FOODS SERVED: "plenty of popcorn for everyone," concessions. ADMISSION: free. ACCOMMODATIONS: in Marion. RESTAURANTS: fast foods, family style, CONTACT: Grant Co. Convention and Visitors Bureau, 215 S. Adams St., Marion, IN 46952, (317) 664-5107.

VILLAGE ART FESTIVAL *second weekend in August,* Nappanee, Elkhart Co., at Amish Acres. Guided tours of the Village, documentary movie, buggy rides, gift shops, mimes, marionettes, puppets, folk singers, fiddle music, barbershop quartets, square dancing, LaMonte's Gray Horse Band, Hoosier Square Dancers, fashion show, and more than 275 artists vying for $3,000 in prizes. FOODS SERVED: Amish style dinner, roast pork, turkey legs, roasted corn on the cob, homemade ice cream, funnel cakes, fruit. ADMISSION: $2.00. ACCOMMODATIONS: motels and hotels, B&B's campgrounds, RV parks. RESTAURANTS: family style. CONTACT: Richard Fletcher, Amish Acres, 1600 W. Market St., Nappanee, IN 46550. 50,000

TURKEY TROT FESTIVAL *first Thursday through Sunday in September,* Montgomery, Daviess Co. at Ruritan Park in recognition of turkey growing in Daviess County. Turkey races, Best-Dressed Turkey Contest, Demolition Derby, Beer Garden, Kids Day, mud volleyball, horse pulls, carnival rides, live country entertainment with stars such as Steve Wariner, Earl Thomas Conley, The Kendalls, Terry Gibb, Mel McDaniel, Barbara Mandrell and Crystal Gayle. FOODS SERVED: lots of barbecued turkey, variety of others. ADMISSION: $5.00 per day or $10.00 season pass. ACCOMMODATIONS: motels and hotels, campgrounds. RESTAURANTS: fast foods, family style. CONTACT: Daviess Co. Chamber of Commerce, Inc., P. O. Box 430, Washington, IN 47501, (812) 254-5262. 13,000

CUMBERLAND COVERED BRIDGE FESTIVAL AND ANTIQUE ENGINE SHOW *first weekend in September,* Matthews, Grant Co. More than 100 craft and flea market exhibits, queen contest, square dancing, 500 antique engines, Senior Citizens Tent, professional entertainment. FOODS SERVED: concessions. ADMISSION: free. ACCOMMODATIONS: in Marion. RESTAURANTS: fast foods, family style. CONTACT: Grant Co. Convention and Visitors Bureau, 215 S. Adams St., Marion, IN 46952, (317) 664-5107.

LAFAYESTA: FAMILY FESTIVAL OF THE ARTS *Labor Day weekend (early September),* West Lafayette, Tippecanoe Co., as a fund-raiser for the Greater Lafayette Museum of Art. Nearly 100 artists' booths and crafts demonstrations including painting, weaving, jewelry, bronzing, tatting, photography, "Sky Train" of 5,000 flying kites, children's activity area where they may try the Art Trek game, spin art, sand bottles, the graffiti wall, scratch art, oogles, and nature paper; tethered balloon rides, live entertainment such as street players, including clowns, Garcia's Flying Tomato Balloon, Raggedy Ann and Andy from Old Indiana, magicians, bluegrass bands, Sunshine Cloggers, Dance Kaleidoscope, middle eastern dancers, Sweet Adelines, magicians, Young People's Dance Theater. FOOD SERVED: "gourmet" local foods, and those of the country featured. ADMISSION: $1.00 for children, $10.00 for two-day family pass. ACCOMMODATIONS: motels and hotels, B&B's, campgrounds, RV parks. RESTAURANTS: fast foods, family, Chinese, Mexican, German. CONTACT: The Greater Lafayette Museum of Art, 101 S. Ninth St., Lafayette, IN 47901, (317) 742-1128. 10,000

LITTLE ITALY FESTIVAL *Labor Day weekend (early September),* Clinton, Vermillion Co., in this community known as "Little Italy". Italian music, dancing, entertainment, and drinking. FOODS SERVED: Italian. ADMISSION: free. ACCOMMODATIONS: motel and hotel, B&B's. RESTAURANTS: fast foods, family, Italian. CONTACT: LIFT, Box 6, Clinton, IN 47842, or the Clinton Chamber of Commerce, P.O. Box 189, Clinton, IN 47842, (317) 832-2239. 100,000

STEAMBOAT DAYS *first weekend after Labor Day (early September),* Jeffersonville, Clark Co., Parade, arts and crafts, talent show, Festival of Music, races, steamboat races and tours, lots of food booths in this city across the Ohio River from Louisville, Kentucky. FOODS SERVED: concessions. ADMISSION: free. ACCOMMODATIONS: motels and hotels, campgrounds. RESTAURANTS: fast foods, family, elegant. CONTACT: Steamboat Days Festival, 1704 Idlewood, Jeffersonville, IN 47130, (812) 949-7267. 500,000

OKTOBERFEST *second and third weekends in September,* Terre Haute, Vigo Co., to simulate the original Oktoberfest of the 1800s in Munich. Arts and crafts, German atmosphere, German music, bands from St. Louis, Chicago, Cincinnati, Cleveland, and Detroit. FOODS SERVED: German. ADMISSION: $1.00. ACCOMMODATIONS: motels and hotels, B&B's, campgrounds, RV parks. RESTAURANTS: fast foods, family,

elegant, German. CONTACT: John Phillips of the German Oberlander Club at (812) 466-9260, or the Terre Haute Convention and Visitors Bureau of Vigo Co., P. O. Box 500, Terre Haute, IN 47808, (812) 234-5555. 20,000

HOOSIER HERITAGE DAYS *third weekend in September,* Sellersburg, Clark Co., at Ivy Tech Campus. Hot Air Balloon Race, fireworks, Antique Car Show, dancing, and much more. ADMISSION: free. ACCOMMODATIONS: motels and hotels, B&B's, campgrounds, RV parks. RESTAURANTS: fast foods, family, elegant. CONTACT: Kathy Copas, 8204 Highway 311, Sellersburg, IN 47172, (812) 246-3301. 25,000

FAIRMOUNT MUSEUM DAYS *last weekend in September,* Fairmount, Grant Co., to honor the memory of Fairmount native James Dean on the date of his death, September 30. 1950s custom and antique car show, "Garfield" cat photo contest, James Dean Look-Alike and Rock Lasso contests, museum and gravesite tours, 50's dance and costume contests, arts and crafts, James Dean Memorial Tribute, showing of James Dean's three major films, Grand Parade, carnival, live entertainment including country-western singers and band, barbershop quartet, Playhouse Dance Studio, high school musicians, gospel singers. FOODS SERVED: concessions and food booths. ADMISSION: free. ACCOMMODATIONS: motels and hotels, campgrounds, RV parks. RESTAURANTS: fast foods, family, elegant, Chinese. CONTACT: Fairmount Historical Museum, Inc., 203 E. Washington St., P.O. Box 92, Fairmount, IN 46928, (317) 948-4776. 10,000

HARVEST HOMECOMING *first two weekends in October,* New Albany, Floyd Co., to celebrate local harvest and to welcome home families and students in this city across the Ohio River from Louisville, Kentucky. Big parade, arts, crafts and food booths fill a four-lane street, live entertainment including big-name stars perform in the Amphitheatre on the Ohio River. ADMISSION: free, charges for some events. ACCOMMODATIONS: motels and hotels, B&B's, campgrounds, RV parks. RESTAURANTS: fast foods, family, elegant. CONTACT: City of New Albany, 1017 Wildwood Lane, New Albany, IN 47150, (812) 945-6321. 320,000

COVERED BRIDGE FESTIVAL *second weekend through third weekend in October,* Rockville, Parke Co. Tours of covered bridges and colorful foliage, arts and crafts, antiques, waterpowered mill, melodrama by Parke Players. FOODS SERVED: "all kinds." ADMISSION: free. ACCOMMODATIONS: motels and hotels, B&B's, campgrounds, RV parks. RESTAURANTS: fast foods, family, elegant. CONTACT: Dee Smith at (317) 569-5226, or the Terre Haute Convention and Visitors Bureau of Vigo Co., P. O. Box 500, Terre Haute, IN 47808, (812) 234-5555. 600,000

IOWA

ST. PAT'S CELEBRATION *weekend closest to St. Patrick's Day (March 17),* Emmetsburg, Palo Alto Co., at St. Pat's Headquarters on Broadway, to celebrate the saint's day and the Irish heritage of local residents. Miss Shamrock Pageant, Diplomat Tea, banquet, parade, dignitaries from Ireland, bagpipe band, Irish dancers from Dublin, Ireland, Emmetsburg's sister city. FOODS SERVED: Irish stew, green beer. ADMISSION: free to most events, charge for beauty pageant and banquet. ACCOMMODATIONS: motels and hotels, campgrounds, RV parks. RESTAURANTS: fast foods, family. CONTACT: St. Patrick's Association, Emmetsburg, IA 50536, (712) 852-4326, or Emmetsburg Chamber of Commerce, 1013 Broadway, Emmetsburg, IA 50536, (712) 852-2283. 10,000

PELLA TULIP TIME *second weekend in May,* Pella, Marion Co., in South Central Iowa, to celebrate the Dutch heritage of Pella residents and to honor the leadership of settler Dominie Hendrick Pieter Scholte. Two parades daily, one in the evening, flower show of fantastic rainbow of tulip colors "in all colors and combinations," tours of the community in open wagons, historical village tours, more than 400 students perform authentic Dutch dances to traditional Dutch folk music in front of the Tulip Tower, street scrubbing, Dutch worship services, Dutch organ music, presentation of Royal Court, antique automobiles, formal tulip gardens. FOODS SERVED: Dutch, American. ADMISSION: free to parade, other events from $3.50 to $5.00. ACCOMMODATIONS: motels and hotels, B&B's, campgrounds, RV parks. RESTAURANTS: fast foods, family, elegant, Dutch. Contact: Pella Chamber of Commerce, 507 Franklin, Pella, IA 50219, (515) 628-4311. 150,000

DUBUQUEFEST *third weekend in May,* Dubuque, Dubuque Co., in the "Tri-state area (with Illinois and Wisconsin)". "Iowa's largest all-arts festival" celebrates "the rich ethnic heritage, historical architecture, and the river attractions of Dubuque on the Mississippi (River), Iowa's oldest and most romantic city." Pops concerts on the Mississippi River by the Dubuque Symphony, juried arts and crafts fair featuring the work of 150 exhibitors, plays, historic house tour, mimes, poetry readings, bike trail, cave, arboretum, children's zoo, puppet shows; entertainment such as the Senior Kitchen Band, five classical ensembles, symphony orchestra, youth ballet, cloggers, Mideast belly dancers, square dancers, clowns, New York's

Lark Quartet. FOODS SERVED: multi-ethnic including German, Malaysian, Greek, Hungarian, Dutch, Chinese, Mexican. ADMISSION: mostly free, charges for theatre performances. ACCOMMODATIONS: motels and hotels, B&B's, campgrounds, RV parks. RESTAURANTS: fast foods, family, elegant, Chinese, Italian, French. CONTACT: DubuqueFest, 422 Loras Blvd., Dubuque, IA 52001, (319) 588-9751. 50,000

TWO RIVERS FESTIVAL *early June*, Des Moines, Polk Co., to celebrate the cultural, ethnic, and historic heritage of Des Moines. Arts and crafts displays, bridge dance, fireworks, bicycle criterium, 10k Foot Race, continuous local entertainment. FOODS SERVED: "wide variety of nationalities serving ethnic foods." ADMISSION: free. ACCOMMODATIONS: motels and hotels, campgrounds, RV parks. RESTAURANTS: fast foods, family, elegant, international. CONTACT: Downtown Des Moines, Inc., 309 Corut Ave., Suite 250, Des Moines, IA 50309, (515) 286-4987. 50,000.

FRONTIER DAYS *first weekend in June*, Fort Dodge, Webster Co., to celebrate Fort Dodge's pioneer heritage. Buckskinner's Rendezvous, black-powder shoot, parade, rodeo, demonstrations of pioneer arts and skills, antique fair; live country, bluegrass, and fiddlers' contest. Frontier Days' motto "sums it all up: 'If you ain't havin' fun, you're doin' it all wrong!'" FOODS SERVED: "frontier and ethnic foods." ADMISSION: $1.00 for Frontier Days button. ACCOMMODATIONS: motels and hotels, B&B's, campgrounds, RV parks. RESTAURANTS: fast foods, family, elegant, Asian. CONTACT: Greater Fort Dodge Chamber of Commerce, Box T, Fort Dodge, IA 50501, (515) 955-5500. 30,000

NORTH IOWA BAND FESTIVAL *first weekend in June*, Mason City, Cerro Gordo Co. High school band concerts, performances by other musical groups, big parade featuring high school bands, queen coronation, street marching competition, movie premieres, appearances by Iowa-born celebrities. FOODS SERVED: concessions. ADMISSION: free. ACCOMMODATIONS: motels and hotels, campgrounds. RESTAURANTS: fast foods, family, elegant, Mexican, Chinese. CONTACT: Mason City Chamber of Commerce, P. O. Box 1128, Mason City, IA 50401, (515) 423-5724. 25,000

GRANT WOOD ART FESTIVAL *second Sunday in June*, Stone City-Anamosa, Jones Co., in "Grant Wood Country," to celebrate the heritage of the Anamosa-born artist, Grant Wood, and the historic region of Stone City. Juried art exhibits including fibers, metals, painting, drawing, photography, pottery, print-making, sculpture, stained glass, and wood; children's and adult's Art Happenings for hands-on experience, demonstrations, blacksmith shop features historical artifacts; replicas and originals of ice wagons used as homes for artists, puppet theatre, guided bus tours of Stone City area, movies of painter Grant Wood and Stone City, entertainers such as folk musicians, musical groups, jugglers, mimes, and a brass band. FOODS SERVED: "lunch stands featuring Iowa beef and pork, refreshments." ADMISSION: ages 14 and over $3.00 badge designed by badge competition winner. ACCOMMODATIONS: motels and hotels, campgrounds, RV parks. RESTAURANTS: fast foods, family. CONTACT: Grant Wood Art Festival, Inc., Box 148, Stone City–Anamosa, IA 52205, (319) 462-3561 or (319) 462-2571. 12,000

GLENN MILLER BIRTHPLACE SOCIETY FESTIVAL *June 12–13*, Clarinda, Page Co., at the Community High School, to honor big band leader Glenn Miller, his music, and his life, which ended tragically and mysteriously while flying from Paris, France to an airfield in England. Films of the famous saxophonist's life and music are presented, Glenn Miller memorabilia are displayed and traded, musical activities abound. ADMISSION: free. ACCOMMO-

DATIONS: motels and hotels, campgrounds. RESTAURANTS: fast foods, family. CONTACT: Wilda Martin of the Glen Miller Birthplace Society at P. O. Box 61, Clarinda, IA 51632 or the Clarinda Chamber of Commerce, 100 S. 15th, Clarinda, IA 51632, (712) 542-2166. 2,000

STURGIS FALLS CELEBRATION *last full weekend in June,* Cedar Falls, Black Hawk Co., to celebrate "our past and our future." Northeast Iowa competitive art show, Sturgis Falls Dixieland Jazz Fest, volksmarch, Big Wheel "500," Civil War group's major artifacts display, talent competition, Fireman's Ball, Turkey Foot Canoe Race, rugby and basketball tournaments, PGA golf tournament, Knights of Columbus horse show, family bicycle ride, teen dance, half marathon, 5k Fun Run, carnival midway, dunking booth, arts and crafts street fair, live entertainment featuring a great variety of jazz from the Maple Street Jazz Band of West Des Moines, IA, to Banu Gibson and the New Orleans Hot Jazz Orchestra, fiddles and guitars, progressive folk music, country-western, 50's, 60's, 70's, and 80's musical specialties, Cedar Falls High School Flute Choir, Sweet Adelines, jazzercise, and drill teams. FOODS SERVED: variety. ADMISSION: free to most events, charges for others. ACCOMMODATIONS: motels and hotels, B&B's, campgrounds, RV parks. RESTAURANTS: fast foods, family, elegant, international. CONTACT: Judith A. Cutler, Sturgis Falls Celebration, Inc., P. O. Box 746, Cedar Falls, IA 50613 or the Cedar Falls Chamber of Commerce, P. O. Box 367, Cedar Falls, IA 50613, (319) 266-3593. 100,000

CLINTON RIVERBOAT DAYS *July 2–5,* Clinton, Clinton Co., at Riverfront Park on the Mississippi River, in "River City America." Boat races and rides, arts and crafts, plays on showboat, carnival, parade, skydivers, professional entertainment, antique car show, mud wrestling, fireworks, tractor pull, tennis tournament. FOODS SERVED: concessions. ADMISSION: $4.00 for badge. ACCOMMODATIONS: mo-

tels and hotels, RV parks. RESTAURANTS: fast foods, family, elegant. CONTACT: Clinton Riverboat Days Committee, P. O. Box 241, Clinton, IA 52732, (319) 243-9400. 15,000

MISSISSIPPI VALLEY BLUES FESTIVAL *first weekend in July,* Davenport, Scott Co., in the Quad Cities area to celebrate the heritage of blues music. Twenty-four hours of continuous blues music featuring national and international blues stars as well as local performers in an outdoor setting on the banks of the Mississippi River. Stars might include the likes of John Lee Hooker, Son Seals, John Hammond, Jr., Memphis Slim, Ron Thompson. For two days prior to the festival, blues are played at different locations throughout Davenport, in addition to blues bands playing on riverboats. FOODS SERVED: specialties of "Quad Cities favorite restaurants." ADMISSION: $2.00 per 12-hour day. ACCOMMODATIONS: motels and hotels, B&B's, campgrounds, RV parks. RESTAURANTS: fast foods, family, elegant, Asian, Mexican, Italian. CONTACT: Gene Hellige, 4130 W. Rusholme, Davenport, IA 52804, (319) 391-2496. 50,000

CZECH FOLK FESTIVAL *third weekend in July,* Traer, Tama Co., on Second Street and at the Traer Memorial Building, to celebrate the Czech heritage of Traer residents. This small town of 1,700 swells to 15,000 for this "old-time festival set around the polka dance, which was born in Bohemia in 1830." Guests are welcome to join in the polkas and songs of old, enjoy Czech culture, the Big parade, Czech and other arts and crafts, entertainment including Jim Kucera and the Vested Czechs, Larry's Concertina Band and "The Number One Polka Band in the U.S.A.," The Czech Lites from Minnesota, Jum Busta Concertina Band, the Alpiners Polka Band, Marc Frana Concertina Sound, The Czech Artists, and the Polka Wind Up. FOODS SERVED: Czech foods and others. ADMISSION: $1.00 per person per day. ACCOMMODATIONS: motels and hotels, campgrounds, RV parks. CONTACT: Traer Czech Folk Fest, 810 First St., Traer, IA 50675 or the Traer Chamber of Commerce, 536 Second St., Traer, IA 50675, (319) 478-8660. 15,000

NORDIC FEST *last full weekend in July,* Decorah, Winneshiek Co., in Northeast Iowa, to celebrate the community's Scandinavian heritage. Scandinavian crafts demonstrations and exhibits, dancing, singing, food demonstrations and booths, Torchlight Parade, bonfire, Troll Walk, antique show and sale, road race, entertainment such as the Dorian Opera Theater's presentation of "Song of Norway," Norwegian folk singer Luther Enstad, and the Leikarring Heimhug folk dance group. FOODS SERVED: Norwegian such as kringla, krumkake, lefse, Sandbakkels, and flatbrød. ADMISSION: free. ACCOMMODATIONS: motels and hotels, B&B's, campgrounds. RESTAURANTS: fast foods, family. Nordic Fest, Inc., Box 364, Decorah, IA 52101, (319) 382-9010, or the Decorah Chamber of Commerce, 101 E. Water St., Decorah, IA 52101, (319) 382-3990. 50,000

BIX ARTS, CRAFTS, AND FOOD FEST *last full weekend in July,* Davenport, Scott Co., to recognize the life of Bix Beiderbecke, "Davenport's claim to jazz fame." Four days of jazz concerts at LeClaire Park on the Mississippi river front, two days of arts, crafts, and food in a seven-block area of downtown, and the Bix 7, a "nationally ranked 7mi. Run." FOODS SERVED: more than forty vendors provide "every type of food imaginable." ADMISSION: free, $6.00 to concert. ACCOMMODATIONS: motels and hotels, B&B's, campgrounds, RV parks. RESTAURANTS: fast foods, family, elegant, Italian, Asian. CONTACT: Downtown Davenport Association, 112 E. Third St., Davenport, IA 52801, (319) 211-1706. 70,000

NATIONAL HOBO CONVENTION *first Saturday in August,* Britt, Hancock Co., to celebrate the hobo way of life.

Hobo Jungle, coronation of King and Queen of Hoboes, parade, carnival, giant flea market, talent show, entertainment such as Night Wing from Offutt Air Force Base, presentation of "Love Rides the Rails," bicycle stunt riders, Taekwondo exhibition. FOODS SERVED: 500 gallons of Mulligan stew served free, concessions. ADMISSION: free. ACCOMMODATIONS: motel, campgrounds, RV parks. RESTAURANTS: fast foods, family. Contact: Britt Chamber of Commerce, P. O. Box 63, Britt, IA 50423, (515) 843-3867. 25,000

ART IN THE PARK *first Sunday in August,* Fort Dodge, Webster Co. at Oleson Park, to recognize the visual and performing arts. Arts and crafts, symphony and chorus in the band shell, Karl King Band, dancing, storytelling, mime, children's activities. FOODS SERVED: concessions. ADMISSION: free. ACCOMMODATIONS: motels and hotels, B&B's, campgrounds, RV parks. RESTAURANTS: fast foods, family, elegant, Asian. CONTACT: Greater Fort Dodge Chamber of Commerce, Box T, Fort Dodge, IA 51501, (515) 955-5500. 15,000

NATIONAL HOT AIR BALLOON CHAMPIONSHIPS *first weekend in August,* Indianola, Warren Co., in the Golden Circle area, to select America's hot air balloon team to compete in the World Hot Air Balloon Championships. Hot air balloons lifting off from the balloon launch site, hot air balloons flying over a target on the launch site, bands perform, fireworks, lip sync contests, local entertainers. FOODS SERVED: concessions. ADMISSION: $1.00. ACCOMMODATIONS: motels and hotels, campgrounds, RV parks. RESTAURANTS: fast foods, family, elegant. CONTACT: National Balloon Championship, Ltd., P. O. Box 346, Indianola, IA 50125, (515) 961-8415, or the Indianola Chamber of Commerce/Development Corp., 515 N. Jefferson, Suite D., Indianola, IA 50125, (515) 961-6269. 300,000

GREAT RIVER DAYS *five days beginning third Wednesday in August,* Muscatine, Muscatine Co., in Riverview Park on the banks of the Mississippi River, to celebrate the community's river heritage and summertime. Venetian boat parade, arts and crafts fair, parade, fireworks, dances, beer garden, antique auction, flea market, carnival, water ski show, antique car show, bingo, carriage rides, sailboat race, children's activities, concerts featuring a variety of music including country-western, rock, polka bands, and local groups. FOODS SERVED: Hispanic, German, old-fashioned barbecue, Iowa pork and beef, desserts, beer garden. ADMISSION: adults $5.00 advance for all five days; $7.00 at the gate. ACCOMMODATIONS: motels and hotels, B&B, campgrounds, RV parks. RESTAURANTS: fast foods, family, elegant, Irish, Chinese, Mexican, Italian, many catfish, Iowa pork and beef. CONTACT: Convention and Visitors Bureau, Great River Days, Ltd., Box 297, Muscatine, IA 52761, (319) 263-8895. 50,000

FAMILY FEST *third weekend in August,* Davenport, Scott Co., at Le Claire Park along the banks of the Mississippi River in the Quad Cities area. This festival is a "thank you" to the Davenport community for watching and listening to KWQC–TV, WOC–AM and KIIK–FM. Quad Cities' Angels minor league baseball game, arts and crafts booths, children's games, beer tent, spectacular fireworks display over the Mississippi River, entertainment such as gospel, country, rock, and nationally known talents Dickey Betts and Mick Taylor in addition to local groups. FOODS SERVED: lots including brats, burgers, cotton candy. ADMISSION: free. ACCOMMODATIONS: motels and hotels. RESTAURANTS: fast foods, family, elegant. CONTACT: KWQC–TV 805 Brady St., Davenport, IA 52808, (319) 383-7000. 20,000

OLD TIME COUNTRY MUSIC FESTIVAL AND PIONEER EXPOSITION OF ARTS AND CRAFTS *Labor Day weekend (early September),* Avoca, Pottawattamie Co., in western Iowa, at the County Fairgrounds. Performers from all over the world come to this festival to play and compete in the championship contests conducted on eight stages simultaneously. Contests include cribbage, "every imaginable acoustic musical instrument" such as accordian, country singer, harmonica, gandy dancer, rag-time piano, spoon and bone, checkers, yodeling, storytelling, whistling, fiddle, banjo, dulcimer, autoharp, and mandolin; other contests in clogging, horseshoeing, yo-yo, square dancing, comedy, songwriting, and hatchet throwing; arts and crafts, pageant show, teepee village, children's activities, gospel shows, and Legends of Our Times. FOODS SERVED: great variety. ADMISSION: $7.00 per day, $20.00 for five days, half price under 13 and over 70. ACCOMMODATIONS: motels and hotels, B&B's, campgrounds, RV parks. RESTAURANTS: fast foods, family, elegant. CONTACT: Bob Everhart, Traditional Country Music Assn., Inc., 106 Navajo, Council Bluffs, IA 51501. 50,000

KANSAS

PANCAKE DAY *Shrove Tuesday, (March),* Liberal, Seward Co., in Southwest Kansas, to acknowledge the annual Pancake Race between ladies of Olney, England and Liberal, Kansas. Ladies of both towns run a 415-yard course, flipping pancakes as they go, with the winner declared over a transatlantic phone call immediately after Liberal, Kansas race is completed. Pancake eating contests, pancake breakfast, parade, children's races, amateur talent contest, entertainers such as Roy Clark, Paul Harvey, Mel McDaniel, and Blue Angels Jets. Pancake Race has been run annually in Olney, England since 1445 and in Liberal, Kansas since 1950. FOODS SERVED: pancakes with adornments of many nationalities. ADMISSION: race free, talent contest $4.00, breakfast $2.00 ACCOMMODATIONS: motels and hotels, campground, RV park. RESTAURANTS: fast foods, family, elegant, Asian, Italian. CONTACT: Liberal Convention and Tourism Bureau, P. O. Box 1626, Liberal, KS 67901-1626, (316) 624-9425. 4,000

ST. PATRICK'S ROAD RACE AND PARADE *Saturday before or on St. Patrick's Day, (March 17),* Aggieville, Manhattan, Riley Co. Parade, men's and ladies' fun run, St. Pat's Road Race (10k) for fourteen age groups, wheelchair division, awards ceremony, and the Vail, Colorado, Precision Lawn Chair Demonstration Team. FOODS SERVED: big barbecue. ADMISSION: Free. ACCOMMODATIONS: motels and hotels, B&B's, campgrounds. RESTAURANTS: fast foods, family, elegant. CONTACT: Aggieville Merchants Association, P. O. Box 1804, Manhattan, KS 66502, (913) 776-8050. 10,000

WICHITA RIVER FESTIVAL *second weekend in May,* Wichita, Sedgwick Co., to celebrate the cultural and recreational resources of Wichita, and featuring "music, madness, and lots of friendly competition." Sundown parade, hot air balloonfest, antique bathtub races, street-side bed races, golf, tennis, and rugby tournaments, 10k River Run, bike race, and the Wichita Symphony Orchestra's Twilight Pops Concerts are examples of more than seventy events. FOODS SERVED: wide variety. ADMISSION: $1.00 button admits to all events. ACCOMMODATIONS: motels and hotels, B&B's, campgrounds, RV parks. RESTAURANTS: fast foods, family, elegant, international. CONTACT: Wichita River Festival, 347 S. Laura, Wichita, KS 67211, (316) 267-2817. 200,000

DOWNTOWN MANHATTAN FUN FESTIVAL *first Saturday in June,* Manhattan, Riley Co., along the 300 and 400 blocks of Poyntz Avenue, as a day of "fam-

ily fun." Parade, horse-and-buggy rides, petting zoo, face painting, children's games and contests, dunking booth, clowns and cartoon characters, musical entertainment such as barbershop, bluegrass, rock 'n' roll, big band, country-western, 50's and 60's, soft rock, classical, and folk music, jugglers, magicians, puppets, jumprope and gymnastics clubs. FOODS SERVED: funnel cakes, Chinese, Mexican, concessions. ADMISSION: free. ACCOMODATIONS: motels and hotels, campgrounds, RV parks. RESTAURANTS: fast foods, family, elegant, Asian, Greek, Italian, Mexican. CONTACT: Manhattan Main Street, 100 N. 4th, Manhattan, KS 66502, (913) 537-9683. 15,000

GOOD OL' DAYS *first weekend in June,* Fort Scott, Bourbon Co., in Southeast Kansas, held annually "just for fun." Recreation of an 1899 street fair featuring more than 200 arts and crafts exhibitors, quilt show, antique show and sale, softball and tennis tournaments, Red Garter Saloon, bed race, ugly truck contest, 10k Fun Run, tours of Fort Scott's restored 1842 military fort, street dances, cloggers, square dancers. FOODS SERVED: barbecue, homemade desserts, all-American. ADMISSION: free, charges for some events. ACCOMMODATIONS: motels and hotels, campgrounds, RV parks. RESTAURANTS: fast foods, family, elegant, Chinese. CONTACT: Good Ol' Days Committee, 20 N. Main, Fort Scott, KS 66701, (316) 223-2334, or the Fort Scott Chamber of Commerce, P. O. Box 205, Fort Scott, KS 66701, (316) 223-3566. 15,000

BEEF EMPIRE DAYS *first weekend in June,* Garden City, Finney Co., in Southwest Kansas, to recognize the beef industry. Live beef and carcass show, beef trivia contest, beef tasting, parade, rodeo, banquet, cutting horse competition, team roping, grandstand judging, golf tournament. FOODS SERVED: several meals, all featuring beef. ADMISSION: free. ACCOMMODATIONS: motels and hotels, B&B's, campgrounds, RV parks. RESTAURANTS: fast foods, family, elegant, Asian, Mexi-

can, Italian. CONTACT: Beef Empire Days, P. O. Box 1197, Garden City, KS 67846, (316) 275-6807. 10,000

SMOKY HILL RIVER FESTIVAL *second full weekend in June*, Salina, Saline Co. Arts and crafts, artists in action, art participation, road and bicycle races, three stages of entertainment including jazz, bluegrass, country, modern music featuring stars such as Maynard Ferguson, Dizzy Gillespie, Mel McDaniels, New Christy Minstrels, Association, Mary Travers, Riders in the Sky, Herbie Mann, Keith Stegal, mimes, puppets, children's theatre. FOODS SERVED: Mexican, German, French, Italian. ADMISION: for all three days, adults $4.00 advance, $5.00 at the gate, children under 12 free. ACCOMMODATIONS: motels and hotels, campgrounds. RESTAURANTS: fast foods, family, Chinese, Mexican, Italian. CONTACT: Lana Jordan, Festival Coordinator, Box 2181, Salina, KS 67402-2181 or the Salina Arts and Humanities Commission, P. O. Box 2181, Salina, KS 67402, (913) 827-4640. 65,000

FESTIVAL INTERNATIONAL *third weekend in June*, Kansas City, Wyandotte Co., to celebrate the "multi-ethnic backgrounds of the community." Ethnic groups host booths with traditional arts, demonstrations, continuous entertainment in the Alpine Garden, music and dance such as the Strawberry Hill Croatian Folk Ensemble, New York's Urban Bush Women, Chicago's Polish Folk Dance Ensemble, Tucson's Mariachi Band, the Aidas Lithuanian Dancers, and The St. Andrew's Pipers and Dancers. FOODS SERVED: Czechoslovakian, American Indian, Croatian, Hispanic, Afro-American, Serbian, Irish, Scottish, Danish, Russian, Polish, Lithuanian, Scandinavian. ADMISION: $3.00 advance, $3.50 at the door. ACCOMMODATIONS: motels and hotels. RESTAURANTS: fast foods, family. CONTACT: Carol Heil of the Kaw Valley Arts Council at (913) 299-0264 or the Convention and Visitors Bureau, Inc., P. O. Box 1576, Kansas City, KS 66117, (913) 321-5800. 15,000

WHEAT FESTIVAL *second week and weekend in July*, Wellington, Sumner Co., in the 'Wheat Capital of the World," 30 miles south of Witchita to celebrate the wheat harvest. Parade, antique custom car show, flower show and contest, queen contest, women's activities including displays and demonstrations, wheat show and contest, children's fair, softball tournament, variety show, live entertainment. FOODS SERVED: First National Bank Free Feed, pancake feed. ADMISSION: free, charges for entertainment and queen contest. ACCOMMODATIONS: motels and hotels, campgrounds, RV parks. RESTAURANTS: fast foods, family, elegant. CONTACT: Wellington Area Chamber of Commerce, 207 S. Washington, Wellington, KS 67152, (316) 326-7466. 10,000

DODGE CITY DAYS AND FORD COUNTY FAIR *last week in July, first weekend in August*, Dodge City, Ford Co., to celebrate the area's western heritage. Arts and crafts festival, dances, cookouts, parades, contests, car shows, fun runs, golf tournament, PRCA rodeo, auctions, auto racing, concerts by entertainers such as Lee Greenwood, Tammy Wynette, Sawyer Brown. FOODS SERVED: beef, concessions. ADMISSION: free, charges for some shows. ACCOMMODATIONS: motels and hotels, campgrounds, RV Parks. RESTAURANTS: fast foods, family, Cantonese, Mexican. CONTACT: Dodge City Chamber of Commerce, P. O. Box 939, Dodge City, KS 67801, (316) 227-3119. 75,000

RENAISSANCE FESTIVAL *Labor Day weekend (early September) and six consecutive weekends following Labor Day*, Kansas City, Wyandotte, Co., as a 16th-century harvest fair. Recreation of a 16th-century English fair including handmade crafts, games, knights in armour performing jousts daily, entertainment on nine stages including jugglers, madrigal singers, magicians, and street performers. FOODS SERVED: old English. ADMISSION: free. ACCOMMODATIONS: motels and hotels. RESTAURANTS: fast foods, family.

CONTACT: Gale Tallis of the Kansas City Art Institute, 4415 Warwick, Kansas City, MO 64111, (816) 561-8005 or the Convention and Visitors Bureau, Inc., P. O. Box 1576, Kansas City, KS 66117, (913) 321-5800. 150,000

WALNUT VALLEY FESTIVAL *third weekend in September,* Winfield, Cowley Co., at the Winfield Fairgrounds. Eight cash-prize contests in the country music and bluegrass fields including the National Finger-Picking Championship, the National Mountain Dulcimer Championship, the Walnut Valley Mandolin Championship, Walnut Valley Old-Time Fiddle Championship, National Flat–Pick Championship, National Hammer Dulcimer Championship, National Bluegrass Banjo Championship, and the International Autoharp Championship; concerts, workshops, arts and crafts fair, camping. Featured performers have included Doc Watson, Mike Cross, New Grass Revival, Berline, Crary & Hickman, Tony Trischka, and Hot Rize. FOODS SERVED: concessions. ADMISSION: charge to some events. ACCOMMODATIONS: motels and hotels, campgrounds, RV parks. RESTAURANTS: fast foods, family. CONTACT: Walnut Valley Association, P. O. Box 245, Winfield, KS 67156, (316) 221-3250. 9,000

MAPLE LEAF FESTIVAL *third weekend in October,* Baldwin City, Douglas Co., to celebrate the fall colors of maple tree foliage and the area's history. More than 250 arts and crafts exhibitors, tours of historic sites, square dancing, airplane rides, 10k Run, pony pull, horseshoe pitching tournament, Street Rod Run, breakfasts on the prairie, carnival, tennis tournament, quilt show, horse-and-buggy rides, continuous country-western and bluegrass music, historical musical "Ballad of Black Jack," Kansas State Chautauqua, international music festival. FOODS SERVED: Navajo and Mexican tacos, steak barbecue. ADMISSION: free, charges to some events. ACCOMMODATIONS: motel, campgrounds. RESTAURANTS: fast foods, family. CONTACT: Maple Leaf Festival Committee, Box 147, Baldwin City, KS 66006, (913) 594-3734 or the Baldwin City Chamber of Commerce, P. O. Box 501, Baldwin City, KS 66006, (913) 594-3464. 20,000

NEEWOLLAH *last week in October,* Independence, Montgomery Co., in Southeast Kansas. "Neewollah" is Halloween spelled backwards in this public celebration of what was once a quasi-religious holiday. Two parades, street acts, carnival, queen's pageant and coronation, musical show with professional performers such as Roy Clark, the Judds, Reba McIntire, Mel Tillis, Williams and Rea. FOODS SERVED: Italian, Mexican, American. ADMISSION: varies by show, average $6.00. ACCOMMODATIONS: motels and hotels, campgrounds, RV parks. RESTAURANTS: fast foods, family, Mexican. CONTACT: Neewollah, Inc., P. O. Box 311, Independence, KS 67301 or the Independence Chamber of Commerce, P. O. Box 386, Independence, KS 67301, (316) 331-1890. 60,000

MICHIGAN

WINTERFEST *first weekend in February,* South Haven, Van Buren Co. Snow sculpting contest, cross-country skiing and sledding, chess tournament, fashion show, children's area, volleyball and softball tournaments, parade, late shopping. FOODS SERVED: nationality featured varies each year. ADMISSION: free. ACCOMMODA-

TIONS: motels and hotels, B&B's, campgrounds, RV parks. RESTAURANTS: fast foods, family, elegant. CONTACT: Greater South Haven Area Chamber of Commerce, 535 Quaker St., South Haven, MI 49090, (616) 637-5171.

NATIONAL TROUT FESTIVAL *last weekend in April*, Kalkaska, Kalkaska Co., in northwestern Michigan, to celebrate the opening day of trout fishing season. Fishing Contest with more than $1,000.00 in prizes for largest brook, rainbow, and brown trout, Crosstrails Arts Council talent show, youth day featuring teen dance and Youth on Parade, 10k and 2mi. runs, children's fishing contest, Grand Royale Parade honoring Vietnam veterans, tug of war, Queen's Ball, Michigan Street Rod Association car show, three- and four-wheel ATV races, model airplane show, midway, One-Man Art Show featuring one well-known artist each year, trolley and helicopter rides, flea market, fireworks. FOODS SERVED: trout and concessions. ADMISSION: free, charges for some contests and events. ACCOMMODATIONS: motels and hotels, B&B, campgrounds, RV parks. RESTAURANTS: fast foods, family, elegant, Mexican, Chinese, Italian. CONTACT: The Greater Kalkaska Area Chamber of Commerce, P. O. Box 291, Kalkaska, MI 49646, (616) 258-9103. 10,000

ALMA HIGHLAND FESTIVAL AND GAMES *Memorial Day weekend, (late May)*, Alma, Gratiot Co., on the Alma College campus, to recognize the Scottish heritage and traditions of many Alma residents. Scottish athletic events, border collie demonstrations, fiddling contest, arts and crafts show, "massed bands," piping, drumming, Ceilidh (Scottish party), Scottish pub. FOODS SERVED: Scottish such as meat pies, haggis, bridies, short bread. ADMISSION: adults $5.00, seniors and students $2.50. ACCOMMODATIONS: motels and hotels, B&B's, campgrounds, college dormitories. RESTAURANTS: fast foods, family. CONTACT: Alma Highland Festival Committee, P. O. Box 506, Alma, MI 48801, (517) 463-5525. 80,000

GARDEN CITY COMMUNITY FLOWER AND GARDEN FESTIVAL *first weekend in June*, Garden City, Wayne Co., in the Metro Detroit area, to celebrate spring flowers in local gardens. Arts and crafts, carnival, parade, Fun Run, golf tournament, gurney race, flea market, musical programs including folk dancers and bands. FOODS SERVED: "various nationalities." ADMISSION: free. ACCOMMODATIONS: motels and hotels. RESTAURANTS: fast foods, family, elegant, Chinese, Italian. CONTACT: Greater Garden City Chamber of Commerce, 6000 Middlebelt Rd., Garden City, MI 48135, (313) 422-4448. 40,000

NATIONAL ASPARAGUS FESTIVAL *second weekend in June*, Hart and Shelby, Oceana Co., in western Michigan, to celebrate the annual asparagus harvest in Oceana County. Art Fair, Asparagus Bake-Off and Recipe Contest, Asparagus Royale Parade featuring more than 100 units, Fireman's Bucket Brigade, kid's parade, Community Coffee Break, round and square dancing, talent show, bingo, entertainment including bluegrass music concert by the McClain Family Band. FOODS SERVED: asparagus in every form imaginable including soup, breads, cookies, asparagus smorgasbord, asparagus luncheon, fresh asparagus, meat entrees, potatoes. ADMISSION: free, asparagus smorgasbord $6.50, concert $6.00. ACCOMMODATIONS: motels and hotels, B&B's, campgrounds, RV parks. RESTAURANTS: family, elegant. CONTACT: National Asparagus Festival of Oceana Co., P. O. Box 117, Shelby, MI 49455, (616) 861-4504, Art Fair (616) 861-4681. (For the National Asparagus Festival Cookbook or a brochure of free recipes write to the same address.) 30,000

FRANKENMUTH BAVARIAN FESTIVAL *second weekend and third week in June*, Frankenmuth, Saginaw Co., at Heritage Park, to celebrate Frankenmuth's German heritage. Dance tent resembling a German "biergarten" open noon to midnight and featuring German dance bands and beverages, arts and crafts, arts and crafts auction, farm tours, parade featuring crowned Bavarian princess, performances by American and international entertainers such as Clay and Sally Hart from the Lawrence Welk Show, the Serendipity Singers, the Martin Christen Duo from Switzerland, Myron Floren, Brenda Byers and the Munich Schuhplattlers have appeared. FOODS SERVED: German beer and foods including bratwurst, roast beef sandwiches on Kummel weck, Bavarian pastries, chicken barbecues, pretzels, other Bavarian foods. ADMISSION: General $3.00, children under 15 free, additional charge for festival show tent. ACCOMMODATIONS: motels and hotels, B&B's, campgrounds, RV parks. RESTAURANTS: fast foods, family, elegant, German, Italian. CONTACT: Frankenmuth Bavarian Festival, 635 Main St., Frankenmuth, MI 48734, (517) 652-8155. 250,000

DETROIT/WINDSOR INTERNATIONAL FREEDOM FESTIVAL *June 19–July 4,* Detroit, MI and Windsor, Ontario, Canada, to celebrate Canada Day, July 1, and American Independence Day, July 4. More than fifty events on both sides of the Canadian–United States border including tugboat races, fun runs, marching bands, a fireworks display over the Detroit River, live concerts and peformances including four days of free concerts with each day having its own theme such as Motown Night, jazz, rock, or country. Past performers have included Chubby Checker, The Spinners, The Contours, J.C. Heard. FOODS SERVED: variety of Canadian and American specialties in addition to concessions. ADMISSION: free. ACCOMMODATIONS: motels and hotels. RESTAURANTS: fast foods, family, elegant, international. CONTACT: Detroit Renaissance Foundation, 100 Renaissance Center, Suite 1760, Detroit, MI 48243, (313) 259-5400. 3,000,000

THREE RIVERS WATER CARNIVAL *third week in June,* Three Rivers, St. Joseph Co. Art in the park, Nostalgia Day, water sports events, carnival midway,

bierfest, flea market, water float parade, demolition derby. FOODS SERVED: ox roast, bratwurst, roast corn, pizza, strawberry feed. ADMISSION: free. ACOMMODATIONS: motels and hotels, campgrounds. RESTAURANTS: fast foods, family, elegant. CONTACT: Three Rivers Area Chamber of Commerce, P. O. Box 279, Three Rivers, MI 49093, (616) 278-8193. 40,000

BELLEVILLE AREA STRAWBERRY FESTIVAL *third weekend in June,* Belleville, Wayne Co., to celebrate the strawberry harvest. Arts and crafts, strawberry food booths, parade, queen pageant, amusement rides, games, antique car show, dancing, musical entertainment such as Herrmann's Royal Lipizzan Stallions Show, Rothchild Rock Band, Country Royal Family, Walt Cieclik and the Musical Ambassadors, and The Misty Blues. FOODS SERVED: variety including strawberry specialties. ADMISSION: free, charge for "major event." ACCOMMODATIONS: motels and hotels, campgrounds, RV parks. RESTAURANTS: fast foods, family, elegant, Chinese. Contact: Belleville Area Chamber of Commerce, 116 Fourth St., Belleville, MI 48111, (313) 697-7151. 80,000

CHESANING SHOWBOAT *second week in July,* Chesaning, Saginaw Co. Arts and crafts fair, Old Home Tour by horse and carriage, dinner boat cruises with entertainment, sidewalk sales, bingo, 10k Road Race, "hilarious" Bed Race, horseshoe pitching contest, antique cars, demonstrations of basket weaving, quilting, and tatting, parade, big-name entertainers have included Tennessee Ernie Ford, Marie Osmond, The Osmond Brothers, Pat Boone, and Debbie Boone. FOODS SERVED: "complete dinners" featuring barbecued or family-style chicken, Swiss steak, or roast beef; pancake and sausage breakfast. ADMISSION: Monday–Thursday, $6.00–$9.50, Friday and Saturday, $8.00–$10.50. ACCOMMODATIONS: motels and hotels, campgrounds. RESTAURANTS: family. CONTACT: Chesaning Chamber of Commerce, 220 E. Broad St., Chesaning, MI 48616, (517) 845-3055. 45,000

NATIONAL CHERRY FESTIVAL *second week in July,* Traverse City, Grand Traverse Co., in "The Cherry Capital of the World," "where seventy percent of the world's red cherries are grown." Three parades, Milk Carton Boat Regatta, cherry cooking contest, cherry pie eating contest, cherry wine competition, cherry smorgasbord luncheon, Bed Race, canoe race, water ski tournament, junior arts and crafts activities, big wheel race, Music on the River dixieland swing, cherry orchard tours, bicycle moto-cross, bingo, midway, sand sculpture and castle building, Governor's Reception, Fun Run, water ski show, fireworks, lots of entertainment including high school bands competition, many concerts such as U.S. Air Force Band of Flight, Golden Garter Revue. FOODS SERVED: cherries in many forms, concessions. ADMISSION: free, charges for few events. ACCOMMODATIONS: motels and hotels, B&B's, campgrounds, RV parks. RESTAURANTS: fast foods, family, elegant. CONTACT: National Cherry Festival, Inc., P.O. Box 141, Traverse City, MI 49684, (616) 947-4230. 350,000

ALPENFEST *third week in July,* Gaylord, Otsego Co., to celebrate summer. Two blocks of Gaylord's main street are blocked off for the festival featuring arts and crafts booths, outdoor cafes where the "World's Largest Coffee Break is held," Burning of the Boog where "people write their troubles on a slip of paper and place it in the Boog which is a 300-pound, ten-foot-high monster, and your troubles go up in smoke when the Boog is burned," carnival, beer tent, queen's pageant, Arts Council-sponsored performances by local arts groups such as the Comic Opera Guild, Art Fairs, Detroit Symphony Orchestra, Songs of Spring and Love, polka bands, and the Gaylord Community Band. FOODS SERVED: Swiss, German, Austrian, Polish, Italian, Asian, French, Greek, American. ADMISSION: free. ACCOMMODATIONS: motels and hotels, B&B, campgrounds, RV park. RESTAURANTS: fast foods, family, elegant, Polish, German,

Greek. CONTACT: Gaylord–Ostego Co. Chamber of Commerce, P.O. Box 513, Gaylord, MI 49735, (517) 732-4000. 40,000

NATIONAL BLUEBERRY FESTIVAL *third Wednesday through third weekend in July,* South Haven, Van Buren Co., in the "Blueberry Capital of the World." Blueberry pie eating contests, windsurfing events, sand castle building contests, bed races, volleyball and golf tournaments, beer tent. FOODS SERVED: "blueberry recipes of all kinds." ADMISSION: free. ACCOMMODATIONS: motels and hotels, B&B's, campgrounds, RV parks. RESTAURANTS: fast foods, family, elegant. CONTACT: Greater South Haven Area Chamber of Commerce, 535 Quaker St., South Haven, MI 49090, (616) 637-5171.

KALAMAZOO COUNTY FLOWERFEST *third weekend in July,* Kalamazoo, Kalamazoo Co., in West Michigan, to honor the Kalamazoo bedding plant industry. Downtown Kalamazoo and cities throughout Kalamazoo County are filled with breathtaking beds of flowers. Garden tours, historic homes tour, fitness walk, picnic in the park, flower shows and seminars, pastel art exhibit, ice cream socials, live entertainment such as a symphony concert, Kalamazoo Big Band, Children's Ethnic Group, blues, jazz, and vesper service. FOODS SERVED: Greek and American, ice cream. ADMISSION: free, fee for tours. ACCOMMODATIONS: motels and hotels, B&B's, campgrounds, RV parks. RESTAURANTS: fast foods, family, elegant, Greek, Mexican, Chinese, Italian. CONTACT: Kalamazoo Co. Convention and Visitors Bureau, 128 N. Kalamazoo Mall, P.O. Box 1169, Kalamazoo, MI 49005, (616) 381-4003. 30,000

HIAWATHA MUSIC CO-OP FESTIVAL *third weekend in July,* Marquette, Marquette Co., at the Tourist Park. Three-day music festival features bluegrass, country, and folk music, food, and beverages. FOODS SERVED: concessions.

ADMISSION: free. ACCOMMODATIONS: motels and hotels, B&B's, campgrounds, RV parks. RESTAURANTS: fast foods, family, elegant, Chinese, Italian, Greek. CONTACT: Brad Veley at (906) 249-3688 or the Marquette Area Chamber of Commerce, 501 S. Front St., Marquette, MI 49855, (906) 226-6591.

PLAINWELL ISLAND CITY FESTIVAL *fourth weekend in July,* Plainwell, Allegan Co., in the Kalamazoo area. Arts and crafts, 5k and 10k races, beer tent, parade, antique cars, kiddie rides, games, street dancing, local bands and singers from Michigan. FOODS SERVED: chicken barbecue, pancake breakfast. ADMISSION: free. ACCOMMODATIONS: motels and hotels, campgrounds, RV parks. RESTAURANTS: fast foods, family, elegant, French. CONTACT: Plainwell Chamber of Commerce, P.O. Box 95, Plainwell, MI 49080, (616) 685-8877. 10,000

HARBOR DAYS *last weekend in July,* Saugatuck–Douglas, Allegan Co., on Lake Michigan, to celebrate the natural wonders of the area. Kite flying, fishing tournaments, parade of decorated boats, performances by Red Barn Theater Summer Stock. ADMISSION: free to most events. ACCOMMODATIONS: motels and hotels, B&B's, campgrounds, RV parks. RESTAURANTS: fast foods, family, elegant, seafood. CONTACT: Saugatuck–Douglas Chamber of Commerce, Inc., P.O. Box 28, Saugatuck, MI 49453, (616) 857-5801. 8,000

DANISH FESTIVAL *third weekend in August,* Greenville, Montcalm Co., to celebrate residents' Danish heritage. Art show, carnival, antique and classic car show, sporting events and demonstrations, parade, children's parade, family games, tavern, dance, and entertainment such as the Danish Festival Players Theatre, the Danish Festival Band, oompah bands, the Danish Festival Singers, a barbershop chorus show, talent show, and bluegrass music show. FOODS SERVED:

"Danish and Danish." ADMISSION: free. ACCOMMODATIONS: motels and hotels, B&B's, campgrounds. RESTAURANTS: fast foods, family, elegant. CONTACT: Danish Festival, 327 S. Lafayette St., Greenville, MI 48838, (616) 754-5697.

MONTREUX DETROIT JAZZ FESTIVAL *September 2–7,* Detroit, Wayne Co., to showcase jazz on a regional, national, and international level. Six days of concerts, performances, and clinics for accomplished students and musicians, which might include stars such as Miles Davis, Howie Smith, Joe Williams, Betty Carter, Sarah Vaughn, Sonny Rollins, Tania Maria, Sadao Watanabe, and Ramsey Lewis. FOODS SERVED: wide range, concessions. ADMISSION: varies by concert. ACCOMMODATIONS: motels and hotels. RESTAURANTS: fast foods, family, elegant. CONTACT: Detroit Renaissance Foundation, 100 Renaissance Center, Suite 1760, Detroit, MI 48243, (313) 259-5400. 357,618

MICHIGAN WINE AND HARVEST FESTIVAL *weekend after Labor Day, (early September),* Kalamazoo, Kalamazoo Co., in West Michigan, to honor Michigan wines. Wine tasting, Annual Bed Race, grape stomping, fine arts and crafts fair, harness racing, midway, footrace, free winery tours, Las Vegas Night, live entertainment all day including jazz, blues, Top 40, and folk music. FOODS SERVED: Michigan products barbecue, ethnic food booths including Chinese, Greek, Mexican, Polish, American. ADMISSION: free. ACCOMMODATIONS: motels and hotels, B&B's, campgrounds, RV parks. RESTAURANTS: fast foods, family, elegant, Greek, Mexican, Chinese, Italian. CONTACT: Kalamazoo Co. Convention and Visitors Bureau, 128 N. Kalamazoo Mall, P. O. Box 1169, Kalamazoo, MI 49005, (616) 381-4003. 220,000

FESTIVAL OF THE PINES *third week in September,* Lake City, Missaukee Co. Art show, Christmas tree judging, wood carving, wood cutting, and archery competitions, polka music and dancing, children's activities, beverage tent. ADMISSION: free. ACCOMMODATIONS: motels and hotels, campgrounds, RV parks. RESTAURANTS: fast foods, family, elegant. CONTACT: Lake City Area Chamber of Commerce, P. O. Box 52, Lake City, MI 49651, (616) 839-4969. 10,000

FESTIVAL OF THE FORKS *third weekend in September,* Albion, Calhoun Co., to commemorate the founding of Albion on the forks of the Kalamazoo River. Arts and crafts, antique show, Trailer Rally, book sale, flea market, 5k and 10k runs, softball tournaments, bed race, pet show, pie eating contest, window displays, Klassic Kanoe Race, River Forks Encampment, canoe jousting, continuous musical entertainment. FOODS SERVED: chicken barbecue, ethnic food booths including Greek, Italian, German, Lithuanian, Mexican, Polish, American. ADMISSION: free. ACCOMMODATIONS: motels and hotels, B&B's, campgrounds, RV parks. RESTAURANTS: fast foods, family, elegant, Cajun, Chinese, Mexican. CONTACT: Greater Albion Chamber of Commerce, P. O. Box 238, Albion, MI 49224, (517) 629-5533. 2,000

TUSCOLA COUNTY PUMPKIN FESTIVAL *first Thursday through the weekend in October,* Caro, Tuscola Co., downtown. Arts and crafts, parade, amusement rides, lip sync program and talent show, Pumpkin Ball, lots of music, pumpkin edibles. FOODS SERVED: pancake supper, pumpkin "goodies," bratwurst, Mexican. ADMISSION: free. ACCOMMODATIONS: motels and hotels, B&B, campground, RV park. RESTAURANTS: fast foods, family, elegant, Italian. CONTACT: Caro Chamber of Commerce, 429 N. State St., Caro, MI 48723, (517) 673-5211. 35,000

OKTOBERFEST *second weekend in October,* South Haven, Van Buren Co., to celebrate fall colors of western Michigan. Art exhibits, color tours, harvest sales, "Taste of South Haven Banquet," children's area, sidewalk sales, fashion show. FOODS SERVED: "variety." ADMISSION: free. ACCOMMODATIONS: motels and hotels, B&B's, campgrounds, RV parks. RESTAURANTS: fast foods, family, elegant. CONTACT: Greater South Haven Area Chamber of Commerce, 535 Quaker St., South Haven, MI 49090, (616) 637-5171.

MINNESOTA

SAINT PAUL WINTER CARNIVAL *last weekend in January through first weekend in February,* St. Paul, Ramsey Co., in the Twin Cities area, to celebrate winter and the Winter Carnival Legend, based on the story that Boreas, King of the Winds, came upon the winter paradise of Minnesota where he proclaimed, "I will make St. Paul the capital of my domains," declaring it "The Realm of Boreas," whose winters are only ended by the arrival of Vulcanus, the God of Fire. Ice carving contest, Winter Garden of snow sculptures on Harriet Island in the Mississippi River featuring master snow craftsmen from Hokkaido, Japan, home of the Sapporo Snow Festival, reenactment of the Legend of Winter Carnival; Snowmobile Speed Run Nationals featuring stock snowmobiles to fun sleds, Snowmobile Formula Challenge including a 200 lap endurance race, Hispanic Winter Fiesta featuring a mariachi band, folk and flamenco dancers, mimes, jugglers, and storytelling, Latin jazz band and flamenco dance band; craft displays, Mexican food; Fine Arts Series in which Rudolf Nureyev and Shirley Jones have performed; 10,000 Lakes International Speedskating Championships, Vulcan Victory Torchlight parade, sleigh and cutter parade featuring antique sleighs and smaller cutters, cross-country ski race, car racing on ice, King Boreas Grande Day Parade. FOODS SERVED: "something for all." ADMISSION: free, charges for some events. ACCOMMODATIONS: motels and hotels. RESTAURANTS: fast foods, family, elegant, international. CONTACT: St. Paul Winter Carnival Association, North Central Life Tower, Suite 600, 445 Minnesota St., St. Paul MN 55101, (612) 297-6953. 1,000,000

FESTIVAL OF NATIONS *last weekend in April or first weekend in May*, St. Paul, Ramsey Co., to celebrate St. Paul's ethnic diversity and unity. Sixty-five ethnic groups provide this festival with a wide range of costumes, demonstrations, cultural exhibits, exciting folk dance performances, international bazaar, ethnic dancers and musicians judged for the festival, guest artists performing mime, vaudeville, clowning, dancing, acrobatics, and comedy. FOODS SERVED: "280 authentic foods" of the sixty-five ethnic groups. ADMISSION: adults $5.00 advance, $6.00 at door; children $4.00. ACCOMMODATIONS: motels and hotels, B&B's, campgrounds. RESTAURANTS: fast foods, family, elegant, international. CONTACT: International Institute of Minnesota, 1694 Como Ave., St. Paul, MN 55108, (612) 647-0191, or the Saint Paul Area Chamber of Commerce, 600 N. Central Tower, 445 Minnesota St., Saint Paul, MN 55101, (612) 293-5000. 75,000

HAGAR'S LUTEFISK FESTIVAL *third Friday in May*, Glenwood, Pope Co., for a fun time during Syttenda Mai Celebration. Great Big Parade, Little Lars and Lena Coronation, troll head contest, live entertainment and Norwegian music, "many fun and humorous events." FOODS SERVED: lutefisk, meatballs, potatoes, beverage. ADMISSION: free, charge for lutefisk dinner (all you can eat), adults $4.00, seniors and students $3.50. ACCOMMODATIONS: motels and hotels, campgrounds. RESTAURANTS: family. CONTACT: Glenwood Chamber of Commerce, 137 E. Minnesota, Ave., Glenwood, MN 56334, (612) 634-3636.

WESTERN FEST *third weekend in June*, Granite Falls, Yellow Medicine Co., in conjunction with the Minnesota State High School Rodeo Championship Finals. Antique and craft flea market, street dance, Grand Parade, 25mi. Bike Race and Tour, beer garden, four rodeo performances. FOODS SERVED: concessions. ADMISSION: free, rodeo tickets adults $4.00, students $2.00. ACCOMMODATIONS: motels and hotels, campgrounds. RESTAURANTS: fast foods, family. CONTACT: Granite Falls Area Chamber of Commerce, P. O. Box 220, Granite Falls, MN 56241, (612) 564-4039. 5,000

WHITE BEAR LAKE AREA MANITOU DAYS *third weekend through fourth week in June*, White Bear Lake, Ramsey and Washington Cos. Grand Parade, sporting events, dances, musical performances, arts and crafts fair. FOODS SERVED: "various." ACCOMMODATIONS: motels and hotels, nearby campgrounds. RESTAURANTS: fast foods, family, elegant, Italian, Chinese. CONTACT: White Bear Lake Area Chamber of Commerce, 2189 Fourth St., White Bear Lake, MN 55110, (612) 429-7666. 15,000

KAFFE FEST *fourth week in June*, Willmar, Kandiyohi Co. Coffee bar, Merrian's midway shows, Parade of Bands, rodeo, Kids Hour of Fun, kiddie parade, concert in the part, Queen's Ball, free coffee at local restaurants, softball tournament, 4–H horse show, Kaffee Fest Parade, Kandy-O-Hi-Lo Chorus Concert, Heritage Day featuring Native American arts, movies, teepees, music, food, and dancing; Jet Ski Race. FOODS SERVED: lots of coffee, pancake feed. ADMISSION: free, charges for queen coronation. ACCOMMODATIONS: motels and hotels, campgrounds, RV parks. RESTAURANTS: fast foods, family, elegant. CONTACT: Willmar Area Chamber of Commerce, P. O. Box 287, Willmar, MN 56201, (612) 235-0300.

LAKE CITY WATER SKI DAYS *last full weekend in June*, Lake City, Wabasha Co., at the Marina and Beach area, "the birthplace of waterskiing." Arts and crafts fair, water ski shows on Lake Pepin, carnival, Venetian Sailboat Parade, Grande Parade, live entertainment such as the Johnny Holm Traveling Fun Show, the Mrozinski Brothers Ensemble Soft Touch Band, storyteller Carol R. McCormick, and Rochester Water Shows. FOODS SERVED: American. ADMISSION: free, purchase button $1.50 for some events. ACCOMMODATIONS: motels and hotels, B&B's, campgrounds, RV parks. RESTAURANTS: fast foods, family. CONTACT: Lake City Chamber of Commerce, P. O. Box 150, Lake City, MN 55041, (612) 345-4123. 40,000

SCANDINAVIAN HJEMKOMST FESTIVAL *last weekend in June,* Fargo ND and Moorhead MN, to celebrate Scandinavian heritage of many Minnesota residents. Street dances, Scandinavian crafts, flags and costumes of the five Scandinavian countries, marching bands from Norway and touring groups from other countries, mini-festivals. FOODS SERVED: Scandinavian. ADMISSION: free. ACCOMMODATIONS: motels and hotels, campgrounds. RESTAURANTS: fast foods, family, elegant, French, Mexican, Chinese. CONTACT: Greater Fargo–Moorhead Convention and Visitors Bureau, Box 719, Moorhead, MN 56560, (701) 237-6134. 30,000

TASTE OF MINNESOTA *July 4th weekend,* St. Paul, Ramsey Co., on the State Capitol grounds. Street festival featuring the culinary arts of Minnesota's forty finest restaurants from tenderloin filets to ethnic foods, Minnesota Orchestra Concert, fireworks show. ADMISSION: free. ACCOMMODATIONS: motels and hotels, B&B's, campgrounds. RESTAURANTS: fast foods, family, elegant, international. CONTACT: Taste of Minnesota, 614 North Central Tower, 445 Minnesota St., St. Paul, MN 55101, (612) 228-0018

WHEELS, WINGS, AND WATER FESTIVAL *mid–July,* St. Cloud, Stearns Co., featuring a transportation theme. Outdoor concerts, craft fairs, raft races, bike races, street dances, parade, 10k Run, water ski show, celebrity entertainment, food festival. FOODS SERVED: German and other international. ADMISSION: free, charges for some events. ACCOMMODATIONS: motels and hotels, B&B's, campgrounds. RESTAURANTS: fast foods, family, elegant, many German. CONTACT: St. Cloud Area Festival Association, P. O. Box 487, St. Cloud, MN 56301, (612) 251-2940.

RIVERFRONT MUSIC FESTIVAL *ten days in mid–July,* Saint Paul, Ramsey Co., in the Twin Cities area. Festival features seven separate entertainment areas with "125 big-name acts" running twelve hours a day for ten days straight; music includes pop, rock, country, jazz, and folk music; circus, carnival rides and games, children's activities, seniors' activities and water shows. FOODS SERVED: concessions. ADMISSION: charge good for one whole day's performances. ACCOMMODATIONS: motels and hotels. RESTAURANTS: fast foods, family, elegant, international. CONTACT: St. Paul Riverfront Music Festival, 614 North Central Tower, 445 Minnesota St., St. Paul MN 55101, (612) 228-0018.

VIENNESE SOMMERFEST *begins Wednesday of second week in July and continues for three weeks,* Minneapolis, Hennepin Co., at the Orchestra Hall–Peavey Plaza. Concerts by orchestras, chamber ensembles, and guest artists performing Viennese and other classical music; Marktplatz on Peavey Plaza features live entertainment on concert evenings, food and drink; films and dancing to Viennese waltzes and polkas. FOODS SERVED: Austrian. ADMISSION: charge. ACCOMMODATIONS: motels and hotels, B&B's, campgrounds, RV parks. RESTAURANTS: fast foods, family, elegant, international. CONTACT: Minnesota Orchestral Association, Orchestra Hall, 1111 Nicollet Mall, Minneapolis, MN 55403, (612) 371-5600.

SINCLAIR LEWIS DAYS *second weekend in July*, Sauk Centre, Stearns Co., to remember, honor, and celebrate the achievements of one-time Sauk Centre resident, author Sinclair Lewis. Wild life art show, chess tournament, car show, road race, trapshoot, parade with more than 100 units, flea market, carnival, high school band concert in the city park bandshell, walk-for-fun. FOODS SERVED: local concessions. ADMISSION: free. ACCOMMODATIONS: motels and hotels, campgrounds, RV parks. RESTAURANTS: fast foods, family, elegant. CONTACT: Sauk Centre Chamber of Commerce, P. O. Box 222, Sauk Centre, MN 56378, (612) 352-5201. 6,000

MINNEAPOLIS AQUATENNIAL *third Friday in July and ten subsequent days*, Minneapolis, Hennepin Co., and at the surrounding lakes and parks, to celebrate the natural and cultural opportunities of Minnesota. Youth and senior art show, Grand Day Parade as a festival kickoff, Family Fun Day includes musicians, mimes, jugglers, and other strolling entertainers, children's games and contests and arts and crafts fair; North American Freestyle Frisbee Championships with 10,000 Frisbees flying, tug of war, River Raft Race with awards given to best-looking and most-original rafts, Rowing Regatta, and Nordic Sprints for Olympic athletes, mobility impaired, or novices, Milk Carton Boat Races, flower and garden show, senior days, youth fishing clinic, torchlight parade, Nicollet Mall Art Fairs, Queen of the Lakes Coronation, maritime party, International Outboard Grand Prix Powerboat Races, Muscle Explosion Body Builders Competition, musical entertainment on five showboats and a floating stage, local boats parade in the Lights Fantastic Boat Parade, sailboard classics racing, sailing regatta, triathlon, water ski extravaganza, Grape Nuts American Bike Festival race through Minneapolis, Minneapple River Run with 2,000 runners, hot air balloon event, Fireworks Finale. FOODS SERVED: fish fry, international. ADMISSION: free. ACCOMMODATIONS: motels and hotels, B&B's, campgrounds, RV parks. RESTAURANTS: fast foods, family, elegant, international. CONTACT: Minneapolis Aquatennial, Commodore Court, 702 Wayzata Blvd., Minneapolis, MN 55403, (612) 377-4621. 2,000,000

ART IN THE PARK *third weekend in July*, Bemidji, Beltrami Co. "Largest juried outdoor arts and crafts festival in North Central Minnesota featuring 150 exhibitors from Minnesota, Wisconsin, Iowa, North Dakota, and South Dakota," variety of live entertainment, demonstrations, children's activities. FOODS SERVED: variety of ethnic foods. ADMISSION: free. ACCOMMODATIONS: motels and hotels. RESTAURANTS: fast foods, family. CONTACT: Bemidji Community Arts Council, 426 Bemidji Ave., Bemidji, MN 56601, (218) 751-7570.

HERITAGEFEST *third weekend in July*, New Ulm, Brown Co., at Twelfth Street North and State Street, to celebrate and promote the German heritage of New Ulm's residents. Arts and crafts exhibit, old-world costumes and ethnic entertainment and folklore, 2mi. and 10k road races, children's race, parade, entertainment on four stages including European performing-groups, jugglers, mimes, magicians, ethnic singers, folk crafts, historical pageant. FOODS SERVED: German foods and beverages. ADMISSION: adults $4.00, children 7–12 $1.50. ACCOMMODATIONS: motels and hotels, campgrounds. RESTAURANTS: family, German. CONTACT: Heritagefest, Inc., P. O. Box 461, New Ulm, MN 56073, (507) 354-8850. 30,000

RIVERTOWN DAYS *fourth weekend in July*, Hastings, Dakota Co., in the Twin Cities area on the Mississippi River. Arts and crafts fair, hot air balloon race, water ski show, carnival, hot air balloon rides, riverboat rides, 10k Run, antique auto show, fishing contest, demolition derby, tennis tournament, swimming olympics, puppets, dance recitals, local bands. FOODS SERVED: multi-national. ADMISSION:

$2.00 button. ACCOMMODATIONS: motels and hotels, B&B, campground. RESTAU-RANTS: fast foods, family, elegant, Chinese, Mexican, Italian. CONTACT: Hastings on the Mississippi Chamber of Commerce, 427 Vermillion, Hastings, MN 55033, (612) 437-6775. 5,000

GLENWOOD WATERAMA *last full weekend in July,* Glenwood, Pope Co. Water ski competition, sailboat regatta, kiddie parade, water ski show, firemen's water fights, Button Dance, softball and golf tournaments, folk art fair and sale, fine arts show and sale, beauty pageants, Lighted Pontoon Parade on Lake Minnewaska, theatre presentations, bicycle marathon race, breakdancing show, innertube regatta, fireworks, parade featuring more than 100 units, Fort Ransom Cavalry Unit presents a program of horsemanship, dances. FOODS SERVED: chicken barbecues, concessions. ADMISSION: $2.00 button. ACCOMMODATIONS: motels and hotels, campgrounds. RESTAURANTS: fast foods, family, elegant. CONTACT: Glenwood Chamber of Commerce, 137 E. Minnesota Ave., Glenwood, MN 56334, (612) 634-3636.

"WE" MINNESOTA COUNTRY MU-SIC FEST *second weekend in August,* Detroit Lakes, Becker Co. Huge outdoor country-music festival featuring at least nine "top-notch country entertainers" such as Alabama, Loretta Lynn, Charlie Daniels, Johnny Cash, Ronnie Milsap, Freddie Fender, Waylon Jennings, Mickey Gilley, Merle Haggard, regional bands, and a "large-scale camp-out." FOODS SERVED: variety of concessions. ADMISSION: advance for four days $33.00, after June 1 $35.00, single-day ticket $20.00, box seats including lunch and back stage privileges for three days, $300.00. ACCOMMODATIONS: on the concert grounds from $25.00 to $100.00 V.I.P. for four days. RESTAURANTS: fast foods, family. CONTACT: We, Inc., Box 1227, Detroit Lakes, MN 56501, (218) 847-1681. 50,000

SONGS OF THE LUMBERJACK *second week in August,* Grand Rapids, Itasca Co., to honor and remember the music of the lumberjack at the Forest History Center. Authentic music of the lumberjack and 1900s period music such as fiddles, Jew's harps, squeeze boxes and mouth organs in the 1900 logging camp at the center. ADMISSION: charge. ACCOMMODATIONS: motels and hotels. RESTAURANTS: fast foods, family. CONTACT: Minnesota Historical Society, Forest History Center, 2609 County Road 76, Grand Rapids, MN 55744, (218) 327-1782.

DEFEAT OF JESSE JAMES DAYS *weekend after Labor Day (early September),* Northfield, Rice Co., to commemorate the defeat in Northfield of the infamous James–Younger Gang. Reenactment of the thwarted bank robbery attempt, queen coronation, beard contest, carnival, P.R.C.A. professional rodeo, bingo, Jesse James Bike Ride race, horse show, radio-controlled airplane fun fly and demonstration, fall fine arts and crafts fair, kiddie parade, Kiddie Karnival, antique tractor pull, crafts show, big wheel races, high school and college football games, Northfield Arts Guild Theater Performance, Cannon Valley Regional Orchestra Performance, bluegrass concerts, Minnesota Street Rod Show. FOODS SERVED: concessions. ADMISSION: purchased buttons required for some events. ACCOMMODATIONS: motels and hotels, RV park. RESTAURANTS: fast foods, family. CONTACT: Northfield Area Chamber of Commerce, P. O. Box 198, Northfield, MN 55057, (507) 645-6321. 120,000

BIG ISLAND RENDEZVOUS AND FESTIVAL *first weekend in October,* Albert Lea, Freeborn Co., at Helmer Myre State Park. Native American art exhibit, pioneer craft skills demonstrations, blackpowder shoot, tomahawk and knife throwing, Tipi Village, traders row, military demonstrations, field kitchen drills and ceremonies, fife and drum, rifle drills, guard mount and flag raising; workshops in primitive camping, blacksmithing, fur-trade skills, military life, voyagers, and visual arts; children's activities such as storytelling, tests of skill, pioneer games, theatre, entertainment; live entertainment including bluegrass, Fiddler's Jamboree, cloggers, open church service, Pony Express Relay, Native American music and dances. FOODS SERVED: fry bread, corn roast, ethnic meats, homemade ice cream and pies. ADMISSION: free. ACCOMMODATIONS: motels and hotels, campgrounds. CONTACT: The Albert Lea Convention and Visitors Bureau, P. O. Box 686, Albert Lea, MN 56007, (507) 373-3938.

OKTOBERFEST *third week in October,* New Ulm, Brown Co., to recognize this traditional German celebration and the German heritage of New Ulm's residents. Continuous German entertainment on two stages. German crafts and costumes. FOODS SERVED: German food and locally brewed beer. ADMISSION: free. ACCOMMODATIONS: motels and hotels, campgrounds. RESTAURANTS: family, German. CONTACT: Concord Singers, P. O. Box 492, New Ulm, MN 56073, (507) 354-8850. 30,000

MISSOURI

STORYTELLING FESTIVAL *last weekend in April or first weekend in May,* St. Louis, St. Louis Co., on the Illinois River at the Jefferson National Expansion Memorial, on the grounds of the Arch. A gathering of storytellers from a variety of disciplines including teachers, librarians, traditional, and professional storytellers and others interested in preserving the art of storytelling. Lectures and symposia, lots of storytelling by aficionados. Visitors have the opportunity to participate. ADMISSION: free. ACCOMMODATIONS: motels and hotels, B&B's, campgrounds, RV parks. RESTAURANTS: fast foods, family, elegant. CONTACT: Nan Kammann at (314) 553-5961 or the St. Louis Convention and Visitors Commission, 10 S. Broadway, Suite 300, St. Louis, MO 63102, (314) 231-5555. 20,000

RICHMOND MUSHROOM FESTIVAL *first weekend in May,* Richmond, Ray Co., in the "Mushroom Capital of the World." Arts and crafts, parade, beer garden with live music. FOODS SERVED: mushrooms by the cup, concessions. ADMISSION: free. RESTAURANTS: fast foods, family, elegant. CONTACT: Richmond

Chamber of Commerce, 114 E. North Main, Richmond, MO 64805, (816) 776-6916. 10,000

INTERNATIONAL FESTIVAL *fourth weekend in May,* St. Louis, St. Louis Co., at Steinburg Rink in Forest Park. At least thirty-five nationalities present their native and authentic music, dance, crafts, and food. FOODS SERVED: specialties of thirty-five nations. ADMISSION: free. ACCOMMODATIONS: motels and hotels, B&B's, campgrounds, RV parks. RESTAURANTS: fast foods, family, elegant. CONTACT: Steve Edison at (314) 997-1445 or the St. Louis Convention and Visitors Commission, 10 S. Broadway, Suite 300, St. Louis, MO 63102, (314) 231-5555.

SCOTT JOPLIN RAGTIME FESTIVAL *first weekend in June,* Sedalia, Pettis Co., to promote and honor the memory of Scott Joplin, and celebrate the "continued enjoyment of ragtime music." Piano competition, dance, symposium, non-stop entertainment at the original Maple Leaf Club site, Champagne Concert at The Liberty Center featuring ragtime standouts such as Renaissance Brass Quintet,

Allegra, John Arpin, Catherine Wilson, St. Louis Ragtimers, Tex Wyndham, Ann Fennessy, David Jasen, David Reffkin, Ian Witcomb, and Richard Hyman. ADMISSION: some performances free, charges for others. ACCOMMODATIONS: motels and hotels, campgrounds, RV parks. RESTAURANTS: fast foods, family, elegant, Chinese, German, Mexican, Greek. CONTACT: Sylvia Thompson, Festival Coordinator, Scott Joplin Commemorative Committee, Inc., P. O. Box 1117, Sedalia, MO 65301 or the Sedalia Area Chamber of Commerce, P. O. Box 1625, Sedalia, MO 65301, (816) 826-2222. 1,500

NATIONAL RAGTIME AND TRADITIONAL JAZZ FESTIVAL *second week in June,* St. Louis, St. Louis Co., at the "Goldenrod Showboat," 400 N. Wharf Street. The historic "Goldenrod Showboat" and adjoining barges house "the world's longest jazz festival" featuring world-renowned jazz artists every night from 6:00 P.M.–1:00 A.M. St. Louis' own St. Louis Ragtimers host this highlight of the jazz musician's and fan's year. ADMISSION: charge. ACCOMMODATIONS: motels and hotels, B&B's, campgrounds, RV parks. RESTAURANTS: fast foods, family, elegant. CONTACT: Dorothy Auble at (314) 621-3311 or the St. Louis Convention and Visitors Commission, 10 S. Broadway, Suite 300, St. Louis, MO 63102, (314) 231-5555.

NATIONAL TOM SAWYER DAYS *week of July 4th,* Hannibal, Marion Co., on the river front in the Mark Twain Region as designated by the Missouri Division of Tourism. National Fence Painting Contest, National Frog Jumping Contest, arts and craft show, pet show, Tomboy Sawyer Competition, parade, Tom and Becky Competition, Tanyard Gardens midnight cruise, mud volleyball, Fun Run, ice cream socials, Huck Finn Raft Race, KIDS Country Cook-off, Governor's Luncheon, mule jumping; beard, bonnet, and moustache competitions, Amateur Ham Radio Operators Club, fireworks. FOODS SERVED: "variety" of local concessions. ADMISSION: free. ACCOMMODATIONS: motels and ho-

tels, B&B's, campgrounds, RV parks. RESTAURANTS: fast foods, family, "semi" elegant. CONTACT: Hannibal Visitors and Convention Bureau, P. O. Box 624, Hannibal, MO 63401, (314) 221-2477. 40,000

VEILED PROPHET FAIR *July 4th weekend,* St. Louis, St. Louis Co., at the Arch grounds, downtown and midtown. Parades, art exhibit, educational and artistic activities, marathons, ethnic dances, air and water events, live music and entertainment. FOODS SERVED: ethnic and concessions. ADMISSION: free. ACCOMMODATIONS: motels and hotels, B&B's, campgrounds, RV parks. RESTAURANTS: fast foods, family, elegant. CONTACT: Veiled Prophet Fair, Inc., One North Taylor Ave., St. Louis, MO 63108, (314) 367-FAIR.

ST. LOUIS STRASSENFEST *fourth weekend in July,* St. Louis, St. Louis Co. Traditional German street festival including oompa bands, German cultural events and German dancing. FOODS SERVED: bratwurst, fresh-baked pretzels, other German food. ADMISSION: free. ACCOMMODATIONS: motels and hotels, B&B's, campgrounds, RV parks. RESTAURANTS: fast foods, family, elegant. CONTACT: Mrs. Lee P. Toberman at (314) 721-7454 or the St. Louis Convention and Visitors Commission, 10 S. Broadway, Suite 300, St. Louis, MO 63102, (314) 231-5555.

JAPANESE FESTIVAL *last weekend in August through first week in September,* St. Louis, St. Louis Co., at the Missouri Botanical Garden on Shaw Boulevard. All aspects of Japanese culture are displayed from Tea Ceremonies to dances, arts and crafts, music, and culinary arts. FOODS SERVED: Japanese. ADMISSION: adults $2.00 weekdays, $3.00 weekends; seniors free weekdays, $1.00 weekends, children 12 and under free. ACCOMMODATIONS: motels and hotels, B&B's, campgrounds, RV parks. RESTAURANTS: fast foods, family, elegant. CONTACT: Missouri Botanical Garden, P. O. Box 299, St. Louis, MO 63166, (314) 577-5100.

SANTA-CALL-GON DAYS *Labor Day weekend (early September),* Independence, Jackson Co., late President Harry Truman's birthplace, to celebrate the meeting of the Santa Fe, Oregon, and California trails. Arts and crafts show, carnival, contests, "commercial-selling spaces," displays, the "Three Trails Shoot Out Gang," and country entertainment. FOODS SERVED: "large variety." ADMISSION: free. ACCOMODATIONS: motels and hotels, B&B, RV parks. RESTAURANTS: fast foods, family, elegant. CONTACT: Independence Chamber of Commerce, P. O. Box 147, Independence, MO 64051, (816) 252-4745. 300,000

SHO-ME SHO-OFF SELEBRATION *third weekend in September,* Poplar Bluff, Butler Co., at the Balley Plaza Shopping Center, to showcase the Poplar Bluff area. Barbecue cooking contest, local and regional country-music groups, other "special events." FOODS SERVED: lots of "southern pork barbecue." ADMISSION: free. ACCOMMODATIONS: motels and hotels, campgrounds, RV parks. RESTAURANTS: fast foods, family. CONTACT: Greater Poplar Bluff Area Chamber of Commerce, P. O. Box 3986, Poplar Bluff, MO 63901, (314) 785-7761. 15,000

BEVO DAY *third or fourth Sunday in September,* St. Louis, St. Louis Co., in the area around Bevo Hill, Gravois, and Morganford. Arts and crafts, antique car display, flea market, rides, parade, 4mi. Run, games, wine garden, continuous entertainment. FOODS SERVED: Italian, Mexican, German, American. ADMISSION: free. ACCOMMODATIONS: motels and hotels, B&B's, campgrounds, RV parks. RESTAURANTS: fast foods, family, elegant. CONTACT: Betty Sanquineete at (314) 352-0141 or the St. Louis Convention and Visitors Commission, 10 S. Broadway, Suite 300, St. Louis, MO 63102, (314) 231-5555.

MEXICO JAYCEES SOYBEAN FESTIVAL *last weekend in September,* Mexico, Audrain Co., to celebrate the soybean harvest. Arts and crafts, Biggest Cockelbur Plant Contest, greased-pig contest, bale bucking contest, cake walks, Outhouse Race, firetruck pull, square dance, 3-wheel pedal race, bicycle drag race, Old Fiddlers Contest, clogging, tug of war, live performances by cloggers, gospel singers, and Miss Missouri. FOODS SERVED: bake sales, concessions. ADMISSION: free. ACCOMMODATIONS: motels and hotels, campground, RV park. RESTAURANTS: fast foods, family, elegant, Chinese. CONTACT: Mexico Jaycees, c/o Mexico Area Chamber of Commerce, P. O. Box 56, Mexico, MO 65265, (314) 581-2765. 10,000

PRAIRIE VIEW FESTIVAL *third weekend in October,* St. Joseph, Buchanan Co., in Northwest Missouri, at the St. Joseph Museum next to the Pony Express Museum. "Living-history festival of 19th-century-style crafts and music." Craftspeople dress in period costumes and demonstrate their crafts skills, juried 19th-century-style music performed by local groups and individuals. FOODS SERVED: local country specialties including funnel cakes, caramel apples, sandwiches. ADMISSION: $2.00 per person. ACCOMMODATIONS: motels and hotels, B&B's, campgrounds, RV parks. RESTAURANTS: fast foods, family, elegant, Chinese, Mexican, Italian. CONTACT: Craft Coordinator, St. Joseph Museum, 11th and Charles St., St. Joseph, MO 64501-2874, (816) 232-8471, or the St. Joseph Area Chamber of Commerce, P. O. Box 1394, St. Joseph, MO 64502, (816) 232-4461. 10,000

AUTUMN HISTORIC FOLKLIFE FESTIVAL *first weekend in November,* Hannibal, Marion Co., in the Mark Twain Historic District of the Mark Twain Region, as designated by the Missouri Division of Tourism, to commemorate Mark Twain's birthday and to remember the traditions of his times. Artists and craftspeople, including those engaging in hobbies or jobs that embody traditional livelihoods of the 1800s, medicine shows, gospel singing extravaganza, Hoop Rolling contest, old-fashioned baking contest, pie and cake auction from baking contest, fiddle and banjo contests, jam sessions, non-denominational church service, "spontaneous square dancing in the streets" at 12:15 Saturday, children's parade, loads of live entertainment including jugglers, puppets, bagpipes, folk dancers, German band, old-time music, Indian dancers, storytellers, open stages for jam sessions. FOODS SERVED: old-time specialties such as chuckwagon stew, cherry and apple fried pies, beer bread and home-made butter, cranberry tea, taffy, bean and cheese soups, baked goods, funnel cakes, Indian fry bread, contemporary concessions. ADMISSION: free. ACCOMMODATIONS: motels and hotels, B&B's, campgrounds, RV parks. RESTAURANTS: fast foods, family, "semi" elegant. CONTACT: Hannibal Arts Council, P. O. Box 1202, Hannibal, MO 63401, (314) 221-6545. 30,000

NEBRASKA

ST. PATRICK'S DAY CELEBRATION *Saturday before St. Patrick's Day (March 17)*, O'Neill, Holt Co., in North-central Nebraska, to celebrate the community's Irish heritage as the "Irish Capital of Nebraska." "World's Largest Shamrock" is painted on main intersection of town, king and queen contest, beard contest, craft show, "large parade," American Legion Award, Irish dances, country-music show, Irish dancers perform in the shamrock. FOODS SERVED: Irish including Mulligan stew. ADMISSION: free, charges for dances and show. ACCOMMODATIONS: motels and hotels, campgrounds. RESTAURANTS: fast foods, family, elegant, Mexican. CONTACT: St. Pat's Booster Club or the O'Neill Area Chamber of Commerce, 315 E. Douglas, O'Neill, NE 68763, (402) 336-2355. 5,000

ARBOR DAY CELEBRATION *weekend following April 22nd*, Nebraska City, Otoe Co., to celebrate Arbor Day. Tree-planting ceremonies, parade, arts festival, craft shows, flea market, fly-in breakfast, long-distance run, environmental awareness games, children's matinee, classic car show. ADMISSION: free. ACCOMMODATIONS: motels and hotels, campgrounds, RV parks. RESTAURANTS: fast foods, family, elegant. CONTACT: Nebraska City Chamber of Commerce. P. O. Box 245, Nebraska City, NE 68410, (402) 873-6654. 7,000

GERMAN HERITAGE DAYS *last weekend in May*, McCook, Red Willow Co., in Southwest Nebraska, to honor the German heritage of McCook's residents. Arts and crafts fair, crowning of royalty, parade, Battle of the Businesses, beer garden, German dancers, square dancers, talent show, firemen's olympics, authentic German musicians perform. FOODS SERVED: German. ADMISSION: free. ACCOMMODATIONS: motels and hotels, campgrounds, RV parks. RESTAURANTS: fast foods, family, elegant. CONTACT: McCook Chamber of Commerce, P. O. Box 337, McCook, NE 69001, (308) 345-3200. 5,000

NEBRASKALAND DAYS *third week in June*, North Platte, Lincoln Co., in West-central Nebraska to celebrate "our western heritage." Amateur art show, chess tournament, senior citizen olympics, rodeos, shoot-outs, road races, outhouse races, two parades, softball, mini-tractor pull, volunteer firefighter water fight, cowboy jackpot bowling, quilting, antique market, melodramas, three evening Grand Stand Shows which have included The Monkees, Roy Clark, gospel singers, and a frontier revue, ethnic entertainment. FOODS SERVED: "all Nebraska ethnic groups" offer food, barbecues. ADMISSION: most events free, charges for some performances. ACCOMMODATIONS: motels and hotels, B&B, campgrounds, RV parks. RESTAURANTS: fast foods, family, private clubs. CONTACT: Nebraskaland Days, P. O. Box 706, North Platte, NE 69101, (308) 532-7939. 100,000

STROMSBURG SWEDISH FESTIVAL
third weekend in June, Stromsburg, Polk Co., to celebrate the Swedish heritage of Stromsburg's residents in "The Swede Capital of Nebraska." Swedish parades, arts and crafts, local entertainment, and costumes, Swedish games. FOODS SERVED: Swedish smorgasbord, traditional Swedish foods. ADMISSION: free. ACCOMMODATIONS: campgrounds, RV parks. Restaurants: fast foods, family. CONTACT: Stromsburg Commercial Club, Stromsburg, NE 68666. 6,000

FUR TRADE DAYS *second weekend in July*, Chadron, Dawes Co., in Pine Ridge country of the Nebraska Panhandle, to recognize local fur trade heritage and the founding of Chadron. "Primitive Rendezvous," authentic costume contest, buffalo-chip throw, parade, 10k Run, softball and horseshoe tournaments, flea market, outdoor cook-off, full boat race, queen contest, flag ceremony featuring flags of twenty-three countries involved in fur trading in the 1800s. FOODS SERVED: barbecue, ice cream social. ADMISSION: free. ACCOMMODATIONS: motels and hotels, campgrounds, RV parks. RESTAURANTS: fast foods, family, western steak houses. CONTACT: Chadron Area Chamber of Commerce, Box 646, Chadron, NE 69337, (308) 432-4401. 10,000

SUMMERFEST CELEBRATION *second weekend in July*, O'Neill, Holt Co., in North-central Nebraska. Art in the Park, antique show, two rodeo performances, "large parade," talent show, Country Showdown, Fun Run, kid's carnival, rodeo queen contest, ice cream social, Irish dan-

cers, puppets. FOODS SERVED: church food booths, funnel cakes, free barbecue. ADMISSION: free, charge for rodeo. ACCOMMODATIONS: motels and hotels, campgrounds. RESTAURANTS: fast foods, family, elegant, Mexican. CONTACT: O'Neill Area Chamber of Commerce, 315 E. Douglas, O'Neill, NE 68763, (402) 336-2355. 10,000

WAYNE CHICKEN SHOW *second weekend in July*, Wayne, Wayne Co., "to pay long overdue tribute to the chicken!" Fun Run for Non-feathered Bipeds, rooster crowing contest, Chicken Flying Meet (fly your own or rent one), arts and crafts fair, roosters and hens on display, National Cluck-Off, Egg Drop and Catch, hardboiled egg eating contest, Chicken Olympecks, balloon release, concessions and games, softball tournament, poetry and essay contest, window displays with chicken decor, parade in which entries are judged on "chicken-ness"; Biggest Midwest Chicken Contest, Chicken Show Hat Contest, and Biggest, Littlest, Prettiest, and Oddest Egg contests. FOODS SERVED: "cheep chicken," free omelet feed. ADMISSION: free. ACCOMMODATIONS: motels and hotels, RV parks. RESTAURANTS: fast foods, family. CONTACT: Wayne Area Chamber of Commerce, P. O. Box 347, Wayne, NE 68787, (402) 375-2240. 3,000

NEBRASKA CZECH FESTIVAL *first full weekend in August*, Wilber, Saline Co., in south-east Nebraska, to honor the "ethnic preservation" of the"Czech people." Art show, children's parade, Czech Parade, travelogue of Czechoslovakia, state and national Czech queen contests, historical pageant, talent contest, quilt show, Duck and Dumpling Run, puppet show, kolache eating contest, Taekwondo Demonstration, All-Nebraska Czech Spectacular, Czech Costume Style Show, quilting and rug making demonstrations, live entertainment including Czech talents such as polka bands, accordian music, dance contests, lots of Czech music and singing. FOODS SERVED: Czechoslovakian roast duck, dumplings, sauerkraut, ko-

laches. ADMISSION: free. ACCOMMODATIONS: motels and hotels (nearby), B&B's, campgrounds, RV parks. RESTAURANTS: fast foods, family, elegant, Czechoslovakian. CONTACT: Irma Ourecky, Box 652, Wilber, NE 68465, (402) 821-2485. 60,000

APPLEJACK FESTIVAL *third weekend in September,* Nebraska City, Otoe Co., to celebrate the apple harvest. Craft show, antique fair, water-barrel fights, Big Wheel and Tricycle Race, parade, marching band contest, queen contest and style show, 10k Run and Fun Run, Flea Show, annual Peru State College vs. Tarkio State College football game, Tri-State Grand Prix of Karting. FOODS SERVED: "anything made with apples," cider and pie garden. ADMISSION: free. ACCOMMODATIONS: motels and hotels, campgrounds, RV parks. RESTAURANTS: fast foods, family, elegant. CONTACT: Nebraska City Chamber of Commerce, P. O. Box 245, Nebraska City, NE 68410, (402) 873-6654. 9,000

OKTOBERFEST *first weekend in October,* Sidney, Cheyenne Co., in western Nebraska, to celebrate a successful harvest and the ethnic backgrounds of Cheyenne County's residents. Art in the Park, craft and flea market, farmers' market, marching bands and field competition, parade, horseshoe pitching, continuous entertainment under large tent featuring performers such as the High Country Cloggers from Denver, Missouri's Matt and Robin Rolf-Show, ethnic dancers and polka bands. FOODS SERVED: German, Swedish, Mexican, Italian. ADMISSION: free. ACCOMMODATIONS: motels and hotels, campgrounds, RV parks. RESTAURANTS: fast foods, family, elegant. CONTACT: Cheyenne Co. Chamber of Commerce, 740 Illinois, Sidney, NE 69162, (308) 254-4444. 18,000

NORTH DAKOTA

WINTER FESTIVAL *third week in February,* Fargo, Cass Co. Dog-sled races, figure skating demonstration, bobsled and sleigh rides, Frisbee contests in the snow, hockey, ski races, wheelchair basketball, Snowball Dance, Scandinavian banquet. FOODS SERVED: Scandinavian and concessions. ADMISSION: free to most events, charges for others. ACCOMMODATIONS: motels and hotels, RV parks. RESTAURANTS: fast foods, family, elegant. CONTACT: Fargo–Moorhead Convention and Visitors Bureau, P. O. Box 2164, Fargo, ND 58107, (701) 237-6134 or (800) 362-3145.

ARTS AND HUMANITIES FESTIVAL *third week in February,* Grand Forks, Grand Forks Co. Film festival, photography and art exhibits, crafts, snow sculpture, theatrical events, dance, concerts.

FOODS SERVED: concessions. ADMISSION: free, charges for concerts. ACCOMMODATIONS: motels and hotels, campgrounds. RESTAURANTS: fast foods, family, elegant. CONTACT: Grand Forks Chamber of Commerce, P. O. Box 1177, Grand Forks, ND 58201, (701) 772-7271.

PIONEER DAYS *weekend before Labor Day (late August),* Bonanzaville, West Fargo, Cass Co., in a re-created early 1900s farming town. Costumed participants demonstrate pioneer life skills such as cooking, soapmaking, horseshoeing, antique tractors, German- and Norwegian-language church services, horse-cart and vintage car rides. FOODS SERVED: home-baked meals at "old-time prices." ADMISSION: free. ACCOMMODATIONS: motels and hotels, RV parks in Fargo. RESTAURANTS: fast foods, family, elegant.

CONTACT: West Fargo Chamber of Commerce, P. O. Box 753, West Fargo, ND 58078, (701) 282-4444.

UNITED TRIBES DAYS *weekend after Labor Day (early September)*, Bismarck, Burleigh Co., at the United Tribes Education and Training Center south of Bismarck. National Indian Singing and Dancing Contest finals, Great Plains Indian Rodeo Association finals, authentic bead and quill work, genuine Indian powwow, slow pitch softball tournament, 10,000m Open Run. FOODS SERVED: Indian such as fry bread; hamburgers, hot dogs. ADMISSION: adults $4.00, children 9 and under free. ACCOMMODATIONS: motels and hotels, camping on grounds, RV parks in Bismarck. RESTAURANTS: fast foods, fam-ily, elegant. CONTACT: United Tribes Education and Training Center, Bismarck, ND 58502 or the Bismarck Area Chamber of Commerce, P. O. Box 1675, Bismarck, ND 58502, (701) 223-5660. 12,000

OKTOBERFEST *third weekend in September*, Bismarck, Burleigh Co. Arts and crafts, parade, queen pageant, dances, biergarten, agricultural show, square dancing. FOODS SERVED: German, concessions. ADMISSION: free, pageant $3.50, dance $3.00. ACCOMMODATIONS: motels and hotels, campgrounds, RV parks. RESTAURANTS: fast foods, family, elegant. CONTACT: Bismarck Area Chamber of Commerce, P. O. Box 1675, Bismarck, ND 58502 (701) 223-5660.

OHIO

WINTERFEST *first weekend in February*, Toledo, Lucas Co. Ice sculpturing around downtown, dog sled races, hot air balloon races, Winter Art Show of the Toledo Art Guild, party in Portside Bazaar, Hot Air Balloon Illumination, Miss Winterfest Competition, Bowling Green Precision Skaters, torchlight cross-country ski, ice sculpture competition, basketball, softball, and volleyball tournaments, free ice skating, children's hands-on art activities, broomball, tennis, and bowling tournaments, golf, triathlon, ice fishing, bike race, Soup-Off competition, fashion show, hockey, entertainment. FOODS SERVED: soup. ADMISSION: free, charges for some events. ACCOMMODATIONS: motels and hotels, B&B's, campgrounds, RV parks. RESTAURANTS: fast foods, family, elegant, international. CONTACT: Greater Toledo Office of Tourism and Conventions, Inc., 218 Huron St., Toledo, OH 43604, (419) 243-8191. 30,000

INTERNATIONAL FESTIVAL *first weekend in May*, Toledo, Lucas Co., at the SeaGate Centre to celebrate all "Toledo area nationalities." Dancing, theatrical productions, musical entertainment, international solos, duets, and dance groups from all countries participating. FOODS SERVED: abundance of international specialties. ADMISSION: advance $3.00, at door $3.50. ACCOMMODATIONS: motels and hotels, B&B's, campgrounds, RV parks. RESTAURANTS: fast foods, family, elegant, international. CONTACT: International Institute at (419) 241-9178 or the Greater Toledo Office of Tourism and Conventions, Inc., 218 Huron St., Toledo, OH 43604, (419) 243-8191. 20,000

MOONSHINE FESTIVAL *Wednesday through Monday of Memorial Day weekend (late May)*, New Straitsville, Perry Co., in the "Moonshine Capital." Arts and crafts,

Moonshine Still, banjo and fiddling contests, Ohio Band of Country Music State Championship, country-music stars, Moonshine Pie and Moonshine Pop, street dancing, parade, midway rides. FOODS SERVED: concessions. ADMISSION: free. ACCOMMODATIONS: (nearby) motels and hotels, campgrounds. RESTAURANTS: fast foods, family. CONTACT: Logan–Hocking Chamber of Commerce, P. O. Box 838, Logan, OH 43138, (614) 385-6836.

HOLY TOLEDO! IT'S SPRING *Memorial Day weekend (late May)*, Toledo, Lucas Co., at the Downtown Riverfront to celebrate the beginning of spring. This three-day rite of spring officially opens the port to recreational boaters, hydroplane races, children's activities, community musical and theatrical productions. FOODS SERVED: "the finest" international. ADMISSION: free. ACCOMMODATIONS: motels and hotels, B&B's, campgrounds, RV parks. RESTAURANTS: fast foods, family, elegant, international. CONTACT: Greater Toledo Office of Tourism and Conventions, Inc., 218 Huron St., Toledo, OH 43604, (419) 243-8191. 50,000

TROY STRAWBERRY FESTIVAL *first full weekend in June*, Troy, Miami Co., on the River Levee. Arts and crafts, athletic events, continuous outdoor entertainment on three stages including "big name" on Saturday night which has included McGuffey Land and The Association. FOODS SERVED: strawberry specialties, variety of other foods. ADMISSION: free. ACCOMMODATIONS: motels and hotels, B&B, campgrounds. RESTAURANTS: fast foods, family, elegant, Chinese. CONTACT: Troy Strawberry Festival, P. O. Box 56, Troy, OH 45373, (513) 339-7714. 125,000

JONATHAN BYE DAYS *second week in June*, Byesville, Guernsey Co., to salute the founder of Byesville. Civil War encampment, reenactment, Military Ball, parade, flea market, arts and crafts, variety of live music. FOODS SERVED: ethnic variety. ADMISSION: free. ACCOMMODA-

TIONS: motels and hotels, B&B, campgrounds, RV parks. RESTAURANTS: fast foods, family, elegant. CONTACT: Cambridge Area Chamber of Commerce, 2250 Southgate Parkway, Cambridge, OH 43725, (614) 439-6688.

FESTIVAL OF THE FISH *third weekend in June*, Vermilion, Lorain Co., at Victory and Exchange parks and the South Shore Shopping Center along the shore of Lake Erie. Carnival throughout this quaint harbor town and historic fishing village. Crazy Craft Boat Race, antique boat show and parade, model boat show at the Great Lakes Museum, queen's pageant, paddle boat and party boat rides, art shows, baking contests, children's games, pet parade, grand parade Sunday, skydivers. FOODS SERVED: Lake Erie fish dinners, fish sandwiches, concessions. ADMISSION: free. ACCOMMODATIONS: motels and hotels, B&B's, campgrounds, RV parks. RESTAURANTS: fast foods, family, elegant. CONTACT: Vermilion Chamber of Commerce, 5488 Liberty, Vermilion, OH 44089, (216) 967-4477. 125,000

INTERNATIONAL WEEK *third weekend through fourth week in June*, Lorain, Lorain Co. Ten full days of fun including Princess Pageant at the Palace Theater, "gigantic International Parade," sacred music, band concert, international festival and bazaar. FOODS SERVED: international, concessions. ADMISSION: free. ACCOMMODATIONS: motels and hotels, B&B's, campgrounds, RV parks. RESTAURANTS: fast foods, family, elegant, international. CONTACT: Greater Lorain Chamber of Commerce, 204 Fifth St., Lorain, OH 44052, (216) 244-2292. 150,000

OHIO SCOTTISH GAMES *fourth Saturday in June*, Oberlin, Lorain Co., at the Oberlin College athletic grounds, to preserve the "traditional Scottish arts in America." Competitions in Highland dancing, piping, drumming, bands, Scottish harp and Scottish heavy athletics, rugby, clan tent displays, Scottish fair with Scottish merchandise and food, Ceilidh (Scottish party). FOODS SERVED: Scottish, American. ADMISSION: adults $7.00, seniors $5.00, children $3.00; Ceilidh $2.00 advance, $3.00 at the door. ACCOMMODATIONS: motels and hotels, B&B's, campgrounds. RESTAURANTS: fast foods, family, elegant. CONTACT: Lorain Co. Visitors Bureau, Inc., 611 Broadway, Lorain, OH 44052, (216) 245-5282. 7,500

DOWNTOWN EUCLID COMMUNITY FESTIVAL *last weekend in June,* Euclid, Cuyahoga Co., near Cleveland at the Shore Civic Centre grounds. Arts and crafts show, auto show, dancing, rides, games, live entertainment such as Phil Dirt and the Dozers rock 'n' roll show, Cedar Point Review, and local amateur and professional groups. FOODS SERVED: those of more than thirty nationalities. ADMISSION: free. ACCOMMODATIONS: motels and hotels, B&B's. RESTAURANTS: fast foods, family, elegant, Chinese, Italian, Slovenian, English. CONTACT: Delores Tocco Tekieli, 5 E. 221st St., Euclid, OH 44123, (216) 261-0261, or the Euclid Chamber of Commerce, 291 E. 222 St., Euclid, OH 44123, (216) 731-9322. 100,000

CROSBY GARDENS FESTIVAL OF THE ARTS *last weekend in June,* Toledo, Lucas Co., at Crosby Gardens, to celebrate the arts in Toledo. Variety of arts and crafts, performing arts such as mimes, clowns, community and area theatrical performances. ADMISSION: free. ACCOMMODATIONS: motels and hotels, B&B's, campgrounds, RV parks. RESTAURANTS: fast foods, family, elegant, international. CONTACT: Crosby Garden Office, 5403 Elmer Dr., Toledo, OH 43604, (419) 536-8365 or the Greater Toledo Office of Tourism and Conventions, Inc., 218 Huron St., Toledo, OH 43604, (419) 243-8191. 40,000

MIDWEST TOBACCO SPITTIN' CHAMPIONSHIP *July 4,* Grafton, Lorain Co., downtown on Main Street. "Top–notch" tobacco chewers compete for prize

money in accuracy and distance events, street festival, Hay Bale Throwing Contest, Jail Bird Run, parade, fireworks. FOODS SERVED: concessions. ADMISSION: free. ACCOMMODATIONS: motels and hotels. RESTAURANTS: family. CONTACT: Lorain Co. Visitors Bureau, Inc., 611 Broadway, Lorain, OH 44052, (216) 245-5282. 8,000

COLUMBIA HOMECOMING AND BLUEBERRY FESTIVAL *July 4th weekend,* Columbia Township, Lorain Co., at Columbia State Park, to celebrate the blueberry harvest. Arts and crafts, blueberry baking contest, horse shows, beauty pageant, parade, live entertainment, fireworks. FOODS SERVED: blueberry concoctions and concessions. ADMISSION: free. ACCOMMODATIONS: motels and hotels, B&B's. RESTAURANTS: family. CONTACT: Lorain Co. Visitors Bureau, Inc., 611 Broadway, Lorain, OH 44052, (216) 245-5282. 20,000

WESTERVILLE MUSIC AND ARTS FESTIVAL *second weekend in July,* Westerville, Franklin Co., at Towers Hall Lawn on the campus of Otterbein College. Juried fine arts and crafts displayed and sold, children's activity tent, storytelling, mime, harpists, theatrical presentations, the Westerville Civic Symphony string quartet and the Tonight Only jazz group. FOOD SERVED: concessions. ADMISSION: free. ACCOMMODATIONS: motels and hotels, campgrounds, RV parks. RESTAURANTS: fast foods, family, elegant, Asian, Mexican. CONTACT: Westerville Area Chamber of Commerce, 5 W. College Ave., Westerville, OH 43081, (614) 882-8917. 20,000

CELINA LAKE FESTIVAL *fourth weekend in July,* Celina, Mercer Co., in the Grand Lake St. Mary's area. Lake and water sports events, antique car parade, antique car show, Grand Parade, triathlon, Queen's pageant, children's contests, sidewalk sales, fireworks, entertainment by the Air Force Band and local groups.

ADMISSION: free, charge for Queen's Pageant. ACCOMMODATIONS: motel, campgrounds, RV parks nearby. RESTAURANTS: fast foods, family, Chinese, Mexican. CONTACT: Celina Area Chamber of Commerce, 226 N. Main St., Celina, OH 45822, (419) 586-2219. 50,000

PRO FOOTBALL HALL OF FAME FESTIVAL *first week in August,* Canton, Stark Co., at Canton Memorial Civic Center and downtown, honoring the year's professional football players to be inducted into the Hall of Fame. Grand Parade, balloon fiesta, Ribs Burn-off, fireworks, Mayor's Breakfast, fashion show luncheon, Enshrinees Civic Dinner, kickoff Sunday parade; celebrities attending include entertainers as well as football players ranging from Glen Campbell to Redd Foxx and Nannette Fabray to former President Gerald Ford and the Budweiser Clydesdale Horses. FOODS SERVED: ribs, luncheons and formal gatherings. ADMISSION: some events free, charges for others. ACCOMMODATIONS: motels and hotels, campgrounds. RESTAURANTS: fast foods, family, elegant. CONTACT: Pro Football Hall of Fame Festival, c/o Greater Canton Chamber of Commerce, P. O. Box 1044, Canton, OH 44701-1044, (216) 456-7253. 300,000

NORTH RIDGEVILLE CORN FESTIVAL *first weekend in August,* North Ridgeville, Lorain Co., featuring fresh-picked Amish-style sweet corn. Arts and crafts, live entertainment, games, demonstrations, rides, and grand parade. FOODS SERVED: Amish-style sweet corn, concessions. ADMISSION: free. CONTACT: North Ridgeville Chamber of Commerce, P. O. Box 172, North Ridgeville, OH 44039, (216) 327-3737. 30,000

THE POTATO FESTIVAL *second weekend in August,* Amherst, Lorain Co., to celebrate the potato crop. Arts and crafts tents, carnival rides and games, BMX Freestyle Show, potato eating contest, potato peeling contest Miss Amherst, Ta-

ter Tot and Golden Ager beauty pageants, big parade, continuous entertainment on stage. FOODS SERVED: more than fifty-five food and beverage booths including potatoes. ADMISSION: free. ACCOMMODATIONS: motels and hotels, campgrounds, RV parks. RESTAURANTS: fast foods, family, elegant. CONTACT: Amherst Area Chamber of Commerce, P. O. Box 2, Amherst, OH 44001, (216) 988-9073. 125,000

SALT FORK ARTS AND CRAFTS FESTIVAL *second weekend in August,* Cambridge, Guernsey Co., at the Cambridge City Park. More than 200 craftspeople display their work, hands-on crafts tent, art judging, puppets, dancing, musical and dramatic performances, classes, lectures. FOODS SERVED: American. ADMISSION: free. ACCOMMODATIONS: motels and hotels, B&B's, campgrounds, RV parks. RESTAURANTS: fast foods, family, elegant, Chinese, Greek. CONTACT: Salt Fork Festival Chairman, Ohio Arts and Crafts Foundation, c/o Cambridge Area Chamber of Commerce, 2250 Southgate Parkway, Cambridge, OH 43725, (614) 439-6688. 60,000

BRATWURST FESTIVAL *second or third weekend in August,* Bucyrus, Crawford Co., in the "Bratwurst Capital of America."* Three parades, arts and craft shows, rides, games, beer gardens. FOODS SERVED: tons and tons of Bucyrus bratwurst roasted on open fires, beer. ADMISSION: free. ACCOMODATIONS: motels and hotels, campgrounds nearby. RESTAURANTS: family. CONTACT: Bucyrus Area Chamber of Commerce, 334 S. Sandusky Ave., Bucyrus, OH 44820, (419) 562-4811.

TOLEDO FESTIVAL: A CELEBRATION OF THE ARTS *Labor Day weekend (early September),* Toledo, Lucas Co., at the downtown river front, to celebrate the visual and performing arts. Four days of visual arts and crafts, waterfront activities, children's art area, fireworks, culinary arts, regional and local entertainers perform on five stages including in the past Lionel Hampton, Rare Silk, Wynton Marsalis, Spyro Gyra, Stanley Jordan, Pat Daily. FOODS SERVED: multi-ethnic specialties. ADMISSION: free. ACCOMMODATIONS: motels and hotels, campgrounds. RESTAURANTS: fast foods, family, elegant, international. CONTACT: Toledo Festival: A Celebration of the Arts, 618 N. Michigan St., Toledo, OH 43624, (419) 255-8968. 550,000

CLINTON COUNTY CORN FESTIVAL *first weekend in September,* Wilmington, Clinton Co. Display of antique machinery, demonstrations of early lifestyles such as making food products, corn olympics, pig races, entertainment. FOODS SERVED: "American." ADMISSION: $1.50 per day or $3.00 weekend pass. ACCOMMODATIONS: motels and hotels, campgrounds, RV parks. RESTAURANTS: fast foods, family. CONTACT: Wilmington Area Chamber of Commerce, 69 N. South St., Wilmington, OH 45177, (513) 382-2737.

PIONEER DAYS FESTIVAL *second weekend in September,* Brownhelm Township, Lorain Co., at Mill Hollow-Bacon Woods Memorial Park. Festival focuses on pioneer life skills, education, demonstrations, and hands-on experiences, and crafts. FOODS SERVED: pioneer emphasis. ADMISSION: free. ACCOMMODATIONS: motels and hotels, campgrounds, RV parks nearby. RESTAURANTS: family. CONTACT: Lorain Co. Visitors Bureau, Inc., 611 Broadway, Lorain, OH 44052, (216) 245-5282. 65,000

OHIO HONEY FESTIVAL *second weekend in September,* Lebanon, Warren Co. World-famous living bee beard, more than 100 arts, crafts, and food booths, continuous live entertainment. FOODS SERVED: honey ice cream, Greek pastries, honey waffles, candy, honey in jars, by the comb, or whipped into honey butter. ADMISSION: free. ACCOMMODATIONS: motels and hotels, campgrounds nearby. RESTAURANTS: family. CONTACT: Ohio

Honey Festival, P. O. Box 192, Lebanon, OH 45036, (513) 932-5142.

ELYRIA APPLE FESTIVAL *third weekend in September,* Lorain, Lorain Co., at Ely Park and downtown Elyria. Old-fashioned street fair, Apple Walk, antique car show, Applethon Race, crowning of Apple Queen, displays by Armed Forces, crafts, children's events. FOODS SERVED: apples, "plenty of good food." ADMISSION: free. ACCOMMODATIONS: motels and hotels, campgrounds, RV parks. RESTAURANTS: fast foods, family, elegant. CONTACT: Lorain Co. Visitors Bureau, 611 Broadway, Lorain, OH 44052, (216) 245-5282. 90,000

RAVENNA BALLOON A-FAIR *third weekend in September,* Ravenna, Portage Co., downtown. Hot air balloon lift-offs, 250 craftspeople display and sell their work, parade. FOODS SERVED: international concessions. ADMISSION: free to downtown, "nominal fee at hot air ballon site." ACCOMMODATIONS: motels and hotels. RESTAURANTS: fast foods, family, elegant. CONTACT: Ravenna Area Chamber of Commerce, 231 W. Main St., Ravenna, OH 44266, (216) 296-3886. 100,000

TIPP CITY MUM FESTIVAL *third weekend in September,* Tipp City, Miami Co., on Main Street and in the City Park, to celebrate the abundance of gorgeous chrysanthemum flowers in bloom. Arts and crafts, flea market, parade, Run for the Mums, metric bike tour, theatrical presentation by the Tipp City Players, comedy and melodrama, and high school band show featuring twenty-five–thirty bands, all with a backdrop of colorful chrysanthemums. FOODS SERVED: concessions. ADMISSION: free, charges for some events. ACCOMMODATIONS: motels and hotels, B&B's. RESTAURANTS: fast foods, family. CONTACT: Tipp City Mum Festival, Inc., P. O. Box 1, Tipp City, OH 45371 or the Tipp City Area Chamber of Commerce, P. O. Box 134, Tipp City, OH 45371, (513) 667-8300. 40,000

JACKSON COUNTY APPLE FESTIVAL *fourth week in September,* Jackson, Jackson Co., downtown, to celebrate the apple harvest. Arts and crafts, street fair featuring rides, games, displays, and contests, four parades, quilt show, car show, Big Wheel Race, Baby Crawling Contest, local and Nashville stars. FOODS SERVED: apple products such as apple butter, apple pies, candy apples, other foods. ADMISSION: free. ACCOMMODATIONS: motels and hotels, campgrounds, RV parks. RESTAURANTS: fast foods, family, elegant. CONTACT: Jackson Co. Apple Festival, Inc., Jackson, OH 45640, (614) 286-1414. 220,000

OHIO PUMPKIN FESTIVAL *fourth weekend in September,* Barnesville, Belmont Co. Giant pumpkin contest, fiddle and hog calling contests, beauty pageants, old car show, arts and crafts show, "spitting contest," apple industry demonstrations, Giant Pumpkin Parade, Tall Tales Contest, beard and moustache contests, Pumpkin Run, midway rides and concessions, antique farm machinery display, quilt show, book sale, procession of antique and classic cars, auction of unclaimed pumpkins, squash, gourds, and other produce, live entertainment including country-western, country rock, and rock'n'roll music. FOODS SERVED: pumpkin pie and ice cream, homemade pies, barbecued steak and chicken, plus more. ADMISSION: free. ACCOMMODATIONS: motel, B&B, campground. RESTAURANTS: fast foods, family. CONTACT: Barnesville Area Chamber of Commerce, P. O. Box 376, Barnesville, OH, (614) 425-2188. 100,000

MIDDFEST INTERNATIONAL *first week in October,* Middletown, Butler Co. Each year a different country is featured including its arts and crafts, music, sporting events, entertainment, and foods, in an effort to create international understanding and trade. Annual events include dart tournament, International Fly-in, Bike Tour, chess tournament, checkers, various distance runs including 10k, 28k, 40k, 52k, 80k, and 100k, and a photogra-phy contest. FOODS SERVED: specialties of featured country and twenty-five other countries. ADMISSION: most events free, entry fees for runs. ACCOMMODATIONS: motels and hotels, campgrounds, RV parks. RESTAURANTS: fast foods, family, elegant, international. CONTACT: Middfest International, One City Centre Plaza, Middletown, OH 45042, (513) 425-7707. 100,000

OHIO SWISS FESTIVAL *first weekend in October,* Sugarcreek, Tuscarawas Co., in this Alpine-design village. Swiss athletic events such as Steinstossen (stone throwing), Schwingfest (Swiss wrestling), yodeling, costumes, parades including kiddies' parade, dancing to several polka bands. FOODS SERVED: tons of Swiss cheese from fifteen plants in the Sugarcreek area, other gourmet foods. ADMISSION: free. ACCOMMODATIONS: motels and hotels, campgrounds nearby. RESTAURANTS: family, Swiss. CONTACT: Ohio Swiss Festival, Box 361, Sugarcreek, OH 44681, (216) 852-4113.

OHIO GOURD SHOW *first full weekend in October,* Mt. Gilead, Morrow Co., at the County Fairgrounds in Central Ohio, to celebrate the fall harvest of gourds. Gourds and gourd craft displays, judging of gourds by classes, Gourd Theatre, parade. ADMISSION: $1.00 per person. ACCOMMODATIONS: motels, campgrounds, RV parks. RESTAURANTS: family. CONTACT: Gourd Show Chairman, Box 274, Mt. Gilead, OH 43338, (419) 946-3302. 10,000

APPLE FESTIVAL *second weekend in October,* Oak Harbor, Ottawa Co., to celebrate the apple harvest. Arts and crafts, literature, children's rides, live entertainment such as Big Band Impact, Pure Quill Deuchmeisters, college groups and high school choirs. FOODS SERVED: apple specialties and "all types." ADMISSION: free. ACCOMMODATIONS: motels and hotels, campgrounds. RESTAURANTS: family, elegant. CONTACT: Oak Harbor Area Chamber of Commerce, 178 W. Water St., Oak Harbor, OH 43449, (419) 898-0479. 10,000

OHIO SAUERKRAUT FESTIVAL *second weekend in October,* Waynesville, Warren Co. Family-oriented folk festival featuring 350 arts and crafts exhibitors, almost continuous folk music and dancing. FOODS SERVED: assorted sauerkraut foods including sauerkraut cookies and bread, sloppy kraut in a pita pocket, sauerkraut pizza, sauerkraut dinners, reuben sandwiches and other sauerkraut sandwiches, candy, donuts. ADMISSION: free. ACCOMMODATIONS: Motels in nearby Lebanon, B&B, campgrounds. RESTAURANTS: family, elegant. CONTACT: Waynesville Area Chamber of Commerce, P. O. Box 281, Waynesville, OH 45068, (513) 897-8855. 200,000

NEW MUSIC FESTIVAL *mid-October,* Bowling Green, Wood Co. at Bowling Green State University, to expose and celebrate art and music of the 1970s and 1980s and the visual arts. Five concerts of new art-music, special concerts by guest artists, panel discussions, workshops, and master classes with guest artists, in conjunction with Bowling Green State University School of Art. Composers and artists from Belgium, Canada, France, Italy, and Switzerland attend, including the merging of art and music in John Cage's recent performance of "Mushrooms et Variationes." ADMISSION: free to public. ACCOMMODATIONS: motels and hotels. RESTAURANTS: fast foods, family, Polynesian. CONTACT: College of Musical Arts, Bowling Green State University, Bowling Green, OH 43403-0290, (419) 372-2181 or the Bowling Green Chamber of Commerce, 139 W. Wooster St., Bowling Green, OH 43402, (419) 353-7945.

OKLAHOMA

AZALEA FESTIVAL *most of April,* Muskogee, Muskogee Co., at Honor Heights Park, to celebrate the spectacular beauty of 70,000 azaleas featuring 600 varieties blooming in a 100-acre park. Parade, rodeo, fly-in, antique car auction, chili cook-off, arts and crafts shows, speedway races, sporting events, concerts and dances. FOODS SERVED: chili, concessions. ADMISSION: free, charges for some events. ACCOMMODATIONS: motels and hotels, campgrounds. RESTAURANTS: fast foods, family, elegant. CONTACT: Muskogee Chamber of Commerce, P. O. Box 797, Muskogee, OK 74401, (918) 682-2401. 700,000

WAYNOKA RATTLESNAKE HUNT *first Sunday after Easter (April),* Waynoka, Woods Co., in the Gypson Hills. Caravans transport participants into the Gypson Hills to hunt rattlesnakes, demonstrations of rattlesnake butchering, selling of meat, and handling snakes, carnival, dance bands. FOODS SERVED: "rattlesnake meat and fast foods." ADMISSION: free. ACCOMMODATIONS: motels and hotels, B&B's, campgrounds, RV parks. RESTAURANTS: fast foods, family, elegant. CONTACT: Austin L. Cue, Box 174, Waynoka, OK 73860, (405) 824-5911.

KOLACHE FESTIVAL *first Saturday in May,* Prague, Lincoln Co., to celebrate the town's birthday. Parade, Czech-costume judging, queen crowning, street dance, Ernie Davis Band. FOODS SERVED: Czechoslovakian. ADMISSION: free. ACCOMMODATIONS: motel, B&B. RESTAURANTS: fast foods, family. CONTACT:

Prague Chamber of Commerce, P. O. Box 223, Prague, OK 74864, (405) 278-8900. 20,000

STILWELL STRAWBERRY FESTIVAL *first or second weekend in May,* Stilwell, Adair Co., to celebrate the strawberry harvest in the "Strawberry Capital of the World." Strawberry Parade, Strawberry Auction, bandstand entertainment, V.I.P. luncheon, queen crowning, "headline" state entertainers. FOODS SERVED: free strawberries and strawberry shortcake. ADMISSION: free. ACCOMMODATIONS: motels and hotels, campgrounds. RESTAURANTS: fast foods, family, elegant. CONTACT: Stilwell Chamber of Commerce, P. O. Box 845, Stilwell, OK 74960, (918) 696-7845.

TULSA INTERNATIONAL MAYFEST *third weekend in May,* Tulsa, Tulsa Co., in northeastern Oklahoma, as a salute to the performing, visual, and literary arts and to downtown Tulsa. Juried art fair featuring 100 artists, mayfest market including arts and crafts, "Artzone" participatory arts for children and adults, theatrical presentations which have included "Three Penny Opera," "Our Town," and "Revenge of the Space Pandas"; entertainers have included Pure Prairie League, Gary Lewis and the Playboys, John Hartford, Oklahoma Sinfonia, and a Woody Guthrie Tribute. FOODS SERVED: Greek, German, Lebanese, Chinese, French, Italian, American. ADMISSION: free. ACCOMMODATIONS: motels and hotels. RESTAURANTS: fast foods, family, elegant. CONTACT: Downtown Tulsa Unlimited, 6 E. Fifth, Suite 200, Tulsa, OK 74103, (918) 583-2617. 400,000

WORLD CHAMPIONSHIP COW CHIP THROWING CONTEST *fourth weekend in May,* Beaver, Beaver Co., at the County Fairgrounds to celebrate Cimarron Territory Days. Cow Chip Throwing Contest, antique, coin, gun, and hobby show, Wild West Shoot Out, black-powder shoot, parade, carnival, children's activities, music shows including area country-western music fest. FOODS SERVED: concessions. ADMISSION: free, $10.00 to participate in Cow Chip Throwing Contest. ACCOMMODATIONS: motels and hotels, campgrounds, RV parks. RESTAURANTS: fast foods, family. CONTACT: Beaver Chamber of Commerce, Box 878, Beaver, OK 73932, (405) 625-4726. 3,500

ITALIAN FESTIVAL *Memorial Day weekend (late May),* McAlester, Pittsburg Co., to celebrate Italian heritage of early residents who came to work the coal mines. Arts and crafts show, rides, concessions, souvenirs. Foods served: 12,000 meatballs, 6,000 sausages, 200 gallons of sauce and spaghetti prepared by the community, which says: "Venitu tutti," or "Come one, come all." ADMISSION: free. ACCOMMODATIONS: motels and hotels, campgrounds, RV parks. RESTAURANTS: fast foods, family, elegant, Italian, Chinese. CONTACT: McAlester Chamber of Commerce, P. O. Box 759, McAlester, OK 74502, (918) 423-2550. 5,000

FESTIVAL DEL PASEO *Memorial Day weekend (late May),* Oklahoma City, Oklahoma Co., on the Paseo at N. W. 30th and Dewey, in Paseo Village, as a festival for the arts and the beginning of summer. Two blocks of 125 artists and craftspeople and their work, two stages with continuous music and 200 performing artists including street performers, jugglers, mimes, unicyclists, dancers, comedians, jazz combos, symphony, dance review, folk dancers, rock bands, folk musicians, and comedy troupes. FOODS SERVED: Native American, Mexican, Vietnamese, German. ADMISSION: free. ACCOMMODATIONS: motels and hotels, B&B's, campgrounds, RV parks. RESTAURANTS: family, Mexican, Italian. CONTACT: Lanny Weisman at (405) 524-1683 or Claude Hall at (405) 528-1222 or the Oklahoma City Chamber of Commerce, One Santa Fe Plaza, Oklahoma City, OK 73102, (405) 278-8900. 50,000

SANTA FE TRAIL DAZE *first weekend in June,* Boise City, Cimarron Co., in the Oklahoma Panhandle, to celebrate "the spirit of the Old West and remind our children of their pioneer heritage." Parade, World Championship Posthole Digging Contest, free bus tour of Santa Fe Trail sites on private lands, tobacco spitting contest, queen coronation, horseshoe pitching and roping contests, antique car show, stagecoach rides, 5k Race, Fun Run and Walk, fiddling contest, Li'l Hombre Rodeo, square dance, Hee-Haw style talent show, barrel racing. FOODS SERVED: free pancake breakfast, free watermelon feed, all-American. ADMISSION: adults $2.00, children 12 and under $1.00. ACCOMMODATIONS: motels and hotels, campgrounds, RV parks. RESTAURANTS: fast foods, family. CONTACT: Boise City Chamber of Commerce, Box 1027, Boise City, OK 73933, (405) 544-3344. 5,000

KIAMICHI OWA-CHITO *third weekend in June,* Idabel, McCurtain Co., at Beavers Bend State Park in the Idabel–Broken Bow area, as a "Festival of the Forest." Canoe races, archery, horseshoe throwing, talent contest, art show, tobacco spitting contest, turkey-owl calling contest, wood carvers, wood turners, log burling, photography show, forestry contests, live entertainment such as gospel singing, fiddling, and major-country stars such as Reba McEntire, Moe Bandy, Janie Fricke, Becky Hobbs, The Shoppe, and bluegrass music. FOODS SERVED: Choctaw Indian, American foods. ADMISSION: free. ACCOMMODATIONS: campgrounds, RV parks, cabins. RESTAURANTS: fast foods, family. CONTACT: Idabel Chamber of Commerce and Agriculture, 13 N. Central, Idabel, OK 74745, (405) 286-3305. 8,000

BLUE GRASS SHOW *July 4th weekend,* Langley, Mayes Co., in the Grand Lake area in the park. Langley calls itself both "The Bluegrass Capital of Oklahoma" and the "Fiddle Capital of the World." A festival of "good fellowship and good music" that features country-western and blue-grass music and attracts both local and international stars such as Merle Haggard and the Lewis Family. FOODS SERVED: international and concessions. ADMISSION: $6.00–$8.00. ACCOMMODATIONS: motels and hotels, campgrounds, RV parks. RESTAURANTS: fast foods, family, elegant. CONTACT: Langley City Hall, Langley, OK 74350, (918) 782-9850. 3,500

GRANT'S BLUEGRASS AND OLD TIME MUSIC FESTIVAL *first Wednesday through Sunday in August,* Hugo, Choctaw Co., at Salt Creek Park. Concerts, 24-hour jam sessions, "all the top names in the Blue Grass Music field" including The Lewis Family, The Johnson Mountain Boys, The New Coon Creek Girls, Signal Mountain, Lonnie Glosson, Bill Grant and Delia Bell, Red Wing, Larry Sparks and the Lonesome Ramblers and Don Wiley and the Louisiana Grass; contests on banjo, mandolin, fiddle, guitar, dobro and bass, with some junior categories, $3,500 in prizes and trophies. FOODS SERVED: cook-outs, American, Mexican, Indian, concessions. ADMISSION: $8.00–$9.00 per day, $32.00 for all five days. ACCOMMODATIONS: motels and hotels, B&B's, campgrounds, RV parks, camping on site. RESTAURANTS: fast foods, family, elegant. CONTACT: Bill and Juarez Grant, Rt. 2, Box 74, Hugo, OK 74743, (405) 326-5598. 20,000

FRONTIER DAYS CELEBRATION *first full week in August,* Tecumseh, Pottawatomie Co. Western heritage entertainment and activities including Frontier Days Rodeo, Miss Frontier Days Pageant, parade, square dancing, 5mi. Run, gospel singing, Little Theater melodrama, tennis tournament. FOODS SERVED: pancake breakfast, concessions. ADMISSION: free, charge for rodeo adults $2.50, children $1.50, under 12 free. ACCOMMODATIONS: motels and hotels, B&B's. RESTAURANTS: fast foods, family. CONTACT: Tecumseh Chamber of Commerce, 114 N. Broadway, Tecumseh, OK 74873, (405) 598-8666.

CHILI BLUEGRASS FESTIVAL *first weekend after Labor Day (early September)*, Tulsa, Tulsa Co., in northeastern Oklahoma. International Chili Society regional cook-off featuring eighty of the best chili-cooking teams in the area, bluegrass banjo and fiddle competition, arts and crafts, nationally renowned bluegrass bands such as Quicksilver, Nashville Bluegrass Band, The Whites, Osborne Brothers, Lost and Found, Skyline and Country Gazette. FOODS SERVED: chili and concessions. ADMISSION: free. ACCOMMODATIONS: motels and hotels. RESTAURANTS: fast food, family, elegant. CONTACT: Downtown Tulsa Unlimited, 6 E. Fifth, Suite 200, Tulsa, OK 74103, (918) 583-2617.

CALF FRY FESTIVAL AND COOK-OFF *third Saturday in September*, Vinita, Craig Co., in Green Country, the "Calf Fry Capital of the World." Calf Fry children's games include egg toss, turtle race, bubble gum blowing, and moseying; adult games such as hairiest legs contest, liar contest, cowboy games, volleyball tournament, tug of war, Frisbee, golf, and horseshoes tournaments, live bands all day, dance where Belle of the Ball is crowned. FOODS SERVED: calf fry lunch and free samples from cook-off teams. ADMISSION: free. ACCOMMODATIONS: motels and hotels, RV parks. RESTAURANTS: fast foods, family. CONTACT: Vinita Chamber of Commerce, P. O. Box 882, Vinita, OK 74301, (918) 256-7133. Note: "Calf fry" according to the Vinita Chamber of Commerce, is "in some areas called mountain oysters. They are actually testicles from a young bull." Vinita probably has few rivals to its claim as the Calf Fry Capital. 7,000

FALL FESTIVAL OF THE ARTS *third weekend in September*, Elk City, Beckham Co. Arts and crafts displayed and sold, hands-on art experiences for children, musical performances, mimes, juggling. FOODS SERVED: native American, Spanish/ Mexican, crepes, American. ADMISSION: free. ACCOMMODATIONS: motels and hotels, campgrounds, RV parks. RESTAU-RANTS: fast foods, family, Chinese, Mexican. CONTACT: Elk City Chamber of Commerce, P. O. Box 972, Elk City, OK 73648, (405) 225-0207. 5,000

CZECH FESTIVAL *first Saturday in October*, Yukon, Canadian Co., in the Greater Oklahoma City area, to celebrate "the Czech heritage of the area" in the "Czech Capital of Oklahoma." Crafts show featuring artists from Oklahoma and the Southwestern U. S., parade, Czech dancers, bandstand under the big tent with polka bands playing polkas and waltzes all day, performances of the Beseda, the Czech National Dance, brass band concert, group singing. Czech records, tapes, dolls, and cookbooks area available with other imported Czech merchandise. FOODS SERVED: kolache and klobasy sandwiches, kolache by the dozen, cold klobasy by the pound, homemade breads and pastries. ADMISSION: free. ACCOMMODATIONS: Oklahoma City. RESTAURANTS: family. CONTACT: Oklahoma Czechs Inc., P. O. Box 850211, Yukon, OK 73085, (405) 354-7573, or the Yukon Chamber of Commerce, 510 Elm, Yukon, OK 73099, (405) 354-3567. 50,000

SORGHUM DAY *fourth Saturday in October*, Wewoka, Seminole Co., on Main Street, to celebrate the area's "territorial past." Arts and crafts shows including needlework, folk art, photo, and quilt shows, biscuit eating contest, beard growing and fiddlers' contests, making and sale of sorghum, tours of the Seminole National Museum, magic show, musical groups all day. FOODS SERVED: "authentic Indian food" and a variety of traditional foods at booths on Main Street. ADMISSION: free. ACCOMMODATIONS: motels and hotels. RESTAURANTS: family. CONTACT: Wewoka Chamber of Commerce, P. O. Box 719, Wewoka, OK 74884, (405) 257-5485. 20,000

CHEESE–SAUSAGE FESTIVAL *last weekend in October or first weekend in November*, Stillwater, Payne Co. More than 140 artists and craftspeople from Oklahoma, Kansas, and Arkansas display their work, cheese and sausage making demonstrations. FOODS SERVED: cheese and sausage products. ADMISSION: free. ACCOMMODATIONS: motels and hotels, RV parks. RESTAURANTS: fast foods, family, elegant. CONTACT: Stillwater Chamber of Commerce, P. O. Box 1687, Stillwater, OK 74078, (405) 372-5573. 10,000

WATONGA CHEESE FESTIVAL *first Friday and Saturday in November,* Watonga, Blaine Co. Art, crafts, and antique shows, cheese tasting, Railroad Swap Meet, flea market, antique cars, horse-drawn carriage rides, Rat Race (fun runs of 1, 3, 6 and 9mi.), pony rides; tours of the Ferguson Museum, Hollytex Carpet Mill, and the Watonga Cheese Factory, two days of continuous entertainment including an old-fashioned melodrama, and musical groups from throughout Oklahoma. FOODS SERVED: "everything you can imagine with cheese." ADMISSION: free. ACCOMMODATIONS: motels and hotels, campground, RV park. RESTAURANTS: fast foods, family. CONTACT: Watonga Chamber of Commerce, Box 537, Watonga, OK 73772, (405) 623-5452. 20,000

SOUTH DAKOTA

ARTS AND CRAFTS FESTIVAL *last weekend in June,* Hot Springs, Fall River Co., in Centennial Park. Variety of arts and crafts, continuous entertainment. FOODS SERVED: food booths. ADMISSION: free. ACCOMMODATIONS: motels and hotels, campgrounds. RESTAURANTS: fast foods, family. CONTACT: Buluah Donnell, Arts and Crafts Committee, Hot Springs, SD 57747, (605) 745-4225.

BLACK HILLS HERITAGE FESTIVAL *fourth weekend in July,* Rapid City, Pennington Co., in the Black Hills, to celebrate Black Hills culture. Arts and crafts fair, traditional Indian Powwow, live entertainment including Indian dances. FOODS SERVED: American Indian, German. ADMISSION: $2.00 per day or $5.00 for whole weekend. ACCOMMODATIONS: motels and hotels, B&B's, campgrounds, RV parks. RESTAURANTS: fast foods, family. CONTACT: Rapid City Convention and Visitors Bureau, P. O. Box 747, Rapid City, SD 57709, (605) 343-1744. 1,000

GOLD DISCOVERY DAYS PAGEANT OF PAHA SAPA (Sacred Land of the Sioux Indians) *last full weekend in July,* Custer, Custer Co., in the Black Hills in "The Buffalo Capital of the World," to remember and celebrate the discovery of gold in the Black Hills. Parade, Little Britches Rodeo, street sales, Gold Rush Run, bingo, Custer State Park Volksmarch, ice cream social; and the Pageant of Paha Sapa in three episodes including the Sacred Land of the Sioux, the coming of the Great Spirit, and the arrival of Custer's expedition and the discovery of gold in 1874, the massacre of Metz's family, and the hanging of Fly Speck Billy, culminating in the creation of a living American flag. FOODS SERVED: "western American." ADMISSION: adults $2.00, children free. ACCOMMODATIONS: motels and hotels, campgrounds, RV parks. RESTAURANTS: fast foods, family, elegant. CONTACT: Custer Co. Chamber of Commerce, 447 Crook St., Custer, SD 57730, (800) 992-9818.

YANKTON RIVERBOAT DAYS *third or fourth weekend in August,* Yankton, Yankton Co., at Riverside Park. Arts festival featuring more than ninety artists and craftspeople from five states, children's art activities including mural painting, plaster necklaces, spatter-painted T-shirts, face painting, buttons, pet extravaganza, water ski show and contests, triathlon, children's parade, arm wrestling championships, political rally, antique and custom auto show, children's events, Bedpan Races by healthcare professionals, antique fashion show, basketball hoop shoot, Kiss the Carp Contest, ice cream social, Bingo Tent, tug of war; live entertainment including Battle of the Bands, The Dakota Dance and Riverboat Show, bluegrass bands, square dancing, open air concert, Riverboat choral presentation. FOODS SERVED: beer garden, "edible art" at many ethnic food booths including kuchen, French pastries, kolaches, creole and southern foods, lefse, bratwurst and sauerkraut, homemade ice cream. ADMISSION: free. ACCOMMODATIONS: motels and hotels, B&B's, campgrounds, RV parks. RESTAURANTS: fast foods, family, elegant, Chinese, Mexican. CONTACT: Yankton Area Chamber of Commerce, P. O. Box 588, Yankton, SD 57078, (605) 665-3636.

FALL FESTIVAL *second weekend in September,* Custer, Custer Co., at Boothill Ranch in the Black Hills in "The Buffalo Capital of the World," to celebrate the arrival of fall. Craft sales, Tri-State Chili Cook-off, black powder competition, live entertainment such as Native Indian dancers, country music, storytelling, cowboy poets. FOODS SERVED: chili. ADMISSION: $.50 per person. ACCOMMODATIONS: motels and hotels, campgrounds, RV parks. RESTAURANTS: fast foods, family, elegant. CONTACT: Custer Co. Chamber of Commerce, 447 Crook St., Custer, SD 57730, (800) 992-9818.

CORN PALACE WEEK *third week in September,* Mitchell, Davison Co., at the "World's Only Corn Palace." Polka fest, carnival rides, games, agricultural exhibits, big-name entertainment such as Bob Hope, Red Skelton, Roger Miller, Mills Brothers. FOODS SERVED: "all nationalities." ADMISSION: $5.00–$13.00. ACCOMMODATIONS: motels and hotels, campgrounds. RESTAURANTS: fast foods, family, elegant. CONTACT: Corn Palace Concessions, P. O. Box 776, Mitchell, SD 57301, (605) 996-5031, or the Mitchell Area Chamber of Commerce, P. O. Box 206, Mitchell, SD 57301, (605) 996-5567. 25,000

WISCONSIN

WINTER FESTIVAL *first full weekend in February,* Cedarburg, Ozaukee Co., in the metropolitan Milwaukee area, "to have fun and frivolity in the midst of long Wisconsin winters." Ice carving, parades, snow man contests, bed races on ice, Alaskan Malamute Weight Pull Contest, chili cook-off, sock hop, barrel races on ice, volleyball and softball tournaments in the snow. FOODS SERVED: pancake breakfast, concessions. ADMISSION: free. ACCOMMODATIONS: motels and hotels, B&B's. RESTAURANTS: fast foods, family, elegant. CONTACT: Cedarburg Chamber of Commerce, P. O. Box 204, Cedarburg, WI 53102, (414) 377-9620. 10,000

WISCONSIN STATE SLED DOG CHAMPIONSHIPS *second weekend in February,* Wisconsin Dells, Sauk Co., at Christmas Mountain Village to celebrate dog sledding. Sled dog races, winter carnival activities including sleigh rides, Torch Light ski Parade, chili cook-off, sled dog weight pull contests, beer and brat tent, bonfire, old-style skydivers, hot air balloons, local radio stations doing live remotes, performances by the Fairfield Fiddlers and nightime duos in the ski chalet. FOODS SERVED: Wisconsin-style chili, beer, brats. ADMISSION: free. ACCOMMODATIONS: motels and hotels, B&B's, campgrounds, RV parks. RESTAURANTS:

fast foods, family, elegant, Italian, Mexican, Chinese, Korean. CONTACT: The Wisconsin Dells Visitor and Convention Bureau, P. O. Box 390, Wisconsin Dells, WI 53965, (608) 254-8088. 10,000

GREAT RIVER FESTIVAL OF THE ARTS *all summer long,* LaCrosse, La Crosse Co., in the Coulee region, to salute jazz, folk music, and dance. Five festivals include Jazz Festival, Traditional Music and Crafts Fest, folk music, crafts demonstrations and sales, dance competitions. FOODS SERVED: "traditional." ADMISSION: varies. ACCOMMODATIONS: motels and hotels, B&B's, campgrounds, RV parks. RESTAURANTS: fast foods, family, elegant, Cajun, Chinese, Italian. CONTACT: Great River Festival of Arts, 119 King St., La Crosse, WI 54601,(608) 785-1433. 25,000

GREAT WISCONSIN DELLS BALLOON RALLY *second weekend after Memorial Day (late May–early June),* near Wisconsin Dells, Sauk Co., at the intersection of Highway 12 and Interstate 90/94 in the Lake Delton area, to celebrate hot air ballooning. Three hot air balloon events including two competition lift-offs, mass ascension, Taste of Wisconsin, local television personalities, and the Joyful Jammers playing jazz, blues, rock 'n' roll. FOODS SERVED: brats, beer, specialties of local restaurants. ADMISSION: free. ACCOMMODATIONS: motels and hotels, B&B's, campgrounds, RV parks. RESTAURANTS: fast foods, family, elegant, Mexican, Chinese, Korean, Italian. CONTACT: The Wisconsin Dells Visitor and Convention Bureau, P. O. Box 390, Wisconsin Dells, WI 53965, (608) 254-8088. 75,000

WALLEYE WEEKEND FESTIVAL AND NATIONAL WALLEYE TOURNAMENT *second weekend in June,* Fond du Lac,Fond du Lac Co., at Lake Winnebago, known as a "walleye factory." "World's Largest Fish Fry" and thirty-nine other events such as the lumberjack show, family land runs, sports olympics, Milk

Carton Boat Race sometimes including the "world's largest," made of 40,000 milk cartons; Saturday Night Shindig, Student Art Exhibit. FOODS SERVED: walleye fish, concessions. ADMISSION: free. ACCOMMODATIONS: motels and hotels, campgrounds, RV space at nearby Fairgrounds. RESTAURANTS: fast foods, family, elegant, international. CONTACT: Fond du Lac Convention and Visitors Bureau, 207 N. Main St., Fond du Lac, WI 54935, (414) 923-3010. 80,000

LAKEFRONT FESTIVAL OF THE ARTS *second weekend in June,* Milwaukee, Milwaukee Co., to celebrate the arts. Arts of all media in an outdoor setting, crafts demonstrations, children's events, music, dancing. FOODS SERVED: local food booths. ADMISSION: $2.00. ACCOMMODATIONS: motels and hotels, B&B's, campgrounds, RV parks. RESTAURANTS: fast foods, family, elegant, international. CONTACT: Milwaukee Art Museum, 750 N. Lincoln Memorial Dr., Milwaukee, WI 53202, (414) 271-9508 or the Greater Milwaukee Convention and Visitors Bureau, Inc., 756 N. Milwaukee St., Milwaukee, WI 53202, (414) 273-3950 or (800) 231-0903. 50,000

MUSKY FESTIVAL *third week in June,* Hayward, Sawyer Co., to celebrate "two world-record muskies." Arts and crafts, fishing contests, parade, pet show, foot race, children's games, juggling, music by the Strategic Air Command Band. FOODS SERVED: "varied." ADMISSION: free. ACCOMMODATIONS: motels and hotels, B&B's, campgrounds, RV parks. RESTAURANTS: fast foods, family, elegant, German. CONTACT: Hayward Chamber of Commerce, P. O. Box 726, Hayward, WI 54843, (715) 634-8662. 10,000

SUMMERFEST *June 25 through July 5,* Milwaukee, Milwaukee Co., downtown and at the Lakefront, to celebrate the sounds of music at "The World's Greatest Music Festival." Jazz, blues, country, big band swing, rock featuring "biggest stars and the rising stars," comedy cabaret, crafts. FOODS SERVED: international. ADMISSION: advance $4.00, at gate $5.00. ACCOMMODATIONS: motels and hotels, B&B's, campgrounds, RV parks. RESTAURANTS: fast foods, family, elegant, international. CONTACT: Bo Black at (414) 273-2680 or the Greater Milwaukee Convention and Visitors Bureau, Inc., 756 N. Milwaukee St., Milwaukee, WI 53202, (414) 273-3950 or (800) 231-0903. 712,000

HODAG COUNTRY FESTIVAL *second weekend in July*, Rhinelander, Oneida Co., at the Hodag "50" Racetrack. Three days of continuous country music by "nationally known performers" which have included Loretta Lynn, Lee Greenwood, Randy Travis, Forester Sisters, Ronnie Prophet, Little Jimmy Dickens, Leo Everette, Margo Smith, and Jim Ed Brown. FOODS SERVED: concessions. ADMISSION: advance weekend tickets $40.00, after May 31 $45.00, at gate $50.00. ACCOMMODATIONS: motels and hotels, campgrounds, camping on grounds. RESTAURANTS: fast foods, family. CONTACT: Hodag Country Festival, 4743 Hwy. 8 E., Rhinelander, WI 54501, (715) 369-3125 or 369-1300. 50,000

BASTILLE DAYS *weekend closest to July 14*, Milwaukee, Milwaukee Co., in East Towne adjacent to the Pfister Hotel. French films, championship bicycle races, Go-Kart Grand Prix, casino, marketplace, French music and theatre, "visit a voyageur encampment." FOODS SERVED: French. ADMISSION: free. ACCOMMODATIONS: motels and hotels, B&B's, campgrounds, RV parks. RESTAURANTS: fast foods, family, elegant, international. CONTACT: Francois Nivaud at (414) 273-8222 or the Greater Milwaukee Convention and Visitors Bureau, Inc., 756 N. Milwaukee St., Milwaukee, WI 53202, (414) 273-3950 or (800) 231-0903. 145,000

PORT WASHINGTON FISH DAY *third Saturday in July*, Port Washington,

Ozaukee Co. Art show, Coast Guard Cutter tours, antique car show, sky divers, 5mi. race, helicopter rides, Stumpfiddle Contest, fire department water fights, fireworks, Martin and Loon Jugglers, Whiskey River Band. FOODS SERVED: fried fish. ADMISSION: free. ACCOMMODATIONS: motels and hotels, B&B's, RV parks. RESTAURANTS: fast foods, family, elegant. CONTACT: Port Washington Chamber of Commerce, 201 N. Franklin St., Port Washington, WI 53704, (414) 284-0900.

FESTA ITALIANA *third weekend in July*, Milwaukee, Milwaukee Co., downtown and on the Lakefront, to celebrate "everything that's Italian." Strolling musicians, traditional Italian dancers, performances on stage, fireworks, high mass on Sunday at noon. FOODS SERVED: Italian delicacies. ADMISSION: advance $4.00, at gate $5.00. ACCOMODATIONS: motels and hotels, B&B's, campgrounds, RV parks. RESTAURANTS: fast foods, family, elegant, international. CONTACT: Paul Iannelli at (414) 963-9613 or the greater Milwaukee Convention and Visitors Bureau, Inc., 756 N. Milwaukee St., Milwaukee, WI 53202, (414) 273-3950 or (800) 231-0903. 151,000

HOLLAND FESTIVAL *last Friday and Saturday in July*, Cedar Grove, Sheboygan Co., in a Dutch community. Take a trip back in time and experience old world Holland in Wisconsin, Dutch parade, Dutch costumes, folk fair, garden show, operetta, Klompen Dansers. FOODS SERVED: woosterbrodjes and other Dutch specialties. ADMISSION: free. ACCOMMODATIONS: motels and hotels, campgrounds nearby. RESTAURANTS: family, Dutch. CONTACT: Holland Festival, Box GD, Cedar Grove, WI 53103, (414) 668-6295 or the Sheboygan Area Convention and Visitors Bureau, Box 687, Sheboygan, WI 53082, (414) 457-9495.

GERMAN FEST *fourth weekend in July*, Milwaukee, Milwaukee Co., downtown and on the Lakefront, to celebrate the

German heritage of many local residents. Cultural exhibits, dancers in German costumes, souvenir booths, big brass bands to contemporary groups. FOODS SERVED: German, with Wisconsin beers and German wines. ADMISSION: advance $4.00, at gate $5.00. ACCOMMODATIONS: motels and hotels, B&B's, campgrounds, RV parks. RESTAURANTS: fast foods, family, elegant, international. CONTACT: Fred Keller at (414) 242-3247 or the Greater Milwaukee Convention and Visitors Bureau, Inc., 756 N. Milwaukee St., Milwaukee, WI 53202, (414) 273-3950 or (800) 231-0903. 80,000

AFRO FEST *first weekend in August,* Milwaukee, Milwaukee Co., to celebrate the Afro-American heritage of many Milwaukee residents. Authentic African village and marketplace, traditional African and contemporary music. FOODS SERVED: Afro-American. ADMISSION: advance $3.50, at gate $4.00. ACCOMMODATIONS: motels and hotels, B&B's, campgrounds, RV parks. RESTAURANTS: fast foods, family, elegant. CONTACT: William Clay at (414) 272-5600 or the Greater Milwaukee Convention and Visitors Bureau, Inc., 756 N. Milwaukee St., Milwaukee, WI 53202, (414) 273-3950 or (800) 231-0903. 26,500

IRISH FEST *second weekend in August,* Milwaukee, Milwaukee Co., to celebrate the preservation of Irish culture. Six stages featuring music from Ireland, parades, bagpipe bands, children's activities, ceili dancing, Irish cultural exhibits, street theatre, clan reunions. FOODS SERVED: Irish. ADMISSION: advance $4.00, at gate $5.00. ACCOMMODATIONS: motels and hotels, B&B's, campgrounds, RV parks. RESTAURANTS: fast foods, family, elegant, international. CONTACT: Ed Ward at (414) 466-6640 or Greater Milwaukee Convention and Visitors Bureau, Inc., 756 N. Milwaukee St., Milwaukee, WI 53202, (414) 273-3950 or (800) 231-0903. 62,600

NORTH HUDSON PEPPER FESTIVAL *second or third weekend in August,* North Hudson, St. Croix Co., at PepperFest Park, to celebrate the community's Italian heritage. Pepper-eating contests, Carp Fishing Contest, Grande Parade, bingo, children's games, spaghetti eating contest, softball tournament, carnival, Bicycle Aerial Trick Team, Italian dance groups, local bands, sound and light shows. FOODS SERVED: Italian including spaghetti and meatballs, Dagoes, sausage, ravioli, hot peppers, stuffed peppers, and more. ADMISSION: $1.00 button good for all three days, $1.50 at gate. ACCOMMODATIONS: motels and hotels, B&B's, campgrounds, RV parks. RESTAURANTS: fast foods, family, elegant. CONTACT: Ben Wopat at (715) 386-9734.

SWEET CORN FESTIVAL *third week in August,* Sun Prairie, Dane Co., to celebrate the corn harvest. Corn-eating contests, midget auto racing, carnival, games, karate exhibitions, magicians, bingo, and stage shows featuring rock 'n' roll bands, all the corn you can put in a tote box for $1.00. FOOD SERVED: brats, hamburgers and sweet corn. ADMISSION: free. ACCOMMODATIONS: motels and hotels. RESTAURANTS: fast foods, family. CONTACT: Sun Prairie Chamber of Commerce, 133 W. Main St., Sun Prairie, WI 53590, (608) 837-4547. 100,000

FIESTA MEXICANA *third weekend in August,* Milwaukee, Milwaukee Co., to celebrate Mexican independence. Colorful customs and costumes, mariachi music. FOODS SERVED: Mexican "spicy sensations." ADMISSION: advance $3.40, at gate $4.50. ACCOMMODATIONS: motels and hotels, B&B's, campgrounds, RV parks. RESTAURANTS: fast foods, family, elegant, international. CONTACT: Oscar Cervera at (414) 278-6682 or the Greater Milwaukee Convention and Visitors Bureau, Inc., 756 N. Milwaukee St., Milwaukee, WI 53202, (414) 273-3950 or (800) 231-0903. 30,000

RUTABAGA FESTIVAL *last weekend in August,* Cumberland, Barron Co., to celebrate the beginning of the rutabaga harvest. Arts and crafts exhibits, parades, carnival, queen coronation, run and other athletic events. FOODS SERVED: mostly Italian. ADMISSION: free. ACCOMMODATIONS: motels and hotels, campgrounds, RV parks. RESTAURANTS: family, Italian. CONTACT: Cumberland Chamber of Commerce, P. O. Box 665, Cumberland, WI 54829, (715) 822-3444. 50,000

POLISH FEST *last weekend in August,* Milwaukee, Milwaukee Co., to celebrate residents' Polish heritage. Polka contests, modern and Polish traditional music and song, regional Polish costumes, outdoor mass and procession, fireworks. FOODS SERVED: Polish. ADMISSION: advance $3.50, at gate $4.50. ACCOMMODATIONS: motels and hotels, B&B's, campgrounds, RV parks. RESTAURANTS: fast foods, family, elegant, international. CONTACT: Richard Gralinski at (414) 225-2603 or Greater Milwaukee Convention and Visitors Bureau, Inc., 756 N. Milwaukee St., Milwaukee, WI 53202, (414) 273-3950 or (800) 231-0903. 44,700

WO-ZHA-WA DAYS FALLS FESTIVAL *second weekend after Labor Day (September),* Wisconsin Dells, Columbia Co., in downtown Wisconsin Dells, to kick off the fall season. Arts and crafts festival, street carnival, 100-unit parade, raffles, local bands in local pubs, beer, and refreshment stands. FOODS SERVED: roast pork and beef, brats, barbecues, roast corn. ADMISSION: free. ACCOMMODATIONS: motels and hotels, B&B's, campgrounds, RV parks. RESTAURANTS: fast foods, family, elegant, Italian, Mexican, Chinese, Korean. CONTACT: Wisconsin Dells Visitor and Convention Bureau, P. O. Box 390, Wisconsin Dells, WI 53965, (608) 254-8088. 100,000

WINE AND HARVEST FESTIVAL *third full weekend in September,* Cedarburg, Ozaukee Co., in the metropolitan Milwaukee area, to celebrate winemaking and the fall harvest. Grape stomping, cherry pit spitting, scarecrow making, art show, craft fair, tailgate antique show, farmers' market, Taste-of-The-Town Food Fair, 5k and 10k runs, dixieland music both afternoons. FOODS SERVED: specialties of local restaurants. ADMISSION: free. ACCOMMODATIONS: motels and hotels, B&B's. RESTAURANTS: fast foods, family, elegant. CONTACT: Cedarburg Chamber of Commerce, P. O. Box 204, Cedarburg, WI 53102, (414) 377-9620. 10,000

POLKA FEST CELEBRATION *first weekend in October,* Wisconsin Dells, Columbia Co. Midwestern polka bands converge on Wisconsin Dells and play in local clubs all weekend long, flea market, beer and brat. FOODS SERVED: German, Polish, Austrian. ADMISSION: advance $2.00, at the door $2.50. ACCOMMODATIONS: motels and hotels, B&B's, campgrounds, RV parks. RESTAURANTS: fast foods, family, elegant, Mexican, Chinese, Italian. CONTACT: The Wisconsin Dells Visitor and Convention Bureau, P. O. Box 390, Wisconsin Dells, WI 53965, (608) 254-8088. 25,000

FALL-O-RAMA *second weekend in October,* Waupaca, Waupaca Co., in the Chain O' Lakes region, to celebrate the fall harvest and color. Arts and crafts, fall color tours by land, air, and water, Apple Festival, hayrides, auto show, square dancers, cloggers, folk singers, storytellers, folk music, other bands. FOODS SERVED: German, Polish, Norwegian, Swedish. ADMISSION: free, $2.50 for folk singing and storytelling. ACCOMMODATIONS: motels and hotels, B&B, campgrounds. RESTAURANTS: fast foods, family, elegant. CONTACT: Waupaca Area Chamber of Commerce, P. O. Box 262, Waupaca, WI 54981, (715) 258-7343. 5,000

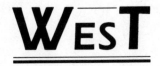

WEST

Alaska / 167	Nevada / 191
California / 169	Oregon / 192
Hawaii / 184	Washington / 197
Idaho / 187	Wyoming / 200
Montana / 188	

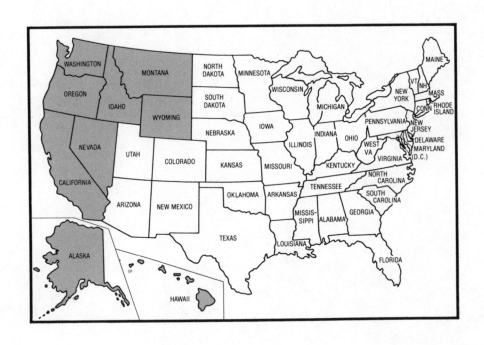

ALASKA

TENT-CITY FESTIVAL *first weekend in February,* Wrangell, commemorating Alaska gold rush days. Long John Contest, 1860–1900 period-costumes fashion show, Shady Lady Fancy Costume Ball and crowning of Tent-City's Shady Lady, sour dough pancake feed, ugly dog contest, family sing-along with crazy hat contest, melodrama by Tent-City Players. "Get out your old hats and shawls, hitch up old Dobin to the sleigh heading for Wrangell, the Lumber Capital of Alaska." FOODS SERVED: pancakes, local food booths. ADMISSION: free. ACCOMMODATIONS: local hotels and inns, city park campgrounds. RESTAURANTS: fast foods and few specialty houses. CONTACT: Wrangell Chamber of Commerce, P. O. Box 49, Wrangell, AK 99929, (907) 874-3327.

CORDOVA ICEWORM FESTIVAL *first full weekend in February,* Cordova, on Prince William Sound, to recognize "winter doldrums." Iceworm Egg Hatch Guessing Contest, iceworm breakfast, arts and crafts, flea market, Blessing of the Fleet and boat parade, survival-suit race, photographic show, cross-cut contest, carnival and concessions, Monte Carlo "Casino", fireworks, bonfire snowshoe/hipboot softball, chili cook-off, beer drinking contest, variety show, Miss Iceworm Contest. FOODS SERVED: hosted buffet at Windsinger Cafe, iceworm breakfast, prime rib feed, chili. ADMISSION: most events free, others vary. ACCOMMODATIONS: hotels, B&B's. RESTAURANTS: family, Chinese, pizza. CONTACT: Cordova Iceworm Festival, P. O. Box 819, Cordova, AK 99574 or the Chamber of Commerce, P. O. Box 99, Cordova, AK 99574, (907) 424-7260.

FUR RENDEZVOUS ("RONDY") *third week in February,* Anchorage. Began as an annual "unplanned" fur trading and carousing event celebrating "the beginning of the end of dark days, frigid nights, and cabin fever." Now includes 130 events such as the famous blanket toss ("originally flipping a trapper into the air so he could scan the horizon for seals, walrus, and whale"), gold and fur auctions, native musicale, World Championship Sled Dog Race, World Dog Weight Pull Championship, Grand Prix and Snow Machine races, hang gliding and parachuting, balloon races, Mr. Alaska Competition, roughhouse boxing, wrist wrestling, curling, arts and crafts, Monte Carlo Night, Miners and Trappers Ball, Alaska Repertory Theatre and Melodrama, board games, outhouse races. FOODS SERVED: wide range of native and local specialties. ADMISSION: many events free, varied costs to others. ACCOMMODATIONS: "elegant hotels to simple lodges," RV parks, hostels. RESTAURANTS: fast foods, family, elegant, international. CONTACT: Anchorage Chamber of Commerce, 415 F. Street, Anchorage, AK 99501-2254, (907) 272-2401 or Anchorage Fur Rendezvous, P. O. Box 773, Anchorage, AK 99510, (907) 277-8615. 200,000

GREAT SITKA HERRING FESTIVAL *mid-March,* Sitka, to celebrate the arrival of spring. "The return of the herring is the surest sign of spring in this area." Events include parade, crab feeds, marine flea market, Blessing of the Fleet, sales, baseball games. FOODS SERVED: lots of crab, others. ADMISSION: free. ACCOMMODATIONS: hotels, B&B's, RV parks. RESTAURANTS: fast foods, family. CONTACT: Sitka Convention and Visitors Bureau, Box 1226, Sitka, AK 99835, (907) 747-5940. 2,000

FAIRBANKS ICE FESTIVAL *Spring Equinox (often third week in March),* Fairbanks, to celebrate the end of winter. Festival of Arts, Annual North American

Sled Dog Championships, body building pageant, Old Time Fiddlers Ball, Fairbanks Kiwanis Ice Festival Luau, Meet the Mushers (mushing is Alaska's official state sport), HIIHTO 45k cross-country ski race and Loppet 18k Race. FOODS SERVED: Aleute, Eskimo, Arctic Indian specialties. ADMISSION: free, charges for some events. ACCOMMODATIONS: motels and hotels, campgrounds, RV parks. RESTAURANTS: fast foods, family, elegant, international. CONTACT: Special Events Director, Fairbanks Chamber of Commerce, P. O. Box 74446, Fairbanks, AK 99707, (907) 452-1105.

LITTLE NORWAY FESTIVAL *weekend closest to May 17*, Petersburg, on Mitkof Island in southeastern Alaska's Wrangell Narrows, to celebrate Norway's Independence Day. Art show, kid's art festival, Sons of Norway Kaffe Hus, natives in Norwegian costume, concession booths on Main Street, Norwegian dancers, pageant, teen dance, Festival Ball, performance by the Mitkoff Mummers. FOODS SERVED: salmon bake, noodle feed, Fish-o-Rama at Petersburg Fisheries Cannery, Norwegian krumkaker, spritz, fish dishes. ADMISSION: some events free, charges for others. ACCOMMODATIONS: motels and hotels, tent–camper area, Forest Service RV park. RESTAURANTS: fast foods, family, seafood. CONTACT: Petersburg Chamber of Commerce, P. O. Box 649, Petersburg, AK 99833, (907) 772-3646.

KODIAK CRAB FESTIVAL *Memorial Day weekend (May)*, Kodiak on Kodiak Island, to celebrate the end of crab season. Blessing of the Fleet, survival-suit races, ultra-marathon and marathon, parade, midway, crab and other food booths, coronation ball. FOODS SERVED: crab, Russian, Filipino, Mexican. ADMISSION: free. ACCOMMODATIONS: motels and hotels, B&B's, campgrounds. RESTAURANTS: fast foods, family, elegant. CONTACT: Kodiak Area Chamber of Commerce, P. O. Box 1485, Kodiak, AK 99615, (907) 486-5557. 12,000

SITKA SUMMER MUSIC FESTIVAL *month of June, Tuesday and Friday evenings*, Sitka, "1,000 miles from any other music center." Founded by proteges of Jascha Heifetz and Gregor Piatigorsky, the festival attracts soloists from all over the world to perform chamber music in the Centennial Building, where a wall of glass behind the stage overlooks Sitka Harbor. Open rehearsals. ADMISSION: charge. ACCOMMODATIONS: hotels, B&B's, RV parks. RESTAURANTS: family. CONTACT: Sitka Summer Music Festival, Box 907, Sitka, AK 99835, (907) 747-6774.

GOLDEN DAYS *third week in July,* Fairbanks, North Star Borough, to celebrate the discovery of gold in Alaska on July 22, 1902 and to honor pioneer and Italian-immigrant Felix Pedro, who made the discovery. Pedro look-alike contest, beard, moustache and hairy leg contest, gaming hall, rededication of the Felix Pedro Monument, air show, Grande Parade, golf tournament, flower show, roving jail, concerts in the park. FOODS SERVED: local food booths. ADMISSION: most events free. ACCOMMODATIONS: motels and hotels, campgrounds, RV hook-ups. RESTAURANTS: fast foods, family, international. CONTACT: Golden Days Manager, Greater Fairbanks Chamber of Commerce, P. O. Box 74446, Fairbanks, AK 99707, (907) 456-6968.

ALASKA DAY FESTIVAL *October 18th,* Sitka-By-The-Sea, once known as "Paris of the Pacific" and the first capital of Alaska. St. Michael's Cathedral houses "one of the world's finest collections of Russian Orthodox ecclesiastical art treasures." Three-day fair with Alaska Day ceremonies at 3:00 P.M. October 18 every year. Flag-raising ceremony commemorating and reenacting the transfer of Alaska from Russia to the United States in 1867; parade featuring period costumes and military bands with the characters of Princess Maksutov, Prince Dimitri, Brigidier General Lovell Rousseau, and the 9th (Manchu) infantry, all portrayed by local residents. Keystone Kops wearing English bobby hats collect fines during the festival from those men who appear on the street beardless and women who are not in costume. FOOD SERVED: local food booths. ADMISSION: free to most events.

ACCOMMODATIONS: motel, hotels, B&B, lighthouse. RESTAURANTS: local specialties, family, elegant. CONTACT: Greater Sitka Chamber of Commerce, P. O. Box 638, Sitka, AK 99835, (907) 747-8604.

CALIFORNIA

NATIONAL DATE FESTIVAL *second Friday to third Friday in February,* Indio, Riverside Co., at the County Fairgrounds, to celebrate the end of the date harvest. Arabian Nights Pageant, Arabian Nights Street Parade, camel and ostrich races, kitchen band contest, flower and garden show, newspaper fold and toss contest, diaper derby, gem and mineral show, demolition derby, 4x4 pull, tractor/truck pull, entertainment such as Lacy J. Dalton, Legends of Rock 'n' Roll, The Robinson Family, Bobby Lynn. FOODS SERVED: lots of dates and wide range of other foods. ADMISSION: adults $4.00, children $2.00. ACCOMMODATIONS: motels and hotels, campgrounds, RV parks. RESTAURANTS: fast foods, family, elegant, many international. CONTACT: National Date Festival, P. O. Drawer NNNN, Indio, CA 92202-9990, (619) 342-8247. 220,000

HOLTVILLE CARROT FESTIVAL *second week in February,* Holtville, Imperial Co., the "Carrot Capital of the World." Carrot recipe cooking contest, parade, tractor pull, arts and crafts, fine arts show, carnival, 4-H and Future Farmers of America livestock show. FOODS SERVED: carrot concoctions, "Mexican and others." ADMISSION: free, except $3.00 to tractor pull. ACCOMMODATIONS: motels and hotels, B&B's campground, RV park. RESTAURANTS: fast foods, family, Mexican. CONTACT: Holtville Chamber of Commerce, P. O. Box 185, Holtville, CA 92250, (619) 356-2923. 5,000

WORLD CHAMPION CRAB RACES *third Sunday in February,* Crescent City, Del Norte Co., "where the redwoods meet the sea," at the County Fairgrounds, to celebrate the crab season and to follow an old custom of fisherman racing their crabs after the fleet comes in. Enter your own crab or rent one to race on a four-foot long plywood raceway, as crabs claw their way. Crab coach categories include media, government, children, and after a long day at the races, the champion wins $100. Band music and Bagpipers (only music heard above the crowds). FOODS SERVED: giant Dungeness crab feed during races. ADMISSION: $1.00 to grounds, $2.00 to race, $1.00 to rent a crab. ACCOMMODATIONS: motels and hotels, B&B's, campgrounds, RV parks. RESTAURANTS: fast foods, family. CONTACT: Events Coordinator, Crescent City–Del Norte Co. Chamber of Commerce, P. O. Box 246, Crescent City, CA 95531, (707) 464-9676. 1,200

SANTA BARBARA INTERNATIONAL FILM FESTIVAL *first week in March,* Santa Barbara, Santa Barbara Co., to honor international filmmaking. Whirlwind of showings, premiers of U. S. and international films, featuring a different country each year, tribute to a film actor, documentaries and archival films, workshops and seminars led by distinguished film industry professionals, Gala Opening Premiere, parties, celebrities everywhere. ADMISSION: varies by event. ACCOMMODATIONS: motels and hotels,

B&B's, campgrounds, RV parks. RESTAURANTS: fast foods, family, elegant, Asian, Mexican, Scandinavian. CONTACT: Santa Barbara Film Festival, 1216 State St., Suite 201, Santa Barbara, CA 93101 at (805) 963-0023 or Santa Barbara Chamber of Commerce, P. O. Box 299, Santa Barbara, CA 93102, (805) 965-3021. 11,000

SNOWFEST! *first week in March,* North Lake Tahoe–Truckee, Placer Co., to celebrate winter in the High Sierra. More than 100 events including parades, ski races, wild game and fish cook-off, craft show, Mr. Lake Tahoe Contest, Dress-Up-Your-Dog Contest, softball on skis, model railroad show, concerts including artists such as Queen Ida, Steve Seskind, and Norton Buffalo, light opera performances by the Truckee Actors Guild. FOODS SERVED: wild game and fish (from the cook-off), western barbecue. ADMISSION: some events free, charges to others. ACCOMMODATIONS: motels and hotels, B&B's, campgrounds. RESTAURANTS: fast foods, family, elegant, continental, Asian, nouvelle. CONTACT: Ruth Schnabel, P. O. Box 7590, Tahoe City, CA 95730, (916) 583-7625. 75,000

WHALE FESTIVAL *third weekend in March,* Mendocino and Fort Bragg, Mendocino Co., on the northern California coast. Marine art show, photo exhibit at Point Arena Lighthouse, orchid show, gem and mineral show, art exhibit, half-marathon, 10k and 2mi. runs. FOODS SERVED: cioppino and wine tastings, lasagna dinner, pancake breakfast. ADMISSION: free, charges for some events. ACCOMMODATIONS: hotels and motels, B&B's, campgrounds, RV parks. RESTAURANTS: family, elegant. CONTACT: Fort Bragg–Mendocino Coast Chamber of Commerce, P. O. Box 1141, Fort Bragg, CA 95437, (707) 964-3153.

SLUG FEST *third Sunday in March,* Monte Rio, Sonoma Co., on the Russian River at the Northwood Restaurant, to cure winter doldrums and liven-up this summer resort area. Slug races (rental of a slug may increase from 5¢ to 10¢ soon), slug cook-off, politicans and local celebrities select champion recipes and devour their favorite slugs. Some luminaries even return the next year! FOODS SERVED: sauteed, baked, boiled, and disguised slugs. ADMISSION: free. ACCOMMODATIONS: motels, B&B's, campgrounds. RESTAURANTS: family, elegant. CONTACT: The Paper, P.O. Box 629, Guerneville, CA 95446, (707) 869-9033. 500

DESERT CAVALCADE PARADE *last weekend in March,* Calexico, Imperial Co., near the California-Mexico border. Reenactment of Captain Juan Bautista de Anza's journey through the Imperial Valley, parade features entries from throughout Imperial Valley and Mexicali, Mexico: Mexican parade, fiesta, dance, mariachis, folkloric dancers from Mexico. FOODS SERVED: Mexican. ADMISSION: free. ACCOMMODATIONS: motels and hotels, campgrounds, RV parks. RESTAURANTS: fast foods, family, elegant, Mexican, Chinese. CONTACT: Desert Cavalcade Association, Calexico Chamber of Commerce, P. O. Box 948, Calexico, CA 92231, (714) 357-1166. 10,000

SAN FRANCISCO FILM FESTIVAL *last week in March through first week in April,* San Francisco, San Francisco Co., at the Kabuki Cinemas in Japantown, at the Castro Theater, and the Palace of Fine Arts Theater. Often ninety movies, thirty-five of which are U. S. premieres, fifty filmmakers, several directors, and a few stars combine with a marathon of parties ranging from a sit-down dinner opening night to dinner at the Palace of Fine Arts with a live telecast of the Academy Awards, free screenings and speeches with Golden Gate Awards to independent and local filmmakers, closing-night festivities, comprising lots of action off-screen as well as on-screen. FOODS SERVED: at parties and dinners. ADMISSION: charge, dinners range from $15.00

to $101.00. ACCOMMODATIONS: motels and hotels, B&B's. RESTAURANTS: fast foods, family, elegant, international. CONTACT: San Francisco International Film Festival, 3501 California St., San Francisco, CA 94118, (415) 762-BASS for tickets, or (415) 221-FILM, or (415) 221-9055 for general information. 4,000.

APPLE BLOSSOM FESTIVAL *first weekend in April*, Sebastopol, Sonoma Co., "The Gravenstein Apple Center." Apple Blossom Parade, Apple Juice Run "down country lanes amid the blossoming orchards with the promised reward of apple juice at the finish line," self-guided tours of apple farms, model railroad show, art show, crafts fair, queen coronation, entertainment such as Billy Daniels, Johnny Ray, and other local talent, dixieland, U.S. Navy Jazz Band, high school and state band concerts. FOODS SERVED: lots of apple desserts, chicken barbecue, pancake breakfast. ADMISSION: free, charge for queen coronation show. ACCOMMODATIONS: motels and hotels, campgrounds nearby. RESTAURANTS: fast foods, family, elegant, continental, Asian, Mexican. Contact: Sebastopol Area Chamber of Commerce, P.O. Box 178, Sebastopol, CA 95472, (707) 823-3032. 25,000

PACIFIC COAST COLLEGIATE JAZZ FESTIVAL *second or third weekend in April*, Berkeley, Alameda Co., at the University of California's Zellerbach Hall, San Francisco Bay area. Big band, combo, and vocal competitions, clinics, seminars, and performance Friday evening by a major artist, such as Gil Evans Orchestra, Hubert Laws, Sonny Rollins, Bill Evans, Phil Woods, George Duke, Bobby McFerrin, Freddie Hubbard. ADMISSION: $10.00–$15.00. ACCOMMODATIONS: motels and hotels, B&B's. RESTAURANTS: fast foods, family, elegant, "All nationalities and all kinds of food available—this is Berkeley!" Contact: U.C. Berkeley Jazz Ensembles, University of California, 91 Student Center, Berkeley, CA 94720, (415) 642-5062. 5,000

CHERRY BLOSSOM FESTIVAL *third and fourth weekends in April*, San Francisco, San Francisco Co., at Japan Center. "Over 2,000 Californians of Japanese descent and performers from Japan participate in most elaborate offering of Japanese culture and customs this side of the Japanese Island of Honshu, capped by crosstown parade on final Sunday." FOODS SERVED: Japanese. ADMISSION: charge. ACCOMMODATIONS: motels and hotels, B&B's. RESTAURANTS: fast foods, family, elegant, international. Contact: San Francisco Convention and Visitors Bureau, 201 Third St., San Francisco, CA 94103, (415) 974-6900. 10,000

CALICO PITCHIN', COOKIN', AND SPITTIN' HULLABALOO *Palm Sunday weekend (April)*, Calico Ghost Town, Yermo, San Bernardino Co., 10 miles from Barstow in the Mojave Desert. Three days of stew cooking, World Tobacco Spitting Championships, campfire programs, California Horseshoe Pitching Tournament, gunfights, flapjack racing, country music. FOODS SERVED: lots of stew. ADMISSION: adults $4.00, juniors $2.00, children free. ACCOMMODATIONS: campground; motels in Barstow. RESTAURANTS: family. Contact: Calico Ghost Town, P.O. Box 638, Yermo, CA 92398, (619) 254-2122.

SANTA BARBARA ARTS FESTIVAL *last week in April through first weekend in May*, Santa Barbara, Santa Barbara Co., to honor the visual and performing arts. Juried art, evening performances of theatre and dance, tours of artists' studios, participation for all ages, literary readings. ADMISSION: varies. ACCOMMODATIONS: motels and hotels, B&B's, campgrounds, RV parks. RESTAURANTS: fast foods, family, elegant, Asian, Mexican, Scandinavian. Contact: Santa Barbara Arts Council, P.O. Box 1267, Santa Barbara, CA 93102 (805) 966-7022 or the Santa Barbara Chamber of Commerce, P.O. Box 299, Santa Barbara, CA 93102, (805) 965-3021. 15,000

BODEGA BAY FISHERMEN'S FESTIVAL *fourth Sunday in April,* Bodega Bay, Sonoma Co., to celebrate the fishing resources of the Pacific Ocean at Bodega Bay. Arts and crafts, U.S. Marine Lab exhibit, fisherman's exhibit, face painting, fishing contest, boat parade and Blessing of the Fleet, Run to the Head and Back, golf tournament, horseshoe contest, bathtub races, kite-flying championships, trapshooting, art show at Bodega Harbor Yacht Club, lots of music including the Carl Thompson Band, U.S. Navy Band, Bob Norman's Dixieland Band, Double Cross Band with Greer Paulsen, the Apple Knockers' Band, and Charlie Krinard, dance. FOODS SERVED: pancake breakfast, fish and chips, barbecued lamb and oysters, popcorn, hot dogs, snow cones. ADMISSION: free. ACCOMMODATIONS: motels and hotels, campgrounds. RESTAURANTS: family, elegant, seafood. Contact: Bodega Bay Area Chamber of Commerce, 555 Highway 1, Bodega Bay, CA 94923, (707) 875-3422. 20,000

SAN DIMAS FESTIVAL OF WESTERN ARTS *last weekend in April,* San Dimas, Los Angeles Co., in the San Gabriel Valley, featuring American Indian and western artists, western dance, Indian dancers, Indian jewelry and crafts, trading post, student art competition, chili cookoff, entertainers such as Gene Autry, Montie Montana, Johnny Grant, and Iron Eyes Cody. FOODS SERVED: American Indian, pancake breakfast, chili. ADMISSION: free, charges for special events. ACCOMMODATIONS: motels and hotels, campgrounds, RV parks. RESTAURANTS: fast foods, family, elegant, Mexican, Japanese, Italian. Contact: San Dimas Festival of Western Arts, Box 146, San Dimas, CA 91773, (714) 599-5374. 6,000

WESTWOOD ART SHOW *first weekend in May and first weekend in October,* Westwood Village, Los Angeles, Los Angeles Co. Arts and crafts, magic shows, marionettes, mimes, live music such as rhythm and blues, pop, jazz with live broadcasting from local jazz station KKGU. FOODS SERVED: Dove Bar ice cream, churros, pretzels, hot dogs. ADMISSION: free. ACCOMMODATIONS: motels and hotels. RESTAURANTS: fast foods, family, elegant, Mexican, Asian, Cajun, Indian. CONTACT: Los Angeles West Chamber of Commerce, 10880 Wilshire Blvd., Los Angeles, CA 90064, (213) 475-4574. 125,000 each show.

CALICO SPRING FESTIVAL *Mother's Day weekend (early May),* Calico Ghost Town, Yermo, San Bernardino Co., 10 miles from Barstow in the Mojave Desert. Old-time bluegrass hootenanny including two-day fiddle, banjo, guitar, and band contests, clogging, square dance, ragtime entertainment. FOODS SERVED: concessions. ADMISSION: adults $4.00, juniors $2.00, children free. ACCOMMODATIONS: motels in Barstow, campground. RESTAURANTS: family. CONTACT: Calico Ghost Town, P.O. Box 638, Yermo, CA 92398, (619) 254-2122.

FAIR OAKS FIESTA *Mother's Day weekend (early May),* Fair Oaks Village Plaza, Sacramento Co. Sun Run foot race, talent show, parade, beauty pageant, Honorary Mayor's Reception, crafts booths, carnival. FOODS SERVED: pancake breakfast, booths featuring Asian, Mexican, Serbian, American foods. ADMISSION: free. RESTAURANTS: fast foods, family, elegant, French, Mexican. CONTACT: Fair Oaks Chamber of Commerce, P.O. Box 352, Fair Oaks, CA 95628, (916) 967-2903. 7,000

CELEBRATE THE ARTS *third weekend in May,* Placerville and other cities and communities, El Dorado Co. in the Gold Country. Week-long event showcasing artists and artisans of the county, special performances and exhibits in local businesses and art galleries, Sierra Symphony in concert, and opening of the season for Theater El Dorado. ADMISSION: free. ACCOMMODATIONS: motels and hotels, B&Bs, campgrounds. RESTAURANTS: fast foods, family. CONTACT: El Dorado Arts Council, 542 Main Street, Placerville, CA 95667, (916) 626-2177.

CAMPBELL WINE AND ARTS MUSIC FESTIVAL *third weekend in May*, Campbell, Santa Clara Co., downtown. Arts and crafts exhibits, wine tasting, local musical entertainment. FOODS SERVED: concessions, local wine. ADMISSION: free. ACCOMMODATIONS: motels and hotels. RESTAURANTS: fast foods, family, elegant. CONTACT: Campbell Chamber of Commerce, 328 E. Campbell Ave., Campbell, CA 95008, (408) 378-6252. 30,000

FIESTA LA BALLONA *third weekend in May*, Culver City, Los Angeles Co., celebrating the early California heritage of La Ballona Valley. Balloon launch, moustache-growing and beauty contests, kiddie parade, family night, arts and crafts, firemen's muster, vintage car display, live entertainment featuring local bands, dance groups, drill teams, and Ronald McDonald. FOODS SERVED: Asian, American Indian, Mexican, Italian. ADMISSION: free. ACCOMMODATIONS: motels and hotels. RESTAURANTS: fast foods, family, elegant, Asian, Mexican, Italian. CONTACT: City of Culver City, 4153 Overland Avenue, Culver City, CA 90230, (213) 202-5855. 20,000

STRAWBERRY FESTIVAL *third weekend in May*, Oxnard, Ventura Co., at Channel Islands Harbor. Strawberry Blonde Contest, waiter's race, arts and crafts, golf and tennis tournaments, pie-eating contest, 10k Run, Tea Dance, Make-Your-Own-Strawberry-Shortcake Booth, dinner dance and gala, continuous entertainment on two stages featuring jazz, contemporary music, and dance troupes, puppets, mimes, jugglers, strolling performers. FOODS SERVED: strawberry shortcake, Cajun, barbecue, "gourmet fair foods." ADMISSION: adults $3.00, seniors and children 5–12 $1.00. ACCOMMODATIONS: motels and hotels, B&Bs, campgrounds, RV parks. RESTAURANTS:

fast foods, family, elegant, Asian, continental, Mexican. CONTACT: Special Events Office, 305 W. Third St., Oxnard, CA 93030, (805) 984-4715 or the Channel Islands Chamber of Commerce, 3886 W. Channel Islands Blvd., Oxnard, CA 93030, (805) 985-2244. 150,000

CALAVERAS COUNTY FAIR AND JUMPING FROG JUBILEE *third full weekend in May*, Angels Camp, Calaveras Co., in the Mother Lode, to celebrate Mark Twain's story "The Celebrated Jumping Frog of Calaveras County." Frog Jump Contest, livestock exhibits, home arts exhibits, carnival, Destruction Derby, music by big-name rock groups. FOODS SERVED: "all kinds." ADMISSION: adults $8.50, varies each day. ACCOMMODATIONS: motels and hotels, B&Bs, campgrounds, RV parks. RESTAURANTS: fast foods, family, elegant. CONTACT: Calaveras County Fairgrounds, P.O. Box 96, Angels Camp, CA 95222, (209) 736-2561. 40,000

RUSSIAN RIVER WINEFEST *third Sunday in May*, Healdsburg, Sonoma Co., on the Russian River. Arts and crafts, jazz and dixieland music, wine tasting. FOODS SERVED: many nationalities. ADMISSION: free. ACCOMMODATIONS: motels and hotels, B&Bs, campgrounds. RESTAURANTS: fast foods, family, elegant. CONTACT: Healdsburg Chamber of Commerce, 217 Healdsburg Ave., Healdsburg, CA 95448, (707) 433-6935. 6,000

MULE DAYS CELEBRATION *Memorial Day weekend (late May)*, Bishop, Inyo Co., at the Tri-County Fairgrounds in the Eastern Sierra Mountains, in the "Mule Capital of the World." Parade features "world's largest non-motorized parade" including hundreds of mules and horses packed as in the old days, mules carrying complete beds, outhouses, bathtubs; Mule Shoeing Contest, mule show, mule races, rodeo events featuring mules, Packer and Mule Scramble, Braying Contest (people mimic mules), naming of

World Champion Mule, arts and crafts festival, country-western music and dances. FOODS SERVED: barbecues, pancake breakfast, concessions. ADMISSION: adults $5.00, children $2.00. ACCOMMODATIONS: motels and hotels, B&B's, campgrounds, RV space at fairgrounds. RESTAURANTS: fast foods, family, elegant, Chinese. CONTACT: Mule Days Committee, Bishop Chamber of Commerce, 690 N. Main St., Bishop CA 93514, (714) 873-8405. 40,000

GRUBSTAKE DAYS *Memorial Day weekend (late May),* Yucca Valley, San Bernardino Co., in the Morongo Basin. Started by miners in the area, festival includes a carnival, horseshoe and golf tournaments, parade, bluegrass festival, tug of war, arm wrestling, antique car show, antique plane show, rock 'n' roll dances, country-western dances. FOODS SERVED: barbecue, pancake breakfast, beer garden, many food booths. ADMISSION: free. ACCOMMODATIONS: motels and hotels, campgrounds, RV parks. RESTAURANTS: fast foods, family, elegant. CONTACT: Yucca Valley Chamber of Commerce, 56020 Santa Fe Trail, Suite B, Yucca Valley, CA 92284, (619) 365-6323. 30,000

FIESTA DE LAS ARTES *Memorial Day weekend (late May) and Labor Day weekend (early September),* Hermosa Beach, Los Angeles Co., downtown at Pier and Hermosa Avenues, in the "Surfing Center of California." 400 artists and craftspeople demonstrate and sell their works at each event with many street musicians, performances on center stage by jugglers, magicians, belly dancers. The Memorial Day weekend features the "collegiate playoffs" for the Playboy Jazz Festival, free face painting and kiddie merry-go-round. FOODS SERVED: Thai, Greek, Mexican, Albanian, Indian, Italian, Chinese. ADMISSION: free. ACCOMMODATIONS: motels and hotels, RV parks nearby. RESTAURANTS: fast foods, family, elegant, lots of seafood, and international. CONTACT: Hermosa Beach Chamber of Commerce, P.O. Box

404, Hermosa Beach, CA 90254, (213) 376-0951. 200,000 each event.

SACRAMENTO DIXIELAND JUBILEE *Memorial Day weekend (late May),* Sacramento, Sacramento Co. at many sites around town, to salute traditional American jazz. Performances by 100 jazz bands from all over the world, including Helen Forrest, Norma Teagarden, Danny Barker, Rosie O'Grady's Goodtime Jazz Band with red hot mama Ruth Crews, many more big and little names in jazz. FOODS SERVED: international. ADMISSION: $45.00 advance, $50.00 that weekend. ACCOMMODATIONS: motels and hotels, B&B's, campgrounds, R V parks. RESTAURANTS: fast foods, family, elegant. CONTACT: Sacramento Dixieland Jubilee, 2787 Del Monte St., W. Sacramento, CA 95691, (916) 372-5277. 200,000

UNION STREET SPRING FESTIVAL *Memorial Day weekend (late May),* San Francisco, San Francisco Co., on Union Street, in the Cow Hollow neighborhood. A Victorian garden party atmosphere prevails through garden cafes, fine arts and crafts, street performers, Uphill Waiter's Race, black-tie Tea Dance, entertainment on three stages including Steve Seskin, Melody Ann and her Rhythm Rascals, Ray Jason, big bands. FOODS SERVED: "gourmet fair foods," California wines. ADMISSION: free. ACCOMMODATIONS: motels and hotels, B&B's. RESTAURANTS: fast foods, family, elegant, international. CONTACT: Terry Pimsleur & Co., 2155 Union St., San Francisco, CA 94123, (415) 346-4446. 90,000

APRICOT FIESTA *last weekend in May,* Patterson, Stanislaus Co., in the San Joaquin Valley, to celebrate the apricot harvest in the "Apricot Capital of the World." Crafts along the streets, balloon rides, afternoon tea, fireworks, old-time fiddlers, "street fun," parade, queen pageant, Little Mr. and Miss Apricot. FOODS SERVED: apricots and their products, barbecue, wine and cheese, Mexican, Chinese, Portuguese. ADMISSION: free, $5.00 for barbecue. ACCOMMODATIONS: motels and hotels, campgrounds. RESTAURANTS: fast foods, family, Chinese, Basque. CONTACT: Patterson Apricot Fiesta, P.O. Box 442, Patterson, CA 95363, (209) 892-3118, or the Patterson–Wesley Chamber of Commerce, P. O. Box 365, Patterson, CA 95363, (209) 892-2821. 12,000

FESTIVAL *first weekend in June,* near Red Bluff at the Sun County Fairgrounds, Tehama Co. Arts and crafts, games, fashion show, country music, fiddlers, country dancers, karate demonstrations, short skits. FOODS SERVED: concessions. ADMISSION: free. ACCOMMODATIONS: motels and hotels, B&B, campgrounds, RV parks. RESTAURANTS: fast foods, family, elegant. CONTACT: Red Bluff–Tehama Co. Chamber of Commerce, P.O. Box 850, Red Bluff, CA 96080, (916) 527-6220. 4,000

SUNNYVALE ART AND WINE FESTIVAL *first full weekend in June,* Sunnyvale, Santa Clara Co., in the Bay Area. 350 artists display and sell their works, six local wineries offer tastings, commemorative glasses sold. FOODS SERVED: Mexican, Chinese, variety of delicacies. ADMISSION: free. ACCOMMODATIONS: motels and hotels, campgrounds, RV parks. CONTACT: Sunnyvale Chamber of Commerce, 499 South Murphy Ave., Sunnyvale, CA 94086, (408) 736-4971. 100,000

SCANDINAVIAN MIDSUMMER FESTIVAL *second or third weekend in June,* Santa Barbara, Santa Barbara Co., at Oak Park. Pageantry of Scandinavian folk dancing and costumes, music, singing, and entertainment of Sweden, Norway, Denmark, and Iceland. FOODS SERVED: Scandinavian. ADMISSION: free. ACCOMMODATIONS: motels and hotels, B&B's, campgrounds, RV parks. RESTAURANTS: fast foods, family, elegant, continental, Asian, Mexican, Scandinavian. CONTACT: Carl R. Lauritsen, President, Scandinavian Council of Santa Barbara at (805) 969-6706 or the Santa Barbara

Chamber of Commerce, P.O. Box 299, Santa Barbara, CA 93102, (805) 965-3021. 1,400

MUSIC IN THE MOUNTAINS SUMMER FESTIVAL *last two weeks in June,* Grass Valley, Nevada Co., in the Sierra foothills. Outdoor picnic and pops concerts, indoor candlelight concerts featuring chamber ensembles, major concerts with chamber orchestra, 100-voice chorale, and guest artists such as Alexander Treger, concertmaster of the Los Angeles Philharmonic, pianist Istvan Nadas, and sopranos Diane Gilfether and Vicky VanDewark. FOODS SERVED: "snacks, beer and wine bar, soft drinks." ADMISSION: $4.00–$15.00. ACCOMMODATIONS: motels and hotels, B&B's, campgrounds, RV parks. RESTAURANTS: fast foods, family, elegant, continental, Asian. CONTACT: Music in the Mountains, P.O. Box 1451, Nevada City, CA 95959. 10,000

NEW NORTH BEACH FAIR *third weekend in June,* San Francisco, San Francisco Co., Grant Avenue and Green Street, in North Beach, to celebrate San Francisco's "historic Italian and Bohemian traditions." Fine arts and crafts show, opera, poetry readings, outdoor cafes, and live music in the streets such as Terry and the Pirates, Terry Dolan, J. C. Burris, The Nuclear Whales Saxophone Orchestra, poets Monte Slow and Whitman McGowan. FOODS SERVED: Italian and California wines. ADMISSION: free. ACCOMMODATIONS: motels and hotels, B&B's. RESTAURANTS: fast foods, family, elegant, international. CONTACT: Terry Pimsleur & Co., 2155 Union St., San Francisco, CA 94123, (415) 346-4446. 60,000

CELTIC FESTIVAL *third weekend in June,* Vallejo, Solano Co., at the County Fairgrounds, in recognition of Celtic culture. Pipe bands, Highland dancing, Scottish and Irish country dancing, singing, fiddling, harping, Scottish and Irish athletics. FOODS SERVED: Scottish, Irish, Welsh, and Cornish foods and beverages. ADMIS-

SION: adults $10.00, children $1.00. AC-COMMODATIONS: motels and hotels, B&B's, campgrounds, RV parks. RESTAU-RANTS: fast foods, family, elegant. CON-TACT: John Dickson, P.O. Box 16281, San Francisco, CA 94116. 25,000

HUCK FINN'S JUBILEE *Father's Day weekend (late June),* Mojave Narrows, Victorville, San Bernardino Co., in the Mojave Desert. Annual recreation of the life and times of Tom Sawyer and Huckleberry Finn with river raft building, fence painting, greased-pole climbing, miracle tonic shows, crafts fair, bluegrass and country music, clogging, Mountain Men Encampment. FOODS SERVED: concessions. AD-MISSION: adults $6.00, juniors $3.00, children free. ACCOMMODATIONS: motels. RESTAURANTS: family. CONTACT: DVT Marketing Enterprises, Inc., P.O. Box 56419, Riverside, CA 92517, (714) 780-8810.

LAKE TAHOE SUMMER MUSIC FESTIVAL *first week after July 4th,* North Lake Tahoe, Placer Co. Symphony, opera and pops concerts featuring the San Francisco Chamber Orchestra. ADMISSION: $10.00–$15.00 per-person per-day. AC-COMMODATIONS: motels and hotels, B&B's, campgrounds, RV parks. RESTAU-RANTS: fast foods, family, elegant, continental, Asian, Cajun, nouvelle. CONTACT: Ruth Schnabel, P.O. Box 7590, Tahoe City, CA 95730, (916) 583-7625. 7,000

EASTER IN JULY LILY FESTIVAL *second weekend in July,* Smith River, Del Norte Co., at the Ship Ashore Resort, to recognize the Easter lily farms of Smith River, which produce 95 percent of the Easter lily bulbs. The lilies are in full bloom in this unique climate, and proceeds from the festival benefit the Rowdy Creek Fish Hatchery, producing four million fingerlings to restore the Smith River steelhead trout and salmon runs. Floats decorated with lilies, fine art show with working artists, crafts show with continuous demonstrations, flea market, bingo,

White Elephant Sale, North Coast Bagpipe Band, Congleton and Buckendahl Band, tours of Rowdy Creek Fish Hatchery, dance, sunrise service, round and square dancing, kids treasure hunt, logging show, floral display and awards. FOODS SERVED: pancake breakfast, international food booths. ADMISSION: free. AC-COMMODATIONS: motel, RV park. RESTAU-RANTS: family. CONTACT: Smith River Kiwanis Club, c/o Ship Ashore, Smith River, CA 95567, (707) 487-3141. 4,000

TWAIN HARTE SUMMER CRAFT FESTIVAL *weekend in mid-July,* Twain Harte, Tuolumne Co., in the Sierras, on the grounds of the Eproson House Restaurant. Country-style crafts for sale, face painting, puppet shows, storytelling, juggling, magicians, bluegrass, jazz, and folk music. FOODS SERVED: sandwiches, beverages. ADMISSION: free. ACCOMMODA-TIONS: motels, B&B's. RESTAURANTS: fast foods, family, elegant. CONTACT: Rich Burleigh, P.O. Box 148, Soulsbyville, CA 95372, (209) 533-3473. 6,000

CARMEL BACH FESTIVAL *mid-July through early August,* Carmel, Monterey Co., at the Sunset Cultural Center. In this beautiful Pacific Coast setting of Carmel-by-the-Sea, you can enjoy twenty-one major concerts, twenty-eight recitals, an opera, lectures, symposia, a master's class, and music camp for children featuring the music of "J.S. Bach and others." Recent soloists have included Cambridge Buskers, Patricia Schuman, Janice Taylor, Karl Markus, Christiane Edinger, Janina Fialkowska. ADMISSION: $15.00–$30.00 individual tickets. ACCOMMODATIONS: motels and hotels. RESTAURANTS: family, elegant. CONTACT: Carmel Bach Festival, Inc., P.O. Box 575, Carmel, CA 93921, (408) 624-1521. 15,000

GILROY GARLIC FESTIVAL *third weekend in July,* Gilroy, Santa Clara Co., on California's Central Coast, to celebrate the garlic harvest in "The Garlic Capital of the World." Gilroy makes this claim because 90 percent of America's garlic is processed in the area, and the garlic aroma that permeates the air as one drives through town is magnified one-hundred-fold during the festival. Will Rogers once described Gilroy as "The only town in America where you can marinate a steak by hanging it on the clothesline." Gourmet Alley features every possible concoction using garlic from calamari, cooked red and green peppers and pepper-steak sandwiches to vegetables con pesto, lobster butter, scampi, and garlic ice cream. The seventy-five food booths use eight tons of garlic during the Festival. Great Garlic Cook-off and Recipe Contest have resulted in two cookbooks, and other attractions include fine arts and crafts, Tour de Garlique bicycle tour, 10k Garlic Gallop, garlic topping contests, Garlic Squeeze Barn Dance, all involving 4,000 volunteers. FOODS SERVED: see above. ADMISSION: adults $5.00, seniors and children free. ACCOMMODATIONS: motels and hotels, B&B's, campgrounds, RV parks. RESTAURANTS: fast foods, family, elegant, Mexican, Italian, Chinese. CONTACT: Gilroy Garlic Festival Association, Inc., P.O. Box 2311, Gilroy, CA 95021, (408) 842-1625. 140,000

SAN ANSELMO ART AND WINE FESTIVAL *third weekend in July,* San Anselmo, Marin Co., on San Anselmo Avenue. Elegant street fair featuring arts and crafts, continuous entertainment including jugglers, magicians, Victorian Circus Theater, Steve Seskin, J. C. Barris, and Terry Dolan and the Acoustic Rangers. FOODS SERVED: "gourmet fair foods," California wines. ADMISSION: free. ACCOMMODATIONS: motels and hotels, B&B's, campgrounds. RESTAURANTS: fast foods, family, elegant. CONTACT: Terry Pimsleur & Co., 2155 Union St., San Francisco, CA 94123, (415) 346-4446. 30,000

SHAKESPEARE AT SAND HARBOR *throughout August,* Incline Village, Washoe Co., Nevada (at California border), Sand Harbor State Park, Lake Tahoe. Twelve evenings of Shakespearean performances by the Valley Institute of Theatre Arts of Saratoga, CA. Works performed include those of Shakespeare and related classics in a natural lakeshore sand amphitheatre. FOODS SERVED: none, but picnic dinners are encouraged. ADMISSION: Adults $8.00, children under 12 $5.00. ACCOMMODATIONS: motels and hotels, B&B's, campgrounds, RV parks. RESTAURANTS: fast foods, family, elegant, international, Creole, California nouvelle. CONTACT: The North Tahoe Fine Arts Council, P.O. Box 18, Tahoe City, CA 95730, (916) 583-9048. 12,000

OLD SPANISH DAYS FIESTA *first week in August,* Santa Barbara, Santa Barbara Co., celebrating Santa Barbara's Hispanic heritage. City-wide five-day celebration with costumed parades, "mercados" (marketplaces), arts and crafts show, country-western music, dancing, free and ticketed theatrical performances, rodeo, traditional Mexican and Spanish folk and classic dancers such as Ballet Español de Los Angeles, musicians such as Carlos Montoya, Herb Alpert and the Tijuana Brass. FOODS SERVED: barbecues, Mexican/Hispanic. ADMISSION: free, charges for some events. ACCOMMODATIONS: motels and hotels, B&B's, campgrounds, RV parks. RESTAURANTS: fast foods, family, elegant, continental, Asian, Mexican, Scandinavian. CONTACT: Old Spanish Days, P.O. Box 1587, Santa Barbara, CA 93102, (805) 962-8101 or the Santa Barbara Chamber of Commerce, P.O. Box 299, Santa Barbara, CA 93102, (805) 965-3021. 175,000

KLAMATH SALMON FESTIVAL AND BOAT RACES *first weekend in August,* Klamath, Del Norte Co., in the Redwood National Park of Northern California. Logging show, beauty pageant, Art in Action, parade, hydro-plane drift-boat rowing, men's and women's rowing races. FOODS SERVED: traditional Indian salmon bake and barbecued New York steak. ADMISSION: free. ACCOMMODATIONS: motels and hotels, B&B's, campgrounds, RV parks. RESTAURANTS: fast foods, family, elegant. CONTACT: "Chub" Morris, P.O. Box 476, Klamath, CA 95548-0476. 7,000

PALO ALTO CELEBRATES THE ARTS *third weekend in August,* Palo Alto, Santa Clara Co., on University Avenue, and home of Stanford University. Fine artists and craftspeople, outdoor cafes with wine tasting, Tea Dance, strolling musicians on beautiful tree-lined University Ave. Entertainers such as David Hardiman's All-Star Big Band, Melody Ann and her Rhythm Rascals, Mist in the Meadow, Steve Seskin, jugglers, clowns. FOODS SERVED: "gourmet fair food" and California wines. ADMISSION: free. ACCOMMODATIONS: motels and hotels, B&B's. RESTAURANTS: fast foods, family, elegant, international. CONTACT: Terry Pimsleur & Co., 2155 Union St., San Francisco, CA 94123, (415) 346-4446. 85,000

MOUNTAIN FESTIVAL *third weekend in August,* Tehachapi, Kern Co. Arts and Crafts Faire, country-western dance, teen dance, fishing derby, PRCA rodeo, parade. FOODS SERVED: pancake breakfast, concessions. ADMISSION: free, charges to Rodeo: adults $6.00, children free; dance $10.00 per couple. ACCOMMODATIONS: motels. RESTAURANTS: fast foods, family. CONTACT: Greater Tehachapi Chamber of Commerce, P.O. Box 401, Tehachapi, CA 93561, (805) 822-4180. 40,000

RUSSIAN RIVER JAZZ FESTIVAL *first weekend in September,* Guerneville, Sonoma Co., at Midway Beach on the Russian River. Two days of great jazz on the beach. Bring a picnic lunch and beach blanket or chairs. Musicians may include Johnny Copeland Blues Band, Amber Skies, Al Dimeola with Larry Coryell, Art Blakey and the Jazz Messingers, Montreux, James Newton Quartet, Diane Schurr, Brasilian Beat. FOODS SERVED: hamburgers and hot dogs, soda, beer. ADMISSION: $17.00–$20.00 per day. ACCOMMODATIONS: motels and hotels, B&B's, campgrounds, RV parks. RESTAURANTS: family, elegant, continental. CON-

TACT: Russian River Jazz Festival, Inc., P.O. Box 763, Guerneville, CA 95446, (707) 887-7720. 5,000

BISHOP HOMECOMING RODEO AND WILD WEST WEEKEND *Labor Day weekend, (early September),* Bishop, Inyo Co., at the Tri-County Fairgrounds in the Eastern Sierra Mountains. Bed races, western parade, PRCA rodeo, queen coronation, and Whiskerino Contest, arts and crafts show, family fun and games day, chili cook-off and dinner, country-western dance, teen dance, carnival, old-timers picnic, local rodeo. FOODS SERVED: chili, pancake breakfast, western barbecue dinner. ADMISSION: adults $6.00–$8.00, children $3.00–$5.00. ACCOMMODATIONS: motels and hotels, B&B's, campgrounds, RV parks. RESTAURANTS: fast foods, family, elegant, Chinese. CONTACT: Bishop Homecoming and Rodeo Association, Bishop Chamber of Commerce, 690 North Main St., Bishop, CA 93514, (619) 873-8405. 30,000

CONCORD FALL FEST *Labor Day weekend (early September),* Concord, Contra Costa Co., at Todos Santos Park. Fine arts and crafts, chili cook-off, celebrity grape stomp, 10k Run, continuous music and entertainment. FOODS SERVED: chili. ADMISSION: free. ACCOMMODATIONS: motels and hotels, B&B's, campgrounds, RV parks. RESTAURANTS: fast foods, family. CONTACT: Terry Pimsleur & Co., 2155 Union St., San Francisco, CA 94123, (415) 346-4446. 40,000

OAKLAND FESTIVAL OF THE ARTS: ARTS EXPLOSION *Labor Day (early September),* Oakland, Alameda Co., in the San Francisco Bay area at Estuary Park. Performing and visual arts including sixteen arts organizations' booths exemplifying Oakland's diverse cultural and ethnic background, participatory events for adults and children, live entertainment such as blues artists Katie Webster, Charles Brown, Maxine Howard and her

Rhythm and Blues Explosion, modern dancers Hassan al Falak with Kent Keyward, Mexican folk dancers Los Danzantes de Alegria, Pete Escovedo and his Orchestra, whistler Jason Serinus. FOODS SERVED: Mexican, Korean, Chinese, Louisiana fancy fine, Texas barbecue, hot dogs. ADMISSION: adults $1.00, children under 12 free. ACCOMMODATIONS: motels and hotels. RESTAURANTS: fast foods, family, elegant, international. CONTACT: Oakland Festival of the Arts, 337 Seventeenth St., Oakland, CA 94612, (415) 444-5588. 16,000

WASCO FESTIVAL OF ROSES *Saturday after Labor Day (September)*, Wasco, Kern Co., celebrating the blooming of hundreds of acres of roses. Rose show, selection of annually-featured rose, parade, art show, rose farm tours, fashion show, Mini Rose Bowl, barn dance, gospel concert, Fun Run, swim meet, beauty pageant. FOODS SERVED: deep-pit barbecue, Sunday Mexican fiesta luncheon sponsored by Wasco Sociedad Progresista Mexicana, pancake breakfast. ADMISSION: free, charge for beauty pageant. ACCOMMODATIONS: motels and hotels. RESTAURANTS: fast foods, family. CONTACT: Wasco Festival of Roses, Inc., 652 E Street, Wasco, CA 93280, (805) 758-2746.

POWWOW DAYS *second weekend in September*, Apple Valley, San Bernardino Co. Indian dancers, parade, dance carnival, stage entertainment, Lovely Leggs and Knobby Knees contests for men, Indian crafts booths, street dancing, beard growing contest. FOODS SERVED: American Indian and other food booths, spaghetti dinner, pancake breakfast. ADMISSION: $3.00 per person. ACCOMMODATIONS: motels and hotels, campgrounds. RESTAURANTS: fast foods, family. CONTACT: Apple Valley Chamber of Commerce, Box 1073, Apple Valley, CA 92037, (619) 247-3202. 25,000

CASTRO VALLEY FALL FESTIVAL *second weekend in September*, Castro Val-

ley, Alameda Co., in the San Francisco Bay area, downtown. One hundred artists and craftspeople sell and demonstrate their work, free health checks, displays of students' art work, three stages of "nonstop free entertainment" including country-western, Latin salsa, American Indian, dixieland, jazz, Mideastern, and folk music, barbershop quartets, jugglers, and acrobats. FOODS SERVED: "multi-ethnic," beer, wine, commemorative glasses sold. ADMISSION: free. ACCOMMODATIONS: motels and hotels, campgrounds, RV parks. RESTAURANTS: fast foods, family, elegant, Asian, French. CONTACT: Castro Valley Chamber of Commerce, P.O. Box 2312, Castro Valley, CA 94546-0312, (415) 537-5300. 70,000

MOUNTAIN VIEW ART AND WINE FESTIVAL *second weekend in September*, Mountain View, Santa Clara Co., on Castro Street. Arts and crafts, musical entertainment from Community School of Music and Art. FOODS SERVED: many nationalities, wine from local wineries, beer. ADMISSION: free, charges for wine and beer tickets. ACCOMMODATIONS: motels and hotels, RV parks. RESTAURANTS: fast foods, family, elegant, Italian, French, Asian. CONTACT: Mountain View Chamber of Commerce, P.O. Box 486, Mountain View, CA 94042, (415) 986-8378. 120,000

16TH OF SEPTEMBER FIESTA *September 16*, Calexico, Imperial Co., in the Imperial Valley near the California–Mexico border, to celebrate Mexican Independence Day. Mexican fiesta, fireworks, mariachis, folkloric dancers from Mexico. FOODS SERVED: Mexican. ADMISSION: free. ACCOMMODATIONS: motels and hotels, campgrounds, RV parks. RESTAURANTS: fast foods, family, elegant, Mexican, Chinese. CONTACT: Calexico Chamber of Commerce, P.O. Box 948, Calexico, CA 92231, (714) 357-1166. 8,000

ART AND WINE FESTIVAL *third weekend in September*, Capitola, Santa Cruz Co., at the Capitola Esplanade. Sale of fine art, live bands including classical, light rock, and jazz, puppet shows. FOODS SERVED: tasting of local wines, variety of food specialties. ADMISSION: free. ACCOMMODATIONS: motels and hotels, B&B's, campgrounds, RV parks. RESTAURANTS: fast foods, family, elegant, local seafood, Mexican. CONTACT: Capitola Chamber of Commerce, P.O. Box 234, Capitola, CA 95010, (408) 688-7351.

MONTEREY JAZZ FESTIVAL *third weekend in September,* Monterey, Monterey Co., at the County Fairgrounds. Five concerts from Friday evening through Sunday evening, featuring the greats of American and international jazz, such as Stephane Grappelli, Tito Puente's Latin Jazz All Stars, John Lee Hooker, Etta James, Rare Silk, Dianne Reeves, Bruce Forman, George Cables, Hank Jones, and Vince Lateano. FOODS SERVED: "all kinds." ADMISSION: about $70.00–$80.00 for all five shows. ACCOMMODATIONS: motels and hotels, B&B's, campgrounds, RV parks. RESTAURANTS: fast foods, family, elegant. CONTACT: Monterey Jazz Festival, P.O. Box JAZZ, Monterey, CA 93942, (408) 373-3366. 50,000

PAN PACIFIC EXPOSITION ART AND WINE FESTIVAL *third weekend in September,* San Francisco, San Francisco Co., on the Marina Green facing San Francisco Bay and the Golden Gate Bridge, to commemorate the 1915 World's Fair held on and near the same site. Fine arts and crafts, high-wheeler bicycle race, vintage fashion show, vaudeville-style review, antique cars, magic shows, musical entertainment such as Bay Area Rapid Brass, Paul Prices, Ragtime Society Orchestra, Hurricane Sam Rudin, William Wizard's Outdoor Magical Extravaganza of 1915, Geoff Palmer's Jazz Explosion. FOODS SERVED: "gourmet fair foods" and California wines. ADMISSION: free. ACCOMMODATIONS: motels and hotels, B&B's. RESTAURANTS: fast foods, family, elegant, international. CONTACT: Terry Pimsleur & Co., 2155 Union St., San Francisco, CA 94123, (415) 346-4446. 25,000

DANISH DAYS *third weekend in September,* Solvang, Santa Barbara Co., in the Santa Ynez Valley, in recognition of Danish heritage of many residents in a quaint Danish village. Danish films, Hans Christian Andersen Story Hour, parade, cloggers, concerts, dinner dance, Estonian Dance Group, roving Danish folk dancers and musicians, Luso American Portuguese Club dance group, Montclair Jazz Choir, gymnasts, Santa Ynez Valley Community Theatre Musical Review Troupe, Air Force Band. FOODS SERVED: Aebleskiver and medisterpølse breakfasts, Food and Wine Fest, lots of Danish foods available. ADMISSION: free. ACCOMMODATIONS: motels and hotels, B&B's, campgrounds, RV parks. RESTAURANTS: fast foods, family, elegant, Danish and other continental, Mexican. CONTACT: Solvang Business Association and Chamber of Commerce, P.O. Box 465, Solvang, CA 93463, (805) 688-3317. 50,000

PACIFIC COAST FOG FEST *fourth weekend in September,* Pacifica, San Mateo Co., on Palmetto Avenue, in recognition of the discovery of San Francisco Bay by Gaspar de Portola. Fine arts and crafts, treks to the discovery site, fog-calling demonstrations, weatherman's contest for the "Fog Capital of the Pacific Coast," continuous entertainment including Nuclear Whales Saxophone Orchestra, Pacific Coast Jazz Band, J. C. Burris, Fog City Ramblers, Steve Seskin and Friends. FOODS SERVED: "gourmet fair food" and fine wine. ADMISSION: free. ACCOMMODATIONS: motels and hotels, B&B's, campgrounds, RV parks. RESTAURANTS: fast foods, family. CONTACT: Terry Pimsleur & Co., 2155 Union St., San Francisco, CA 94123, (415) 346-4446. 30,000

SANTA CLARA ARTS AND WINE FESTIVAL *last weekend in September,* Santa Clara, Santa Clara Co., in Central Park, to celebrate the grape harvest. Many local artists exhibit, strolling musicians, continuous live music featuring light rock and country music, wine tasting. FOODS SERVED: thirty food booths featuring Mexican, Portuguese, "various Asian groups and much more." ADMISSION: free, charges for wine tickets and wine glasses. ACCOMMODATIONS: motels and hotels, B&B. RESTAURANTS: fast foods, family, elegant, many international. CONTACT: Santa Clara Chamber of Commerce, P.O. Box 387, Santa Clara, CA 95052, (408) 296-6863. 10,000

VALLEY OF THE MOON VINTAGE FESTIVAL *last weekend in September,* Sonoma, Sonoma Co., in the Valley of the Moon, site of California's first vineyards. Sponsors' Wine Tasting Party at historic barracks of General Vallejo, Blessing of the Grapes at Mission San Francisco de Solano, reenactment of the Vallejo–Haraszthy wedding, wine tasting in Sonoma's historic Plaza, grape stomp contest, games, continuous music in the plaza, Vintage Ball with music of the 40's. FOODS SERVED: local wines and commemorative glasses sold, spaghetti, local sausages, corn, other concessions. ADMISSION: free. ACCOMMODATIONS: motels and hotels, B&B's. RESTAURANTS: fast foods, family, elegant, continental, Chinese, Mexican. CONTACT: Vintage Festival Board, P.O. Box 652, Sonoma, CA 95476, (707) 938-4722, or Sonoma Valley Chamber of Commerce, 453 First St., E., Sonoma, CA 95476, (707) 996-1033. 15,000

COLUMBUS DAY CELEBRATION *first week in October to Columbus Day (October 12),* San Francisco, San Francisco, Co., in North Beach and Fisherman's Wharf. San Francisco's Italian community commemorates Columbus' discovery of America with a Queen Isabella coronation, civic ceremonies, pageant reenacting Columbus' landing, procession of Madonna del Lume and Blessing of the Fishing Fleet celebrating centuries-old Sicilian folk rite venerating the patroness of fishermen with Mass at Church of Saints Peter and Paul followed by a march to Fisherman's Wharf for blessing. ADMISSION: free. ACCOMMODATIONS: motels and hotels. RESTAURANTS: fast foods, family, elegant, international.

CONTACT: San Francisco Convention and Visitors Bureau, 201 Third St., San Francisco, CA 94103, (415) 974-6900. 10,000

AUTUMN JUBILEE *first weekend in October,* North Lake Tahoe–Truckee, Placer Co., to celebrate the fall season in the High Sierra. Firefighters muster and parade, food and wine tasting, dances, concerts, Oktoberfest, western bands. FOODS SERVED: local delicacies, western barbecue. ADMISSION: varies by event. ACCOMMODATIONS: motels and hotels, B&B's, campgrounds, RV parks. RESTAURANTS: fast foods, family, elegant, continental, Asian, Cajun, nouvelle. CONTACT: Ruth Schnabel, P.O. Box 7590, Tahoe City, CA 95730, (916) 583-7625. 7,000

ITALIAN AMERICAN CULTURE FESTIVAL *first weekend in October,* San Jose, Santa Clara Co., at the County Fairgrounds, in recognition of Columbus Day. Arts and crafts, continuous entertainment, from performances by Opera San Jose directed by former diva Irene Dalis to tarantella dances, street dancing, entertainers such as Frankie Fanelli, Ree Burnell and local well known performers, Catholic Mass, bocce ball. FOODS SERVED: lots of Italian food booths. ADMISSION: free. ACCOMMODATIONS: motels and hotels, B&B's, campgrounds, RV parks. RESTAURANTS: fast foods, family, elegant, Spanish, Italian, Asian. CONTACT: Italian American Heritage Foundation, 425 No. 4th Street, San Jose, CA 95112, (408) 293-7122. 200,000

FESTA ITALIANA *week before Columbus Day (October 12),* Santa Barbara, Santa Barbara Co., to celebrate Columbus Day. Reenactment of Columbus' landing takes place on the beach, Italian Mass, music by Tony DeBruno's Orchestra, dancing, lots of Italian food. FOODS SERVED: home-cooked pasta, peppers, sausage, sweets. ADMISSION: free. ACCOMMODATIONS: motels and hotels, B&B's, campgrounds, RV parks. RESTAURANTS: fast foods, family, elegant, Asian,

Mexican, Scandinavian. CONTACT: Frank Raso at (805) 964-5959, Italian–American Boot Club, 3970 La Colina Rd., Santa Barbara, CA 93110 10,000

JAZZ AND ALL THAT ART ON FILLMORE *Columbus Day weekend (October 12)*, San Francisco, San Francisco Co., on "upper" Fillmore Street, to "celebrate 'The Fillmore's' historical jazz reputation." "The only outdoor jazz festival in San Francisco's prestigious Pacific Heights and Upper Fillmore Districts" includes top-name jazz performers such as Richie Cole, Mary Stallings, Dick Whittington, Bruce Forman, Bill DeLisle and the Blazing Redheads, fine arts and crafts, fashion show. FOODS SERVED: food and wine pavilions. ADMISSION: free. ACCOMMODATIONS: motels and hotels, B&B's. RESTAURANTS: fast foods, family, international. CONTACT: Terry Pimsleur & Co., 2155 Union St., San Francisco, CA 94123, (415) 346-4446. 30,000

CALICO DAYS *Columbus Day weekend (near October 12)*, Calico Ghost Town, Yermo, San Bernardino Co., 10 miles from Barstow in the Mojave Desert. Wild West 1880s celebration features parade, National Gunfight Stunt Championships, old prospectors burro run, raw-egg toss, searching for nickels in a haystack, stilt races, 1880s fashions. ADMISSION: adults $4.00, juniors $2.00, children free. ACCOMMODATIONS: campground, motels in Barstow. RESTAURANTS: family. CONTACT: Calico Ghost Town, P.O. Box 638, Yermo, CA 92398, (619) 254-2122.

BRUSSELS SPROUT FESTIVAL *second weekend in October*, Santa Cruz, Santa Cruz Co., at the Santa Cruz Beach Boardwalk, "to gain some respect for poor brussels sprouts." brussels sprouts cooking demonstrations, Sprout Toss, live entertainment including jazz, bluegrass, blues, free brussels sprouts for first 5,000 families, sprout testing. FOODS SERVED: sprouts tempura, marinated sprouts, sprout pizza, sprout ice cream and more. ADMISSION: free. ACCOMMODATIONS: mo-tels and hotels, B&B's, campgrounds, RV parks. RESTAURANTS: fast foods, family, elegant. CONTACT: Santa Cruz Beach Boardwalk, Santa Cruz Seaside Co., 400 Beach St., Santa Cruz, CA 95060-5491, (408) 423-5590. 5,000

GOLETA VALLEY DAYS *second full week in October*, Goleta, Santa Barbara Co., in a center for orchid (cymbidium) ranches. Chili cook-off, Fiddlers Convention, hoedown, arts and crafts fair, orchid show, parade, lemon-meringue-pie baking contest, band concert, square dance, Depot Day, tours. FOODS SERVED: chili, lemon meringue pie, lots of others. ADMISSION: free. ACCOMMODATIONS: motels and hotels, campgrounds. RESTAURANTS: fast foods, family, elegant. CONTACT: Goleta Chamber of Commerce, P.O. Box 781, Goleta, CA 93116, (805) 967-4618.

RIVERBANK CHEESE AND WINE EXPOSITION *second weekend in October*, Riverbank, Stanislaus Co., in the Modesto area. Eight blocks of street festival featuring arts and crafts, lots of live entertainment. FOODS SERVED: international booths, wine and cheese. ADMISSION: free, $12.50 to Cheese and Wine Tasting. ACCOMMODATIONS: RV parks. RESTAURANTS: fast foods, family. CONTACT: Riverbank Chamber of Commerce, 3237 Santa Fe St., Riverbank, CA 95367, (209) 869-4541. 80,000

HALF MOON BAY PUMPKIN FESTIVAL *third weekend in October*, Half Moon Bay, San Mateo Co., to celebrate the pumpkin harvest. Great Pumpkin Parade, Masquerade Ball, pumpkin pie eating contest, fine arts and handmade crafts, live entertainment by Mist in the Meadow, Dorahim Chakoor, Saxophone Quartet, and the Pumpkin Carvers. FOODS SERVED: Pumpkins! ADMISSION: free. ACCOMMODATIONS: motels and hotels, B&B's, campgrounds, RV parks. RESTAURANTS: fast foods, family, elegant. CONTACT: Half Moon Bay Coastside Chamber of Commerce, 225 S. Cabrillo, Half Moon Bay, CA 94019, (415) 726-5202. 150,000

HANGTOWN JAZZ JUBILEE *third Sunday in October,* Placerville, El Dorado Co., in the Gold Country. Traditional jazz bands from all over northern California play at various locations on Main Street. ADMISSION: adults advance $7.50, day of event $10.00. ACCOMMODATIONS: motels and hotels, B&B's, campgrounds. RESTAURANTS: fast foods, family. CONTACT: El Dorado Co. Chamber of Commerce, 542 Main St., Placerville, CA 95667, (916) 626-2344. 1,200

BORREGO DAYS DESERT FESTIVAL *last weekend in October,* Borrego Springs, San Diego Co., near the Anza Borrego Desert State Park, in recognition of the beginning of winter in the desert. Arts and crafts, queen selection, dances, chili cook-off, parade, talent show, desert tours conducted by State Park. FOODS SERVED: barbecue, chili, others. ADMISSION: free. ACCOMMODATIONS: motels and hotels, campgrounds, RV parks. RESTAURANTS: elegant, Chinese, Mexican. CONTACT: Borrego Springs Chamber of Commerce, P.O. Box 66, Borrego Springs, CA 92004, (714) 767-5555. 4,000

FINE ARTS FESTIVAL *first full weekend in November,* Calico Ghost Town, Yermo, San Bernardino Co., 10 miles from Barstow in the Mojave Desert. At least eighty of the West's foremost artists display and sell their work, art auctions, country and bluegrass music. ADMISSION: $3.00 per car. ACCOMMODATIONS: campground, motels in Barstow. RESTAURANTS: family. CONTACT: Calico Ghost Town, P.O. Box 638, Yermo, CA 92398, (619) 254-2122.

AUBURN CRAFT FESTIVAL AND CHRISTMAS MARKETPLACE *second weekend in November,* Auburn, Placer Co., at the County Fairgrounds in the Sierra Foothills. Arts and crafts by 150 artists and craftspeople, two stages with continuous entertainment of elves, bluegrass, jazz, jugglers, and folk music. FOODS SERVED: "wide variety." ADMISSION: adults $1.50, children 12 and under free. ACCOMMODATIONS: motels and hotels, B&B's, RV parks. RESTAURANTS: fast foods, family, elegant. CONTACT: Rich Burleigh, P.O. Box 148, Soulsbyville, CA 95372, (209) 533-3473. 6,000

BRAWLEY CATTLE CALL *second weekend in November,* Brawley, Imperial Co., in the Imperial Valley, as a salute to the cattle industry. Beef cook-off, bluegrass music with Casey Tibbs, the Lone Ranger, Wayne Northrup, Cal Worthington, and usually Hollywood stars, western parade, PRCA rodeo, western dances. FOODS SERVED: chuckwagon breakfast, deep-pit beef barbecue, Mexican food. ADMISSION: free, charges for rodeo and some events. ACCOMMODATIONS: motels and hotels, B&B's, campgrounds, FV parks. RESTAURANTS: fast foods, family, elegant. CONTACT: Cattle Call Committee, Brawley Chamber of Commerce, P.O. Box 218, Brawley, CA 92227, (619) 344-3160. 50,000

SONORA CHRISTMAS CRAFT FESTIVAL *Thanksgiving weekend (November),* Sonora, Tuolumne Co., at the Mother Lode Fairgrounds. 250 artists present their works, children's stories and songs, Santa and his elves, magicians, jugglers, jazz, bluegrass, rock, reggae, carolers, folk music on three stages. FOODS SERVED: wide variety including Asian, continental, Mexican. ADMISSION: adults $2.50, children 12 and under free. ACCOMMODATIONS: motels and hotels, B&B's, RV parks. RESTAURANTS: fast foods, family, elegant. CONTACT: Rich Burleigh, P.O. Box 148, Soulsbyville, CA 95372, (209) 533-3473. 12,000

HAWAII

NARCISSUS FESTIVAL *January 10–March 1*, Honolulu, Oahu in celebration of the Chinese New Year. Queen pageant, coronation ball, Chinese cooking demonstration, Chinatown Open House with lion dances, firecrackers, food booths, arts and crafts. FOODS SERVED: Chinese, Hawaiian. ADMISSION: free. ACCOMMODATIONS: motels and hotels, B&B's, condominiums. RESTAURANTS: fast foods, family, elegant, Asian, Polynesian. CONTACT: Welton Won at (808) 533-3181 or the Hawaii Visitors Bureau, Waikiki Business Plaza, Suite 801, 2270 Kalakaua Ave., Honolulu, HI 96815, (808) 923-1811.

CHERRY BLOSSOM FESTIVAL *January 14–April 4*, Honolulu, Oahu. Japanese cultural celebration that includes a fun run, song contest, Japanese cultural show, music concert, queen pageant, coronation ball. ADMISSION: free. ACCOMMODATIONS: motels and hotels, B&B's, condominiums. RESTAURANTS: fast foods, family, elegant, Asian, Polynesian. CONTACT: Alan Okimoto at (808) 945-3545 or the Hawaii Visitors Bureau, Waikiki Business Plaza, Suite 801, 2270 Kalakaua Ave., Honolulu, HI 96815, (808) 923-1811.

CAPTAIN COOK FESTIVAL *third weekend in February*, Waimea, Kauai. Waimea town party with refreshments, entertainment, canoe race, reenactment of Captain Cook's landing and a 7.4 mi. run. ADMISSION: free. ACCOMMODATIONS: motels and hotels, condominiums, campgrounds. RESTAURANTS: fast foods, family, elegant, Asian, Polynesian. CONTACT: Sylvia Dobry at (808) 338-1226 or the Hawaii Visitors Bureau, Waikiki Business Plaza, Suite 801, 2270 Kalakaua Ave., Honolulu, HI 96815, (808) 923-1811.

MERRIE MONARCH FESTIVAL AND CONCERT AT KA'AUEA *third weekend and fourth week in April*, Hilo, Hawaii. Full week of hula competitions among Hawaii's best hula halau (schools) including both ancient and modern dances, other Hawaiian festivities. The Concert at Ka'auea is a major outdoor concert featuring Hawaiian folk music and dance, and is held in front of the Volcanoes Art Center, Hawaii Volcanoes National Park, Hawaii. ADMISSION: charges. ACCOMMODATIONS: motels and hotels, B&B's, campgrounds, condominiums. RESTAURANTS: fast foods, family, elegant, Asian, Polynesian. CONTACT: Merrie Monarch Festival. Call Dorothy Thompson at (808) 935-9168 and for the Concert at Ka'auea call Marsha Erickson at (808) 967-7179 or the Hawaii Visitors Bureau, Waikiki Business Plaza, Suite 801, 2270 Kalakaua Ave., Honolulu, HI 96815, (808) 923-1811.

FESTIVAL OF THE PACIFIC *first week in June*, Honolulu, Oahu. Athletic tournaments, music, songs, and dance of the multi-ethnic people of the Pacific, including presentation of forty flags of the Pacific area. ADMISSION: free, charges for some events. ACCOMMODATIONS: motels and hotels, B&B's, campgrounds, condominiums. RESTAURANTS: fast foods, family, elegant, Asian, Polynesian. CONTACT: Harry Cooper at (808) 883-0026 or the Hawaii Visitors Bureau, Waikiki Business Plaza, Suite 801, 2270 Kalakaua Ave., Honolulu, HI 96815, (808) 923-1811.

GOTCHA PRO SURF CHAMPIONSHIPS *second week and weekend in June*, Sandy Beach, Oahu. Summer surfing festival featuring many water and beach events including board, body, and skin surfing, skate boarding, BMX bike contests, bikini contests with contestants from twelve countries and $33,000 in prize money. ADMISSION: free, charges for some events. ACCOMMODATIONS: motels and hotels, campgrounds. RESTAURANTS: fast foods, family, elegant. CONTACT:

Randy Rarick at (808) 638-7266 or the Hawaii Visitors Bureau, Waikiki Business Plaza, Suite 801, 2270 Kalakaua Ave., Honolulu, HI 96815, (808) 923-1811.

KING KAMEHAMEHA CELEBRATION *June 11,* all islands. State holiday honoring Kamehameha the Great, Hawaii's first monarch. Oahu Island features a lei draping ceremony at statue site, Civic Center, downtown Honolulu. Waikiki features a parade with floral floats, pageantry, bands, and a ho'olaule'a (street party). On Hawaii Island the entire day features Hawaiian entertainment, crafts demonstrations and exhibits, food booths at Coconut Island, Hilo. Kauai Island presents a parade, ho'olaule'a, arts and crafts, at the Kihue and Kukui Grove Shopping Center. FOODS SERVED: Hawaiian concessions. ADMISSION: free. ACCOMMODATIONS: motels and hotels, condominiums. RESTAURANTS: fast foods, family, elegant, international. CONTACT: Hawaii Visitors Bureau, Waikiki Business Plaza, Suite 801, 2270 Kalakaua Ave., Honolulu, HI 96815, (808) 923-1811.

ESTABLISHMENT DAY CULTURAL FESTIVAL *last weekend in June,* Kawaihae, Hawaii. Ancient hula and workshops in lei-making, Hawaiian language, and other ancient skills. FOODS SERVED: Hawaiian. ADMISSION: charge. ACCOMMODATIONS: motels and hotels. RESTAURANTS: fast foods, family, elegant. CONTACT: Pu'ukohala Heiau at (808) 882-7218 or the Hawaii Visitors Bureau, Waikiki Business Plaza, Suite 801, 2270 Kalakaua Ave., Honolulu, HI 96815, (808) 923-1811.

PRINCE LOT HULA FESTIVAL *third Saturday in July,* Honolulu, Oahu, at Moanalua Gardens. Hawaii's best hula schools gather to perform authentic ancient and modern hula; games, arts and crafts exhibits and demonstrations. FOODS SERVED: Hawaiian. ADMISSION: charges for some events. ACCOMMODATIONS: motels and hotels, B&B's, condominiums. RESTAURANTS: fast foods, family, elegant,

Asian, Polynesian. CONTACT: Moanalua Gardens, 1401 Mahiole, Honolulu, HI 96819, (808) 839-5334 or the Hawaii Visitors Bureau, Waikiki Business Plaza, Suite 801, 2270 Kalakaua Ave., Honolulu, HI 96815, (808) 923-1811.

MACADAMIA NUT HARVEST FESTIVAL *second weekend and third week in August,* Honokaa, Hawaii, to celebrate the macadamia nut harvest. Golf and baseball tournaments, cross-country run, ethnic nights jamboree, entertainment, parade. FOODS SERVED: macadamia nuts and Hawaiian specialties. ADMISSION: free, charges to some events. ACCOMMODATIONS: motels and hotels. RESTAURANTS: fast foods, family, elegant. CONTACT: Clarence Garcia at (808) 775-7792 or the Hawaii Visitors Bureau, Waikiki Business Plaza, Suite 801, 2270 Kalakaua Ave., Honolulu, HI 96815, (808) 923-1811.

OKINAWAN FESTIVAL *Labor Day weekend (early September),* Honolulu, Oahu at Thomas Square. Exciting dances, arts and crafts exhibits and demonstrations, food booths, and "Kachashi," a dance contest involving volunteers from the audience. FOODS SERVED: Okinawan specialties. ADMISSION: free. ACCOMMODATIONS: motels and hotels, B&B's, condominiums. RESTAURANTS: fast foods, family, elegant, Asian, Polynesian. CONTACT: Richard Fukuhara at (808) 546-8119 or the Hawaii Visitors Bureau, Waikiki Business Plaza, Suite 801, 2270 Kalakaua Ave., Honolulu, HI 96815, (808) 923-1811.

ALOHA WEEK FESTIVALS *fourth week in September,* all islands. Hawaiian pageantry, canoe races, Ho'olaule'a (street parties), parades, a variety of entertainment everywhere, and a Royal Ball in Honolulu. Oahu's parade is the fourth Saturday in Honolulu. FOODS SERVED: Hawaiian concessions. ADMISSION: many events free, charges for others. ACCOMMODATIONS: motels and hotels, condominiums, campgrounds. RESTAURANTS: fast foods, family, elegant, international. CON-TACT: each island for details or: Aloha Week, 750 Amana St., Suite 111-A, Honolulu, HI 96814, (808) 944-8857 or the Hawaii Visitors Bureau, Waikiki Business Plaza, Suite 801, 2270 Kalakaua Ave., Honolulu, HI 96815, (808) 923-1811.

KANIKAPILA (LET'S PLAY MUSIC) *mid–October,* Honolulu, Oahu, at Andrews Amphitheatre. Festival of Hawaiian music featuring singers, musicians, and dancers from four islands. ADMISSION: charge. AC-COMMODATIONS: motels and hotels, B&B's, condominiums. RESTAURANTS: fast foods, family, elegant, Asian, Polynesian. CONTACT: University of Hawaii Bureau of Student Activities, 2411 Dole St., Honolulu, HI 96822, (808) 948-8178 or the Hawaii Visitors Bureau, Waikiki Business Plaza, Suite 801, 2270 Kalakaua Ave., Honolulu, HI 96815, (808) 923-1811.

KAMEHAMEHA SCHOOLS FESTIVAL *fourth Saturday in October,* Kamehameha Schools, Oahu. An old-style Hawaiian festival featuring continuous hula, Hawaiian, and contemporary entertainment by prominent Hawaiian entertainers, arts and crafts, Hawaiian children's games, with participation of the people of five islands. FOODS SERVED: variety of specialties from all five islands. ADMISSION: charge. ACCOMMODATIONS: motels and hotels. RESTAURANTS: family. CONTACT: Sherlyn Franklin at (808) 842-8663 or the Hawaii Visitors Bureau, Waikiki Business Plaza, Suite 801, 2270 Kalakaua Ave., Honolulu, HI 96815, (808) 923-1811.

KONA COFFEE FESTIVAL *first weekend in November,* Kailua–Kona, Hawaii, to celebrate the harvest of the "only U.S. commercially grown coffee," Queen contest, parade, recipe contest, arts and crafts, entertainment. FOODS SERVED: multi-ethnic. ADMISSION: free. ACCOMMODATIONS: motels and hotels, B&B's. RESTAURANTS: family, elegant. CONTACT: Alan Pratt at (808) 879-4577 or the Hawaii Visitors Bureau, Waikiki Business Plaza, Suite 801, 2270 Kalakaua Ave., Honolulu, HI 96815, (808) 923-1811.

NA MELE O'MAUI FESTIVAL *first weekend in November,* Kaanapali and Lahaina, Maui. A celebration of "Hawaiiana" through Hawaii's arts, crafts, dances, music, and a luau at several hotels in the towns of Kaanapali and Lahaina. FOODS SERVED: Hawaiian. ADMISSION: varies. ACCOMMODATIONS: motels and hotels, condominiums. RESTAURANTS: fast foods, family, elegant, Asian, Polynesian. CONTACT: Betsy Kinau at (808) 879-4577 or the Hawaii Visitors Bureau, Waikiki Business Plaza, Suite 801, 2270 Kalakaua Ave., Honolulu, HI 96815, (808) 923-1181.

HAWAII INTERNATIONAL FILM FESTIVAL *last weekend in November and first week in December,* Honolulu, Oahu. Cross-cultural films by award-winning filmmakers from Asia, the Pacific, and the U.S. ADMISSION: charges. ACCOMMODATIONS: motels and hotels, B&B's, condominiums. RESTAURANTS: fast foods, family, elegant, Asian, Polynesian. CONTACT: Jeannette Paulson at (808) 944-7203, the East West Center Public Affairs at (808) 944-7200, or the Hawaii Visitors Bureau, Waikiki Business Plaza, Suite 801, 2270 Kalakaua Ave., Honolulu, HI 96815, (808) 923-1181.

IDAHO

WINTER FESTIVAL *third weekend in January,* Grangeville, Idaho Co., on the Camas Prairie, to celebrate winter. Snowmobile races, downhill and cross-country ski races, snow sculptures, talent show, square dance, art show, 3-wheeler and 4-wheeler races, torchlight ski parade, snowshoe races, bingo. FOODS SERVED: free chili feed. ADMISSION: varies by event. ACCOMMODATIONS: motels and hotels, campgrounds. RESTAURANTS: fast foods, family, Chinese. CONTACT: Grangeville Chamber of Commerce, P.O. Box 212, Grangeville, ID 83530, (208) 983-0460. 2,000

McCALL WINTER CARNIVAL *last weekend in January through first weekend in February,* McCall, Valley Co. Ice sculptures, art show, downhill and cross-country skiing, McCall lighting ceremony and torchlight parade, fireworks, queen crowning, teen dance, carnival, parade, snowmobile races, snowman building contest, Arts and Crafts Fair, Idaho State Snow Sculpting Competition, casino nite, Snowflake Ball, ice fishing clinic, beard and shaving contests, cabaret concert, sleigh rides to view sculptures, Poker Run, square dance, children's masquerade. FOODS SERVED: chili feed, others available. ADMISSION: varies by event, some events free. ACCOMMODATIONS: motels and hotels, B&B's, RV parks. RESTAURANTS: fast foods, family, elegant, continental, Mexican, seafood. CONTACT: McCall Area Chamber of Commerce, Box D, McCall, ID 83638, (208) 634-7631. 30,000

DOGWOOD FESTIVAL *last week in April through first week in May,* Lewiston, Nez Perce Co., the "Seaport of Idaho," and Clarkston, Washington. Fair, River Run, parades, dogwood tree planting, antique show and sale, golf and tennis tournaments, historical walking tour, dance concerts, art contests, art show, luncheons, garden tours, folk art celebrations, concerts, barbershop harmony, puppet shows. FOODS SERVED: concessions. ADMISSION: free to most events, charges for others. ACCOMMODATIONS: motels and hotels, campgrounds. RESTAURANTS: fast foods, family, elegant. CONTACT: Sharon Hatch at Lewis Clark State College, Artists' Series, 6th Street and 8th Ave., Lewiston, ID 83501, (208) 799-2243 or Greater Lewiston Chamber of Commerce, 2207 E. Main St., Lewiston, ID 83501, (208) 743-3531. 7,000

PAYETTE APPLE BLOSSOM FESTIVAL *first week in May,* Payette, Payette Co., in the Western Treasure Valley, to celebrate the blooming of spring apple blossoms. Queen coronation, community dance, children's old-fashioned races, golf tournament, ice cream social, carnival, Apple Blossom Run, parade, fire chief hose competition, outhouse races, Arts in the Park, historic home tour. FOODS SERVED: barbecue in the park, pancake breakfast, homemade ice cream. ADMISSION: free. ACCOMMODATIONS: RV parks. RESTAURANTS: fast foods, family. CONTACT: Payette Chamber of Commerce, 700 Center Ave., Payette, ID 83661, (208) 642-2362. 10,000

NATIONAL OLDTIME FIDDLERS' CONTEST *third full week in June,* Weiser, Washington Co. "Non-stop fiddling all week," preliminaries and national championships, workshops, parade, arts and crafts booths, sidewalk sales, and the music of 325 fiddlers of ages from 3-92 from thirty states and Canada. FOODS SERVED: barbecue and concessions. ADMISSION: $1.50–$9.00. ACCOMMODATIONS: motels and hotels, campgrounds. RESTAURANTS: fast foods, family. CONTACT: National Oldtime Fiddlers' Contest, c/o Weiser Chamber of Commerce, 8 E.

Idaho St., Weiser, ID 83672, (208) 549-1890. 15,000

ART ON THE GREEN *July 31–August 2*, Coeur d'Alene, Kootenai Co., at North Idaho College. More than 100 artists-in-action booths, juried show, cash prizes of $3,500. Demonstrations include glassblowing, stained glass, drawing, painting, pottery, fiberwork, and weaving; musical, theatrical, and dance performances, children's section for creative expression, artshop classes for ages 4 through 15. FOODS SERVED: "variety." ADMISSION: free. ACCOMMODATIONS: motels and hotels, B&B's, campgrounds, RV parks. RESTAURANTS: fast foods, family, elegant. CONTACT: Citizens Council for the Arts, c/o Flammia and Solomon, P.O. Box 1117, Coeur d'Alene, ID 83814, (208) 667-3561 or the Chamber of Commerce, P.O. Box 850, Coeur d'Alene, ID 83814, (208) 664-3194. 25,000

PEND OREILLE ARTS COUNCIL'S ARTS AND CRAFTS FESTIVAL *second weekend in August*, Sandpoint, Bonner Co., at the City Beach, celebrating local artists' talents. Continuous live entertainment such as the Jazz Dogs, Jerry Luther–the Hooey Man with trained wooden ducks, the Average Brothers, and Jamie and the G-Spots; "custom handmade fine art and crafts." FOODS SERVED: "quality fast foods." ADMISSION: free. ACCOMMODATIONS: motels and hotels, B&B's, campgrounds, RV parks. RESTAURANTS: fast foods, family, elegant, continental, Chinese. CONTACT: Pend Oreille Arts Council, P.O. Box 1694, Sandpoint, ID

83864, or The Greater Sandpoint Chamber of Commerce, P.O. Box 928, Sandpoint, ID 83864, (208) 263-2161. 4,000

IDAHO HUCKLEBERRY FESTIVAL *second weekend in August*, Priest River, Bonner Co., at City Park, to salute Idaho huckleberries. Arts and crafts, 6 mi. Fun Run, Soap Box Derby, grand parade, kiddies' parade, firemen's water fights, face painting, huckleberry bake-off, contests and games, local country-western, gospel, fiddle, and folk music. FOODS SERVED: huckleberry pancake breakfast, barbecue, German sausages, huckleberry milk shakes. ADMISSION: free. ACCOMMODATIONS: motels and hotels, B&B's, campgrounds, RV parks. RESTAURANTS: fast foods, family. CONTACT: Idaho Huckleberry Association, P.O. Box 182, Priest River, ID 83856, (208) 448-1401.

McCALL SUMMER ARTS AND CRAFTS FAIR "LOVE IN THE ARTS" *fourth weekend in August*, McCall, Valley Co., on the lake at Mill Park. McCall is the home of the next teacher in space, Barbara Morgen and is "100 miles north of Boise up in the mountains." More than seventy-five fine arts and crafts booths, fair on the lake including wind surfing, sail boating, theatre arts and music. FOODS SERVED: Italian and Mexican. ADMISSION: free. ACCOMMODATIONS: motels and hotels, campgrounds, RV parks. RESTAURANTS: fast foods, family, elegant. CONTACT: Edna Lunt, McCall Artisans Association, P.O. Box 1659, McCall, ID 83638, (208) 634-2418.

MONTANA

WHITEFISH WINTER CARNIVAL *first weekend in February*, Whitefish and The Big Mountain, Flathead Co. Three-day celebration of winter featuring "roy-

alty," torchlight skiing and fireworks at nearby Big Mountain Ski Resort, parade, winter games. FOODS SERVED: banquets, buffets, luncheons, breakfasts. ADMIS-

SION: free, charges for meal related events. ACCOMMODATIONS: motels and hotels, resorts. RESTAURANTS: fast foods, family, elegant. CONTACT: Whitefish Chamber of Commerce, Box 1309, Whitefish, MT 59937, (406) 862-3501.

FLATHEAD CHERRY BLOSSOM FESTIVAL *first weekend in May,* Flathead, Lake Co., to celebrate cherry blossom time, with participation by the many cherry orchardists and growers. Cherry blossom viewing, open houses at three community clubs, antique car parade featuring Cherry Queen and Cherry King candidates, talent show, entertainment by Ronan High School Choral/Theatrical Group, Montana Fiddlers, barbershop quartets, Flathead Valley Jazz Society. FOODS SERVED: lunches at community clubs featuring cherry desserts. ADMISSION: free. ACCOMMODATIONS: motels and hotels, B&B's, campgrounds, RV parks. RESTAURANTS: fast foods, family, elegant, French, Mexican, German, Italian, Chinese. CONTACT: Flathead Valley Lions Club, c/o Don Patterson, East Lake Shore, Bigfork, MT 59911, (406) 982-3316.

RED LODGE MUSIC FESTIVAL *early June for nine days,* Red Lodge, Carbon Co., at the northeast entrance to Yellowstone National Park. During the day faculty of thirty musicians from major symphonies and music schools throughout the U.S. provide instruction and seminars for 175 students from the Pacific Northwest. In the evening, the faculty performs at the Red Lodge Civic Center. ADMISSION: charge. ACCOMMODATIONS: motels and hotels, campgrounds, RV parks. RESTAURANTS: family, elegant. CONTACT: Bob Moran, Coordinator, Box 1089, Red Lodge, MT 59068, (406) 446-1905 or the Red Lodge Area Chamber of Commerce, P.O. Box 998, Red Lodge, MT 59068, (406) 446-1718. 2,000

ART IN WASHOE PARK *third weekend in July,* Anaconda, Deer Lodge Co., in

southwestern Montana. Arts and crafts, children's activities, live musical entertainment such as the Last Chance Dixieland Jazz Band, Aleph Movement Theatre (mime), Chip Jasmin, Patchwork Puppett Company, ragtime pianist Dan Battleson, and bluegrass band Homemade Jam. FOODS SERVED: international. ADMISSION: $2.00 button. ACCOMMODATIONS: motels and hotels, campgrounds, RV parks. RESTAURANTS: fast foods, family, elegant, Asian. CONTACT: Copper Village Museum and Arts Center, 110 E. Eighth, Anaconda, MT 59711 or the Anaconda Chamber of Commerce, P.O. Box 757, Anaconda, MT 58711, (406) 563-2400. 20,000

LIBBY LOGGER DAYS *third weekend in July,* Libby, Lincoln Co., in Kootenai Country, to recognize lumber as "one of the main industries of Montana," and to show off the beauty of the area. Raft race in homemade rafts down the Kootenai River, bed race down main street, Montana Lumberjack Championships, Bull of the Woods competition, marathon race, Ma and Pa Relay, children's games, parade. FOODS SERVED: pancake breakfast, barbecued chicken, concessions. ADMISSION: $4.00 button admits to all events. ACCOMMODATIONS: motels and hotels, B&B's, campgrounds, RV parks. RESTAURANTS: fast foods, family, elegant. CONTACT: Libby Area Chamber of Commerce, P.O. Box 767, Libby, MT 59923, (406) 293-3832. 5,000

LEWIS AND CLARK EXPEDITION FESTIVAL *last full weekend in July,* Cut Bank, Glacier Co., to remember the expedition of Lewis and Clark. Annual Chili Cook-off, art auction, log-cutting contest, 3k, 5k, and 10k runs, pie throwing contest, dunking booth, antique car show, district softball tournament, Crazy Days, horse show, tug of war, beauty pageant, parades, dance, flag ceremony. FOODS SERVED: barbecue, concessions. ADMISSION: $3.00 admits to barbecue and all other events except dance. ACCOMMODATIONS: motels and hotels, campground,

RV park. RESTAURANTS: fast foods, family. CONTACT: Cut Bank Area Chamber of Commerce, P.O. Box 1243, Cut Bank, MT 59427, (406) 873-4041.

FESTIVAL OF NATIONS *first Saturday in August*, Red Lodge, Carbon Co., at the northeast entrance to Yellowstone National Park, on the Beartooth Highway, rated as "the most scenic in North America by Charles Kuralt," according to locals. Nine-day festival in which each day features the customs, arts and crafts, music, and food of a different "old world" country whose residents settled in this early mining town. Nations included are Scotland, Yugoslavia, England, Ireland, Germany, Scandinavia, Finland, Italy. Activities include arts and crafts exhibits, foreign exhibits, flower show and doll display, folk dancing and music, while local restaurants feature the foods of the country honored each day. FOODS SERVED: those of each nation on its day. ADMISSION: free. ACCOMMODATIONS: motels and hotels, campgrounds, RV parks. RESTAURANTS: family, elegant. CONTACT: Bob Moran, Coordinator, Box 1089, Red Lodge, MT 59068, (406) 446-1905, or the Red Lodge Area Chamber of Commerce, P.O. Box 998, Red Lodge, MT 59068, (406) 446-1718. 20,000

CROW FAIR *third weekend in August*, Crow Agency Reservation, as an eight-day Northern Plains Indian celebration featuring parades, hand games, craft displays, nightly rodeos. FOODS SERVED: Indian foods and concessions. ADMISSION: free, charge for rodeo. ACCOMMODATIONS: campgrounds. CONTACT: Dale Old Horn or Joe Medicine Crow, Big Horn College, Crow Agency, MT 59022, (406) 638-2228.

HERITAGE OF THE YELLOWSTONE FOLKLIFE FESTIVAL *Labor Day weekend (early September)*, Billings, Yellowstone Co., at Eastern Montana College. Cowgirl poetry, basketweaving, saddlemaking, drumming, beadwork, children's activities, spinning, horsehair hitching, rawhide braiding, horse packing, willow basket weaving, Indian drum making, water dowsing, Crow stick games, strolling fiddlers. German Brass Band, kids tent for leather tooling, cowboy cooking and games, calf roping, Saturday evening concert featuring traditional music and cowboy poetry. FOODS SERVED: traditional, Native American, Dutch, Norwegian, Yugoslavian, Hispanic, Chinese, Montana ranch, Hutterite, Scottish, H'mong (Laotian), German, Welsh. ADMISSION: free. ACCOMMODATIONS: motels and hotels, campgrounds. RESTAURANTS: fast foods, family. CONTACT: Western Heritage Center, 2822 Montana Ave., Billings, MT 59101, (406) 256-6809.

NORDICFEST *third week in September*, Libby, Lincoln Co., in Kootenai Country, to celebrate Scandinavian heritage of local residents. Arts and crafts, Swedish Varpa Championship, horseshoes, soccer match, Trail Run, Fjord Horse Show, parade, Heritage Museum display, Scandinavian dancers and costumes, continuous entertainment including melodrama, Gordon Tracis, "foremost Scandinavian dance teacher," the Tordenskjold Chorus, Wooden Shoe Dancers, Lundin Family Fiddlers, St. John's Bell Choir, Treasure Tones and Norwegian dancers. FOODS SERVED: Scandinavian foods at dinner, food booths. ADMISSION: free, charge to melodrama, dinner from $4.50–$8.50. ACCOMMODATIONS: motels and hotels, B&B's, RV parks. RESTAURANTS: fast foods, family, elegant, Scandinavian. CONTACT: June McMahon, Box 1070, Libby, MT 59923, (406) 293-8573 or the Libby Area Chamber of Commerce, P.O. Box 767, Libby, MT 59923, (406) 293-3832. 10,000

HERBSTFEST *fourth weekend in September*, Laurel, Yellowstone Co., in the Billings area. Traditional German harvest festival featuring German tasting tea, vintage style show, free dance, teen dance, pageant, parade. Bierstube, and fourteen bands and performing groups, such as the

Al Holman Polkatoons, Betty Rydell, "Polka King" Frank Yankovic and the Verne Meisner Band. FOODS SERVED: German, other foods. ADMISSION: adults $5.00, children $1.00, good for both days.

ACCOMMODATIONS: motels and hotels, campground. RESTAURANTS: fast foods, family, Chinese. CONTACT: Laurel Chamber of Commerce, P.O. Box 395, Laurel, MT 59044, (406) 628-8105.

NEVADA

ELKS HELLDORADO DAYS *first ten days in May*, Las Vegas, Clark Co., at the Thomas and Mack Center, as a good old western celebration. Eight P.R.C.A. rodeo performances, carnival midway, Whiskerino Contest, Helldorado Queen Contest, street dances, continuous western music. FOODS SERVED: "six days of barbecue," concessions. ADMISSION: free, charge for rodeo adults $10.00, children, $7.00; family nights, family of five $25.00. ACCOMMODATIONS: motels and hotels, campgrounds, RV parks. RESTAURANTS: fast foods, family, elegant. CONTACT: B.P.O. Elks #1468, 900 Las Vegas Blvd. No., Las Vegas, NV 89101, (702) 385-1221. 200,000

BASQUE FESTIVAL *second weekend in June*, Winnemucca, Humboldt Co., at the City Park. Basque parade, traditional Basque games of strength such as weight lifting and carrying, wood chopping, tugs of war, Catholic mass, dancing, sheep and hog herding contests, performances by the Boise, Elko, and Winnemucca dancers, big dance at the fairgrounds, sheepherder bread contest, Irriatze Contest, Jota Dancing, Bota Bag Wine Drinking Contest, junior games of strength. FOODS SERVED: Basque including barbecue, bar. ADMISSION: $10.00–$12.00 per person per day, including picnic. ACCOMMODATIONS: motels and hotels, B&B's, campgrounds, RV parks. RESTAURANTS: fast foods, family, elegant, Basque. CONTACT: Humboldt Co. Chamber of Commerce, Nixon Building, Winnemucca, NV 89445, (702) 623-2225. 10,000

FESTIVAL RENO *six weekends from third weekend in June through fourth weekend in July*. Locals and visitors alike gather for six weekends of food festivals, parades, gaming tournaments, sports tournaments, music and dancing in the streets; casinos have booths on sidewalks, music. FOODS SERVED: Cajun, country, Mexican, American foods with a different theme each weekend. ADMISSION: free. ACCOMMODATIONS: motels and hotels, B&B's, campgrounds, RV parks. RESTAURANTS: fast foods, family, elegant, international. CONTACT: Reno–Sparks Convention and Visitors Authority, P. O. Box 837, Reno, NV 89504, 1-800-FOR-RENO.

DIXIELAND JAZZ FESTIVAL *first week in July*, Sparks, Washoe Co., at John Ascuaga's Nugget. Three in-house performance locations with ten bands performing under one roof, featuring continuous day and evening performances for three days by internationally know jazz luminaries. ADMISSION: charges to some events. ACCOMMODATIONS: motels and hotels, B&B's, campgrounds, RV parks. RESTAURANTS: fast foods, family, elegant, international. CONTACT: John Ascuaga's Nugget, 1100 Nugget Ave., Sparks, NV 89431, at (702) 356-3300 or the Reno–Sparks Convention and Visitors Authority, P.O. Box 837, Reno, NV 89504, 1-800-FOR-RENO.

TOMBOLA *second weekend in July*, Reno, Washoe Co., at Pickett Park. Tombola (village fair) features western handmade crafts and art show, horseback rides, Bertha the Performing Elephant (she's everywhere in Reno), and Basque feast to benefit the Washoe Medical Center. FOODS SERVED: barbecued lamb, salads, breads, wine, soft drinks. ADMISSION: free, donation for meal. ACCOMMODATIONS: motels and hotels, B&B's, campgrounds, RV parks. RESTAURANTS: fast foods, family, elegant, international. CONTACT: Zazpiak Bat Basque Club of Reno at (702) 785-4166 or the Reno-Sparks Convention and Visitors Authority, P.O. Box 837, Reno, NV 89504, 1-800-FOR-RENO.

ELY BASQUE CLUB FESTIVAL *third weekend in July,* Ely, White Pine Co., to preserve and celebrate Basque traditions and culture. Basque parade in Ely, games and contests of strength including weight lifting and carrying, Jota dance contests, Basque yell contests, wood-chopping and sheep-hooking contests, dance exhibitions, lamb auction, bread baking contest, dancing until 3:00 a.m., field mass Sunday, live entertainment. FOODS SERVED: twelve lambs cooked over open-spit for a meal of lamb, Basque beans, salads, chorizo, wine, rolls, soft drinks, "all you can eat." ADMISSION: adults $10.00, children under 12 $5.00. ACCOMMODATIONS: motels and hotels, campgrounds, RV parks. RESTAURANTS: family, elegant, Basque, Mexican, Italian. CONTACT: White Pine Chamber of Commerce, P.O. Box 239, Ely, NV 89301, (702) 289-8877. 1,000

RENO BASQUE FESTIVAL *second Sunday in August,* Reno, Washoe Co., at the Reno Livestock Event Center. Traditional Basque games of strength such as sokatira (5-man tug of war), sheep dog relays, National 3-man Weight-carrying Relay Championships, intricate Basque dances, and traditional feast. FOODS SERVED: deep-pit barbecued lamb, bean salads, breads, wine, soft drinks. ADMISSION: free, charge for meal. ACCOMMODATIONS: motels and hotels, B&B's, campgrounds, RV parks. RESTAURANTS: fast foods, family, elegant, international. CONTACT: (702) 331-2010 or the Reno–Sparks Convention and Visitors Authority, P.O. Box 837, Reno, NV 89504, 1-800-FOR-RENO.

WORLD'S INTERNATIONAL WHISTLE-OFF *fourth weekend in August,* Carson City, Carson City Co., to preserve and foster the art of whistling. Outdoor whistling competition "open to any individual or duet who can whistle a tune with some degree of skill without aid of a musical contrivance." Categories of melodic whistling include classical, popular, novelty, and duet. FOODS SERVED: international food boths. ADMISSION: free. ACCOMMODATIONS: motels and hotels, B&B's, campgrounds, RV parks. RESTAURANTS: fast foods, family, elegant, Basque, Asian, Italian, Mexican. CONTACT: Carson City Chamber of Commerce, 1191 S. Carson St., Carson City, NV 89701, (702) 882-1565. 10,000

OREGON

OREGON SHAKESPEAREAN FESTIVAL *February 20–October 31,* Ashland, Jackson Co., in southern Oregon. Eleven productions on three magnificent stages, including three Shakespearean works and eight by other classic and contemporary writers annually, performances Tuesday through Sunday, matinees and evenings.

Backstage tours, Festival Noons for lectures and concerts, institute classes for Shakespearean study, and Summer Seminar for High School Juniors, child-care available. Advance reservations necessary. ADMISSION: $10.00–$17.00 with lower prices for children, previews, and members, bargain packages. Writing for brochure is highly recommended for schedule and ticket-order form. Processing of ticket orders begins in early November of year preceding season. ACCOMMODATIONS: motels and hotels, B&B's, hostel, campgrounds. RESTAURANTS: fast foods, family, elegant, French, Italian, Mexican, Polish. CONTACT: Oregon Shakespearean Festival, Box 158, Ashland, OR 97520, (503) 482-4331. 320,000

NEWPORT SEAFOOD AND WINE FESTIVAL *third weekend in February,* Newport, Lincoln Co., on the Pacific Coast. Local seafood and wines from Oregon, Washington, and California are featured at 111 seafood and wine booths, crafts, antique show, car show and sale, beer garden, live entertainment such as the Portland Dixieland Jazz Band, oompah bands or rock and western music. FOODS SERVED: Oregon seafood, wines, and other specialties. ADMISSION: $2.00 plus charges for tastes. ACCOMMODATIONS: motels and hotels, B&B's, campgrounds, RV parks. RESTAURANTS: fast foods, family, elegant, seafood. CONTACT: Newport Chamber of Commerce, 555 S. W. Coast Highway, Newport, OR 97365, (503) 265-8801. 17,000

TILLAMOOK COUNTY MID-WINTER FESTIVAL *first weekend in March,* Tillamook, Tillamook Co., at the County Fairgrounds. Arts and crafts, beer garden, dancing, games for children, polka bands, Tyrolean Dancers. FOODS SERVED: "variety" and breakfast from 1:00 A.M. until 3:00 A.M. ADMISSION: $2.00 button admits to all events. ACCOMMODATIONS: motels and hotels, B&B's, campgrounds, RV parks. RESTAURANTS: fast foods, family, elegant, international. CONTACT: Tillamook Co. Chamber of Commerce, 3705 Hwy. 101 N., Tillamook, OR 97141, (503) 842-7525. 8,000

PEAR BLOSSOM FESTIVAL *second weekend in April,* Medford, Jackson Co., to celebrate the springtime blooming of pear trees and the rich fruit crops of the area. Arts and crafts, 13mi. Pear Blossom Run, bicycle races, parade saluting fruit growing industry. ADMISSION: free. ACCOMMODATIONS: motels and hotels, campgrounds. RESTAURANTS: fast foods, family, elegant. CONTACT: Medford Visitors and Convention Bureau, 304 S. Central Medford, OR 97501, (503) 772-6293.

RHODODENDRON FESTIVAL *third weekend in May,* Florence, Lane Co., on the Oregon Coast, to celebrate the profuse blooming of rhododendrons. Arts and crafts show, working art studio, dance, golf tournament, quilt display, vendor's corner, aerobic Dance-A-Thon, Soap Box Derby, row boat races, junior parade, rhododendron show including azaleas, children's program, tug of war, photo display, open-art studio, sail board races, Kiwanis Sportspectacular for preschool children, Eugene Topless Auto and Lane Mustang Club auto displays, dances, Rhody Run including 5,000m and 10,000m runs, display aircraft, grand parade, Silver Trails Slug Race, helicopter rides, carnival. FOODS SERVED: All-you-can-eat breakfast of pancakes and eggs for $2.50, Elks Lodge Rhody Breakfast, homemade snacks. ADMISSION: free. ACCOMMODATIONS: motels and hotels, B&B's, campgrounds, RV parks. RESTAURANTS: fast foods, family, elegant, Cajun, Mexican, Chinese, Italian. CONTACT: Florence Area Chamber of Commerce, P.O. Box 712, Florence, OR 97439, (503) 997-3128. 25,000

BOATNIK FESTIVAL *third or fourth weekend in May,* Grants Pass, Josephine Co. Hydro-jet boat races, parade, carnival, crafts fair, water-ski and sky-diving exhibitions, dancing, marathon run. FOODS SERVED: local concessions. ADMISSION: free. ACCOMMODATIONS: motels and hotels, B&B's, campgrounds, RV parks. RESTAURANTS: fast foods, family, elegant. Grant's Pass–Josephine Co. Chamber of Commerce, P.O. Box 970, Grants Pass, OR 97526, (503) 476-7717 or 1-800-547-5927. 4,000

PORTLAND ROSE FESTIVAL *first Friday in June and ten days following,* Portland, Multnomah Co., on both sides of the Willamette River. Three parades of which the Grand Floral Parade is the largest, rose show and competition, woodcarving show, dances, displays, musical and theatrical events, art show, ski exhibition, Indian Powwows, boat races, concerts, tennis tournament, queen selection, drag races, runs, three carnivals, fireworks, Coast Guard and Canadian ships on display. FOODS SERVED: concessions. ADMISSION: free. ACCOMMODATIONS: motels and hotels, B&B's, campgrounds, RV parks. RESTAURANTS: fast foods, family, elegant. CONTACT: Greater Portland Convention and Visitors Association, Inc., 26 S. W. Salmon, Portland, OR 97204, (503) 222-2223. 200,000

LEBANON STRAWBERRY FESTIVAL *first long weekend in June,* Lebanon, Linn Co., to honor the strawberry, "a major agricultural crop of the area." Parades, exhibits, dances, and the "world's largest strawberry shortcake—more than 6,000 pounds of it." FOODS SERVED: strawberries and strawberry shortcake. ADMISSION: free. ACCOMMODATIONS: motels and hotels, campgrounds. RESTAURANTS: fast foods, family. CONTACT: Lebanon Chamber of Commerce, 1040 Park St., Lebanon, OR 97355, (503) 258-7164.

PHIL SHERIDAN DAYS *third weekend in June,* Sheridan, Yamhill Co. Junior and grand parades, rodeo, art show, antique car show, carnival, craft booths, sled dog races, All Class Reunion, Timber Carnival, dances 8k Road Run, firemen's competition, softball tournament. FOODS SERVED: chicken barbecue and food booths. ADMISSION: free. ACCOMMODATIONS: motels and hotels, campgrounds, RV parks. RESTAURANTS: fast foods, family. CONTACT: Phil Sheridan Days, Inc., P.O. Box 225, Sheridan, OR 97378, (503) 843-3165. 10,000

ROOSTER CROW FESTIVAL *fourth Saturday in June,* Rogue River, Jackson Co., to duplicate a coal-miners celebration in Wales. Rooster crowing competition, mini-marathon (2mi.), arts and crafts, parade. FOODS SERVED: local food booths. ADMISSION: free. ACCOMMODATIONS: motels and hotels, campgrounds, RV parks. RESTAURANTS: fast foods, family, elegant. CONTACT: Rogue River Chamber of Commerce, P.O. Box 457, Rogue River, OR 97537, (503) 582-0242. 2,500

OREGON BACH FESTIVAL *last Sunday in June through second Sunday in July,* Eugene, Lane Co., on the University of Oregon campus and at the Hult Center for the Performing Arts. The works of Bach and other classics are performed during this two-week series of orchestra and choral concerts featuring nationally acclaimed guest artists. ADMISSION: charge. ACCOMMODATIONS: motels and hotels, B&B's, campgrounds, RV parks. RESTAURANTS: fast foods, family, elegant, international. CONTACT: University of Oregon School of Music, Eugene, OR 97403, (503) 686-3761 or the Eugene Area Chamber of Commerce, P.O. Box 1107, Eugene, OR 97401, (503) 484-1314. 2,000

WESTERN DAYS *week of July 4th,* Monmouth–Independence, Polk Co. Firefighters muster, parade and children's parade. Carnival booths, miniature sailboat regatta, Grants Pass Cavemen, Royal Canadian Mounted Police Bicycle Drill Team, Mexican fiesta, pet show, talent show, dunk tank, children's arts and crafts, tennis and softball tournaments, tug of war, square dancers, frog jumping race, balloon games, apple swing, River Parade, raft and canoe races, old-fashioned games, old-fashioned band concert, auction, 4mi. run, bike race, mini-marathon, croquet matches, live entertainment including Portland Rose Jazz Band, Portland Brass Quintet, country-western, pops, ragtime music and old-time fiddlers, dance groups, community chorus, 234th Army Band, round dancing, queen's court. FOODS SERVED: Mexican, barbecue, concessions. ADMISSION: free. ACCOMMODATIONS: motels and hotels, B&B's. RESTAURANTS:

fast foods, family, Mexican. CONTACT: Monmouth–Independence Chamber of Commerce, P.O. Box 401, Monmouth, OR 97361, (503) 838-4268. 20,000

FESTIVAL CORVALLIS—MIDSUMMER MUSIC *middle two weeks in July,* Corvallis, Benton Co., at the LaSells Stewart Center and Bruce Starker Arts Park in the Willamette Valley. "Musical performances to suit all tastes" such as the Pacific Northwest Ballet, classical guitarist Neil Ancher Roan, Woody Hite Big Band, performers from "A Prairie Home Companion," The Nashville Bluegrass Band, and Queen Ida. FOODS SERVED: concessions. ADMISSION: $6.00. ACCOMMODATIONS: motels and hotels, B&B's, RV parks. RESTAURANTS: fast foods, family, elegant, Mexican, Chinese, Italian. CONTACT: Vickie Audette, P.O. Box 258, Corvallis, OR 97339 or the Corvallis Area Chamber of Commerce, 420 N.W. 2nd, Corvallis, OR 97330, (503) 757-1505.

OBON ODORI (Obon Festival) *third Saturday in July,* Ontario, Malheur Co., in the Treasure Valley, at the Buddhist Temple. "A Festival of Joy" in "celebration of consideration for one's ancestors and the sacrifices they made for the betterment of future generations." Japanese dancing, flower arranging, evening auction, Japanese clothing, tours of the Temple, audience participation in Japanese folk dancing, displays of Japanese folk craft, dolls, and imports are showcased. FOODS SERVED: authentic Japanese, "not Americanized," such as teriyaki chicken, sunomono salad, tempura. ADMISSION: free. ACCOMMODATIONS: motels and hotels, RV parks. RESTAURANTS: fast foods, family. CONTACT: Ore–Idaho Buddhist Temple, 286 S.E. 4th, Ontario, OR 97914 or the Ontario Chamber of Commerce, 173 S.W. 1st, Ontario, OR 97914, (503) 889-8012.

SALEM ART FAIR AND FESTIVAL *third full weekend in July,* Salem, Marion Co., at Bush's Pasture Park, to celebrate the arts. More than 200 artists and crafts-people display and sell their creations, 5k Fun Run, children's participatory art area, children's parade, tours of the Bush House Museum, two fine arts exhibits, folk arts, demonstrations of arts and crafts, continuous live entertainment such as children's theatre, Army band, bluegrass, African, Latin, jazz, clogging, big band sounds, concert band, bagpipes, and others. FOODS SERVED: variety of local specialties. ADMISSION: free. ACCOMMODATIONS: motels and hotels, B&B's, RV park. RESTAURANTS: fast foods, family, elegant. CONTACT: Salem Art Association, 600 Mission S.E., Salem, OR 97302, (503) 581-2228 or the Salem Area Chamber of Commerce, 220 Cottage St., N.E., Salem, OR 97301, (503) 581-4325. 100,000

RENAISSANCE ARTS FESTIVAL *third or fourth weekend in July,* Grants Pass, Josephine Co., at Riverside Park, to celebrate the arts. Arts and crafts booths, on-site painting and crafts design, Renaissance Sport Show, live Renaissance entertainment by local and other southern Oregonians. FOODS SERVED: local food booths. ADMISSION: free. ACCOMMODATIONS: motels and hotels, B&B's, campgrounds, RV parks. RESTAURANTS: fast foods, family, elegant. CONTACT: Gary Davisson at (503) 476-1555 or the Grants Pass–Josephine Co. Chamber of Commerce, P.O. Box 970, Grants Pass, OR 97526, (503) 476-7717 or 1-800-547-5927. 2,000

MT. HOOD FESTIVAL OF JAZZ *first weekend in August,* Gresham, Multnomah Co., with the magnificent backdrop of Mt. Hood. Nationally renowned jazz artists such as Dave Brubeck, Dizzie Gillespie, Spyro Gyra, Carmen McRae, and Stan Getz have gathered to perform and collaborate in this outdoor festival of music. FOODS SERVED: Ten of Gresham's best restaurants offer delicacies at food booths, beer and wine. ADMISSION: $17.50–$25.00 per day. ACCOMMODATIONS: motels and hotels, campgrounds, RV parks. RESTAURANTS: fast foods, family, elegant, international. CONTACT:

Gresham Chamber of Commerce, 150 W. Powell, Gresham, OR 97030, (503) 665-1131.

WILD BLACKBERRY FESTIVAL *first or second weekend in August,* Cave Junction, Josephine Co., to celebrate the blackberry harvest. Arts and crafts booths, games, dance, live entertainment. FOODS SERVED: everything made with blackberries. ADMISSION: free. ACCOMMODATIONS: motels and hotels, campgrounds, RV parks. RESTAURANTS: fast foods, family, elegant. CONTACT: Larry La Vada of the Blackberry Association, P.O. Box 1077, Cave Junction, OR 97523 at (503) 592-4631 or the Grants Pass–Josephine Co. Chamber of Commerce, P.O. Box 970, Grants Pass, OR 97526, (503) 476-7717 or 1-800-547-5927.

JUNCTION CITY SCANDINAVIAN FESTIVAL *second week in August,* Junction City, Lane Co., with each of four days honoring a different country including Denmark, Finland, Norway, and Sweden. Residents wear costumes and some enter costume fashion show, Ol' Haven Beer Garden, Scandia 10k Run, bus farm tours, historical museum, Scandinavian handwork and arts and crafts, singing and dancing. FOODS SERVED: breakfast and dinner daily, Scandinavian food booths. ADMISSION: free. ACCOMMODATIONS: motels and hotels in Eugene, RV park on site. RESTAURANTS: fast foods, family, others in Eugene. CONTACT: Scandinavian Festival Association, P.O. Box 5, Junction City, OR 97448, (503) 998-3300. 15,000

DEPOE BAY SALMON BAKE *third Saturday in September,* Depoe Bay, Lincoln Co., at Fogarty Creek State Park 3 miles from Depoe Bay, which calls itself both the "Whale Watching Capital of the Oregon Coast" and the "World's Smallest Harbor." This event celebrates the seasonal abundance of coho salmon, and is truly an orgy of feasting on salmon. FOODS SERVED: 2,500 pounds of fresh salmon are roasted Indian-style on alder stakes over a 100-foot long fire line and served with coleslaw, garlic bread, ice cream and beverage. ADMISSION: adults $7.00, children under 12 $3.00 (prices subject to change until July 1.) ACCOMMODATIONS: motels and hotels, B&B's, campgrounds, RV parks. CONTACT: Depoe Bay Chamber of Commerce, Box 21, Depoe Bay, OR 97341, (503) 765-2889. 2,500

PENDLETON ROUND-UP AND HAPPY CANYON *third week and weekend in September,* Pendleton, Umatilla Co., "The Hub of Eastern Oregon." In a seventy-five-year-old tradition of celebrating the harvest, six American Indian tribes and other locals converge on Pendleton for six days of "The Fastest Moving Rodeo in America!", the Westward Ho! Parade featuring a history in non-motorized transportation including ox teams, Mormon carts, pack trains, and stage coaches; the Happy Canyon night pageant transports the visitor into the past experiences of Indian forefathers and culture, Happy Canyon Dance Hall features dancing, entertainment, and other western frontier-town activities, concerts, kids day, Indian beauty pageants, Dress-Up Parade, Tribal Ceremonial Dancing Contest, Main Street Cowboy Show. FOODS SERVED: "western" including cowboy breakfasts, barbecue, concessions. ADMISSION: many events free, charges for Round-up and Happy Canyon from $5.00-$10.00. ACCOMMODATIONS: motels and hotels, B&B's, campgrounds (tent and camping space on grounds), RV parks, private homes. RESTAURANTS: fast foods, family, elegant. CONTACT: Pendleton Round-up Association, P.O. Box 609, Pendleton, OR 97801, (503) 276-2553, inside Oregon 1-800-824-2603, outside Oregon 1-800-524-2984.

CORVALLIS FALL FESTIVAL *last weekend in September,* Corvallis, Benton Co., at Central Park in the Willamette Valley. Arts and crafts booths, wine and beer gardens, continuous live entertainment including Neil Gladstone, Nightwhale, The Chantrelles, Marysville Cloggers, Balaton Marimba Band, Oregon Dance Company, mimes, and choral performances. FOODS SERVED: Chinese, Mexican, seafood, natural foods, American. ADMISSION: free. ACCOMMODATIONS: motels and hotels, B&B's, RV parks. RESTAURANTS: fast foods, family, elegant,

Chinese, Mexican, Italian. CONTACT: Fall Festival Committee, Corvallis Area Chamber of Commerce, 420 N.W. 2nd, Corvallis, OR 97330, (503) 757-1505. 8,000

WASHINGTON

RAIN OR SHINE JAZZ FESTIVAL *Presidents' Day weekend (mid-February),* Aberdeen, Grays Harbor Co., on the Olympic Peninsula. Jazz music presentations which have included the Hume St. Preservation Jazz Band #405, Phoenix Jazzers from Vancouver, British Columbia; Portland, Oregon's Stumptown Jazz, Seattle, Washington's Uptown Lowdown Jazz Band, the Electric Park Jazz Band, San Francisco's South Frisco Jazz Band, Dr. Joh's Medicine Show, and the Coos Bay Clambake (band). ADMISSION: $25.00 for entire festival. ACCOMMODATIONS: motels and hotels, B&B's, campgrounds, RV parks. RESTAURANTS: fast foods, family, elegant. CONTACT: Greg Jones or Gary Knowles at the Jazz Hotline (206) 533-2910 or the Grays Harbor Chamber of Commerce, P.O. Box 450, Aberdeen, WA 98520, (206) 532-1924. 500

RHODODENDRON FESTIVAL *second through third weekends in May,* Port Townsend, Jefferson Co., on Puget Sound, to celebrate the blooming of the rhododendron, Washington's state flower. Grand parade, 7.5mi. Rhody Run, trike race, bed race, beard growing contest, Pet Parade, children's parade, high school band concerts. ADMISSION: free. ACCOMMODATIONS: motels and hotels, B&B's, campgrounds, RV parks. RESTAURANTS: fast foods, family, elegant. CONTACT: Port Townsend Chamber of Commerce, 2437 Simms Way, Port Townsend, WA 98368, (206) 385-2722. 10,000

VIKING FEST *weekend closest to May 17,* Poulsbo, Kitsap Co., to celebrate Norway's independence. Arts and crafts fair, parade, carnival, photography show, Rowers Race across the sound, lutefisk eating contest, chowder cook-off, road race, flea market, live entertainment at the Waterfront Pavillion including Scottish and Irish ballads, North Kitsap Jazz Ensemble, Sweet Adelines, Buz Whitley's Big Band music, Free Wheel Stunt Biking, Sol Feggio Quartet, Scottish Curachan Pipes and Drums, Scandinavian Dancers, cloggers, square dancers. FOODS SERVED: Scandinavian, Indian, German, American, pancake breakfast, Sons of Norway Scandinavian luncheon. ADMISSION: free, charge for photography show. ACCOMMODATIONS: motels, campgrounds, RV parks. RESTAURANTS: fast foods, family, elegant, German, Italian, Scandinavian, Mexican. CONTACT: Greater Poulsbo Chamber of Commerce, P.O. Box 1963, Poulsbo, WA 98370, (206) 779-4848. 40,000

WALLA WALLA HOT AIR BALLOON STAMPEDE *third weekend in May,* Walla Walla, Walla Walla Co., at the high school. Nearly fifty hot air balloons participate in three scheduled flights, arts and crafts shows, wine tasting, games, kite flying demonstrations, Japanese cultural programs, Sportech Fun Run, volleyball tournament, skydiving, Mideastern dancing by the Troupe Azure, square dancing, modern dance by the Dance Foundation, and the Wa-Hi Band in concert. FOODS SERVED: ROTC breakfast, Japanese yaki soba and teriyaki beef, hot dogs, dietetic foods. ADMISSION: free. ACCOMMODATIONS: motels and hotels, B&B, campground, RV parks. RESTAURANTS:

fast foods, family, elegant, Mexican, Ethiopian, Chinese, continental. CONTACT: Walla Walla Chamber of Commerce, P.O. Box 644, Walla Walla, WA 99362, (509) 525-0850. 12,000

SKI TO SEA FESTIVAL *third Sunday through fourth weekend in May,* Bellingham, Whatcom Co. Art show, junior parade, grand parade, sea race. FOODS SERVED: concessions. ADMISSION: free. ACCOMMODATIONS: motels and hotels, B&B's, campgrounds, RV parks. RESTAURANTS: fast foods, family, elegant. CONTACT: Whatcom Bellingham-Whatcom Co. Visitors Convention Bureau, P.O. Box 340, Bellingham, WA 98227, (206) 671-3990.

MOSES LAKE SPRING FESTIVAL *Memorial Day weekend (late May),* Moses Lake, Grant Co., in the Columbia River Basin. Arts and crafts, sidewalk sales, carnival, bed races, torchlight boat parade, 10k and 5k fun runs, antique classic cars, swimming, ATV races, kiddies parade, Tri-State 3rd Avenue Mile Race, moonlight parade, Mud Race, triathlon, fireworks. Air Band Competition. FOODS SERVED: variety. ADMISSION: free. ACCOMMODATIONS: motels and hotels, campgrounds, RV parks. RESTAURANTS: fast foods, family, elegant, Asian, Italian. CONTACT: Moses Lake Spring Festival, P.O. Box 1231, Moses Lake, WA 98837, (509) 765-8248. 30,000

NORTHWEST FOLKLIFE FESTIVAL *Memorial Day weekend (late May),* Seattle, King Co., at the Seattle Center in the Puget Sound area, to celebrate the "traditional, folk, and ethnic heritage of the Pacific Northwest." The Seattle Center is the site of the 1962 World's Fair and the Space Needle, with beautiful grounds. More than 5,000 participants from the American Northwest and British Columbia show their crafts and perform traditional music and dance on nineteen stages, the Folklife Crafts Marketplace showcases 150 artisans' handmade goods, the Uncommon Market sells commercial products of folk origin, International Foods Walkway with thirty ethnic food booths, Traditional America Project demonstrates early building and homemaking skills, liars contest, dance and music workshops, international folk dancing, evening concerts and "The Roadhouse swings with dancing and calling 'till midnight," gospel concerts, children's programs, Cajun, bluegrass, folk, blues, ballads, country-western, string bands, and Native American music. Ethnic dances are performed representing Africa, Bulgaria, Cambodia, Cuba, England, Finland, Thailand, Philippines, and many other countries. FOODS SERVED: specialities of thirty countries. ADMISSION: free. ACCOMMODATIONS: motels and hotels. RESTAURANTS: fast foods, family, elegant, international. CONTACT: Seattle-King Co. Convention and Visitors Bureau, 666 Stewart St., Seattle, WA 98101, (206) 447-4240. 150,000

GREEK FESTIVAL *Memorial Day weekend (late May),* Soap Lake, Grant Co., in the Columbia River Basin. Parade, ladies' mud wrestling, men's knee judging, Greek folk dancers, flea market, children's rides, street entertainment, the Whistling Midgets, and Bonnie Guitar. FOODS SERVED: Sunday Greek dinner. ADMISSION: free, dinner—adults $8.00, children and senior citizens $6.00. ACCOMMODATIONS: motels and hotels, campgrounds, RV parks. RESTAURANTS: fast foods, family. CONTACT: Maxine Lyerly at (509) 246-0426 or the Soap Lake Chamber of Commerce, P.O. Box 433, Soap Lake, WA 98851, (509) 246-1821. 2,000

SKANDIA MIDSOMMAR FEST *second Sunday in June,* Poulsbo, Kitsap Co., at Frank Raab Park in the Puget Sound area, to celebrate the Nordic heritage of many residents and a traditional old country midsommar. Old-time Scandinavian dancing, Nordic arts and crafts show, parade, traditional pole-raising, folk dancing, Scandinavian costumes, fiddlers, continuous outdoor entertainment. FOODS SERVED: Scandinavian. ADMISSION: adults $3.00. ACCOMMODATIONS: motels and hotels, RV park. RESTAURANTS: fast foods, family, Chinese, Italian, Mexican. CONTACT: Greater Poulsbo Chamber of Commerce, P.O. Box 1063, Poulsbo, WA 98370, (206) 779-4848.

BERRY-DAIRY DAYS *third Wednesday through Friday in June,* Burlington, Skagit Co., to celebrate the strawberry harvest. Lawnmower races, fun run, grand parade, sidewalk sale, fireworks, salmon barbecue, Mexican music. FOODS SERVED: strawberry shortcake, Mexican food, others. ADMISSION: free. ACCOMMODATIONS: motels and hotels, B&B's, campgrounds, RV parks. RESTAURANTS: fast foods, family, elegant. CONTACT: Burlington Chamber of Commerce, P.O. Box 522, Burlington, WA 98233, (206) 757-1121. 20,000

SEDRO WOOLLEY LOGGERODEO *five days including July 4th,* Sedro Woolley, Skagit Co., in the Skagit Valley, a tradition since 1898. Grand parade, log show, foot race, rodeo, carnival, crafts, lawnmower races, firemen's muster, kiddies' parade, community picnic, Bluegrass Jamboree. FOODS SERVED: "all types." ADMISSION: free, charges for rodeo and log show. ACCOMMODATIONS: motels and hotels, campgrounds, RV parks. RESTAURANTS: fast foods, family. CONTACT: Sedro Woolley Chamber of Commerce, 714 Metcalf St., Sedro Woolley, WA 98284, (206) 855-0770. 30,000

CAPITAL LAKEFAIR *second weekend in July,* Olympia, Thurston Co., to celebrate the recreational attributes of Capital Lake. Water ski tournament, YMCA Sports Festival including swimming, cycling, track, basketball, soccer and weights events, carnival, queen coronation, U.S. Navy ships, midway, tennis, volleyball, and soccer tournaments, drum and bugle corps competition, Crafts on the Sound, parachute jump, grand twilight parade, square dance, chess tournament, piano competition, boat races, fireworks, bed races, outboard hydro regatta; live entertainment such as George Barner and

the Trendsetters of "Louie Louie" fame, Black Hills Shufflers swing dancing, hard rock of Van Halen, modern country, Olympia Jazz Society Big Band, Sweet Adelines Quartet, Affinity, Paragon, The Edge and its "high-energy positive image rock," performances by the Abbey Players, Olympia Kitchen Band, the tapdancing Sheri Schmidt Dancers, traditional Sousa Band music, and local new wave and rock bands; ATV Grand National Championships including three-wheel vehicles with all-amateur and all-pro days. FOODS SERVED: concessions. ADMISSION: free. ACCOMMODATIONS: motels and hotels, B&B's, campgrounds, RV parks. RESTAURANTS: fast foods, family, elegant, Asian, Mexican. CONTACT: Capital Lakefair, Inc., P.O. Box 1427, Olympia, WA 98507, (206) 357-3362. 100,000

WALLA WALLA SWEET ONION FESTIVAL *third weekend in July,* Walla Walla, Walla Walla Co., at the Fort Walla Walla Museum, to celebrate the Walla Walla sweet onion season. Onion cooking contests, onion slicing contests, Onion Shot Put Throw using double headed onions, onion competition between Walla Walla, Texas, and Vidalia sweet onions, appearances by the Walla Walla Sweets costumed ensemble, tours of Fort Walla Walla Museum Complex. FOODS SERVED: onion dishes, Italian, chili, raw onions, dietetic foods. ADMISSION: $1.00. ACCOMMODATIONS: motels and hotels, B&B, campground, RV parks. RESTAURANTS: fast foods, family, elegant, Mexican, Ethiopian, Chinese, continental. CONTACT: Walla Walla Chamber of Commerce, P.O. Box 644, Walla Walla, WA 99362, (509) 525-0850.

LOGGERS JUBILEE *second weekend in August,* Morton, Lewis Co., to salute the logging industry. Competitive logging skills, arts and crafts festival, parades. FOODS SERVED: concessions. ADMISSION: between $4.50–$6.00. ACCOMMODATIONS: motels and hotels, B&B's, campgrounds, RV parks. RESTAURANTS: fast foods, family. CONTACT: Morton Chamber of Commerce, P.O. Box 10, Morton, WA 98356, (206) 496-5123. 10,000

OMAK STAMPEDE AND WORLD FAMOUS SUICIDE RACE *second weekend in August,* Omak, Okanogan Co., at Omak East Side Park. Suicide Race (on horses down a hill), western art show and auction, PRCA Rodeo, "traditional 100 village Indian encampment with traditional dancing and gaming," carnival, kiddies' parade, grand parade, two big rodeo dances; Walk and Trot Fun Run 5k and 10k races. FOODS SERVED: Indian, cowboy barbecue, concessions. ADMISSION: free, charge for rodeo from $4.00–$10.00. ACCOMMODATIONS: motels and hotels, campgrounds, RV parks. RESTAURANTS: fast foods, family, elegant, Chinese. CONTACT: Omak Stampede, Inc., P.O. Box 2028, Omak, WA 98841, (509) 826-1983. 20,000

CHIEF SEATTLE DAYS *third weekend in August,* Suquamish, Kitsap Co., honoring Chief Seattle, for whom the city of Seattle is named. Indian arts and crafts sales, Indian powwow, Indian war canoe races, Indian dancing, Indian Princess Contest, Indian drummers, Indian dancers, Indian storytellers. FOODS SERVED: "mainly Indian foods." ADMISSION: free. ACCOMMODATIONS: motels. CONTACT: Charles Sigo, Coordinator, Suquamish Tribe, P.O. Box 498, Suquamish, WA 98392, (206) 598-3311.

WOODEN BOAT FESTIVAL *weekend after Labor Day (early September),* Port Townsend, Jefferson Co., on the Olympic Peninsula, to celebrate wooden boats and maritime history. Regattas, schooner races, 150 boats on display, classes, workshops, demonstrations, maritime films, children's programs, sail cruises aboard traditional schooners, bagpipes, gospel music, steel-drum bands, fiddlers, dances. FOODS SERVED: German, French, American, Chinese, Mexican. ADMISSION: $5.00 per day, $10.00 for three days. ACCOMMODATIONS: motels and hotels, B&B's, campgrounds, RV parks. RESTAURANTS: fast foods, family, elegant. CONTACT: Mary L. Dietz, Wooden Boat Foundation, 637 Water St., Port Townsend, WA 98368, (206) 385-3628 or the Port Townsend Chamber of Commerce, 2437 Simms Way, Port Townsend, WA 98368, (206) 385-2722. 10,000

WYOMING

CULTURAL FESTIVAL *first Saturday in May,* Rock Springs, Sweetwater Co., in the Red Desert, to celebrate "the diversity of cultures in the area." Arts and crafts display, music, dance, and cultural activities of Greece, Germany, Mexico, Scotland, American Indian, Italy, and Basque cultures. FOODS SERVED: specialties of nations and cultures represented. ADMISSION: adults $1.00, children and senior citizens $.50. ACCOMMODATIONS: motels and hotels, campground. RESTAURANTS: fast foods, family, elegant. CONTACT: Jean Wade, YWCA of Sweetwater County, P.O. Box 1667, Rock Springs, WY 82901, (307) 362-7923. 5,000

ENCAMPMENT WOODCHOPPERS JAMBOREE *third full weekend in June,* Encampment, Carbon Co., in the Saratoga–Platte Valley, to celebrate the timber industry in southern Carbon County. Timber Carnival includes woodchopping contests and lumberjack competition, parade, rodeo, melodrama performed by Grand Encampment Opera Company, street dance. FOODS SERVED: western barbecue, beans, hamburgers, hot dogs. ADMISSION: free to parade, charges for all other events. ACCOMMODATIONS: motel, RV park, others in Saratoga. RESTAURANTS: family, others in Saratoga. CONTACT: Saratoga–Platte Valley Chamber of Commerce, P.O. Box 1095, Saratoga, WY 82331, (307) 326-8855. 4,000

FLAMING GORGE DAYS *late June through early July,* Green River, Sweetwater Co., to celebrate the summer. Parade, flea market, relay race, adults' and children's games, concerts which have included Eddie Rabbit, Mickey Gilley, Johnny Lee, Mel Tillis, and The Association. FOODS SERVED: Mexican, Greek. ADMISSION: $8.00–$12.00. ACCOMMODATIONS: motels and hotels, campgrounds, RV parks. RESTAURANTS: fast foods, family, elegant. CONTACT: Green River Chamber of Commerce, 1450 Uinta Dr., Green River, WY 82935, (307) 875-5711. 10,000

LANDER PIONEER DAYS *July 4th weekend,* Lander, Fremont Co., to celebrate Wyoming's "pioneer background." Shrine circus, Red Dog Bike Races, carnival, children's games, "Men and Women (Jointly) Open Slow Pitch Invitational," Pioneer Museum open house, melodrama, half-marathon race, Pageant of the Old West Parade, rodeo, Barn Dance, fireworks, Pore Devils Shade Tree Auto Display and swap meet. FOODS SERVED: barbecue, concessions. ADMISSION: free, charges for some events. ACCOMMODATIONS: motels and hotels, B&B's, campgrounds, RV parks. RESTAURANTS: fast foods, family, elegant, international. CONTACT: Lander Area Chamber of Commerce, 160 N. First, Lander, WY 82520, (307) 332-3892. 14,000

GRAND TETON MUSIC FESTIVAL *all summer beginning July 9,* Teton Village, Teton Co., near Jackson, at the Teton Music Festival Hall. Grand Teton Symphony Orchestra, made up of artists from outstanding orchestras throughout the country, performs chamber, pops, solos, and other renditions on weekdays, and as a full orchestra on Saturday nights. ADMISSION: charge. ACCOMMODATIONS: motels and hotels, B&B's, campgrounds, RV parks. RESTAURANTS: fast foods, family, elegant, international. CONTACT: Jackson

Hole Area Chamber of Commerce, P.O. Box E, Jackson, WY 83001, (307) 733-3316.

WORLD OPEN ATLATL CHAMPIONSHIPS, CRAFTS FAIR, AND COMMUNITY TROUT FRY *third Saturday in July,* Saratoga, Carbon Co., "where the trout leap in Main Street" to celebrate "Ice Age technology and (Saratoga–Platte) Valley history." Flint-knapping demonstration, Atlatl Contest featuring professional and amateur archaeologists from throughout the country, parade, crafts fair, trout fry. FOODS SERVED: fried trout, Saratoga chips (fried potatoes), baked beans. ADMISSION: free, Trout Fry $4.50. ACCOMMODATIONS: motels and hotels, B&B, campgrounds, RV parks. RESTAURANTS: family, Mexican, Italian. CONTACT: Saratoga–Platte Valley Chamber of Commerce, P.O. Box 1095, Saratoga, WY 82331, (307) 326-8855. 500

CHEYENNE FRONTIER DAYS *last full week in July,* Cheyenne, Laramie Co., to celebrate the old west. Parades, rodeos, chuckwagon races, "night shows with top-name entertainment," which have included The Judds, Nitty Gritty Dirt Band, Exile, Johnny Cafferty and the Beaver Brown Band, and Johnny Cash. FOODS SERVED: free pancake breakfasts, concessions. ADMISSION: free to some events, charges for others. ACCOMMODATIONS: motels and hotels, campgrounds, RV parks. RESTAURANTS: fast foods, family. CONTACT: Cheyenne Chamber of Commerce, P.O. Box 1147, Cheyenne, WY 82003, (307) 638-3388. 40,000

LANDER VALLEY APPLE FESTIVAL *third or fourth weekend in August,* Lander, Fremont Co., at Jaycee Park, to celebrate Wyoming's apple harvest. Arts and crafts festival, triathlon race, fiddler's contest, chili cook-off, apple pie contest, apple carving contest, kids' parade, performances by the Fremont County Wyoming Fiddlers Association and the Missoula (Montana) Children's Theatre. FOODS

SERVED: pancake breakfast, concessions. ADMISSION: free. ACCOMMODATIONS: motels and hotels, B&B's, campgrounds, RV parks. RESTAURANTS: fast foods, family, elegant, Mexican, Chinese. CONTACT: Lander Area Chamber of Commerce, 160 N. First, Lander, WY 82520, (307) 332-3892. 2,000

SOUTHWEST

Arizona / 205

Colorado / 208

New Mexico / 212

Texas / 215

Utah / 225

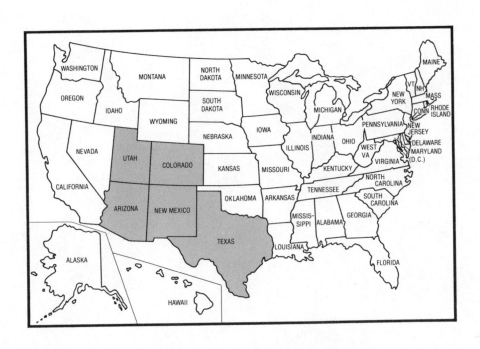

GOLD RUSH DAYS *second weekend in February,* Wickenburg, Maricopa Co. Gold panning, mucking and drilling contest, beard growing contest, parade, arts and crafts show, carnival, old-fashioned melodrama, cowboy dance, old-timers rodeo, booth displays, "free stage entertainment," Budweiser Clydesdale horses. FOODS SERVED: food concessions, cowboy barbecue. ADMISSION: most events free, charges for rodeo, dance, and gold panning. ACCOMMODATIONS: motels and hotels, campgrounds, RV parks. RESTAURANTS: fast foods, family, elegant. CONTACT: Wickenburg Chamber of Commerce, Drawer CC, Wickenburg, AZ 85358, (602) 684-7524. 20,000

LOST DUTCHMAN DAYS *last weekend in February,* Apache Junction, Pinal Co., 25 miles east of Phoenix at the foot of the Superstition Mountains and the "gateway to the Salt River chain of lakes." Arts and crafts show and sale (including local turquoise), dances, three-day rodeo, carnival, talent show, tennis, shuffleboard and horseshoe tournaments, parade. FOODS SERVED: barbecue. ADMISSION: most events free. ACCOMMODATIONS: motels and hotels, campgrounds, RV parks. RESTAURANTS: fast foods, family. CONTACT: Apache Junior Chamber of Commerce, P.O. Box 1747, Apache Junction, AZ 85220, (602) 982-3141. 45,000

COOLIDGE COTTON FESTIVAL *first weekend in March,* Coolidge, in San Carlos Park at Central Avenue, Pinal Co. Bale rolling contest, carnival, go-cart races, banjo picking contest, chicken drop contest in which "tickets are sold on squares like a giant checkerboard while a rooster is kept in a box to work up his frustrations; upon his release, the owner of the first square on which he drops his calling card is the big winner." Arts and crafts, dances, volleyball tournaments, bike and 10k races, live local entertainment. FOODS SERVED: international food booths. ADMISSION: free. ACCOMMODATIONS: hotels and motels, RV parks. RESTAURANTS: fast foods, family. CONTACT: Coolidge Chamber of Commerce, 320 W. Central, Coolidge, AZ 85228, (602) 723-3009. 5,000

TOMBSTONE TERRITORIAL DAYS *first weekend in March,* Tombstone, Cochise Co. Parade, rodeo, melodrama shows, art festival, fast-draw contest, reenactment of historical events, 1880 fashion show, old-time fiddlers. Similar events occur in Tombstone during "Wyatt Earp Days" on Memorial Day weekend, "Wild West Days" on Labor Day weekend, and "Heldorado Days" on the third weekend in October. ADMISSION: free. FOODS SERVED: western and concessions. ACCOMMODATIONS: motels, campgrounds. RESTAURANTS: family. CONTACT: Tombstone Tourism Association, Box 917, Tombstone, AZ 85638, (602) 457-2202.

TUCSON FESTIVAL *three weekends in April,* Tucson, Pima Co., in celebration of Tucson's multi-cultural heritage. Four festivals combine to form the unusual celebration hosted by the people of Tucson and the Tucson Festival Society. Events include Pioneer Days featuring a two-day living history celebration featuring cavalry, mountain men, music, transportation, and period costumes of Tucson's early days, crafts, tent city. San Xavier Pageant and Fiesta celebrates region's origins as represented in the O'Odham culture and the arrival of the Christian faith through the Catholic Church. At Mission San Xavier del Bac, the Fiesta begins with traditional Hohono O'Odham dances, mariachis, traditional Indian music and dance, historical reenactments of priests and Spanish colonialists arriving, bonfires, fireworks, horsemanship. The Fiesta del Presidio in and around the Tucson Museum of Art complex provides dancing by and for audiences, on-site muralists competition, Mexican charreada (rodeo), and visits to historic homes in the El Presidio district, children's parade, Mexican fiesta. The Children's Writing Festival is a competition among students to draw or write in poetry- or story-form their interpretations of Tucson's history. Two days of almost-continuous celebration of local and regional folk music and arts comprise the Tucson Folk Festival, which also includes workshops on storytelling, folk dancing, non-stop bluegrass, gospel, fiddling, ragtime, acoustic blues, barbershop quartets, clogging, and country swing dancing. Entertainers include Lalo Guerrero, Yaqui Matachine Performers and Deer Dancers, mariachis, Folklorico Dancers, Tohono O'Odham Dancers, Silver Coronet Band, Katie Lee, White Mountain Apache Crown Dancers. FOODS SERVED: wide range of southwestern specialties such as Mexican, Anglo, Yaqui, Chinese, Apache, Tohono O'Odham Indian. ADMISSION: free. ACCOMMODATIONS: motels and hotels, B&B's, campgrounds, RV parks. RESTAURANTS: fast foods, family, elegant, lots of Mexican, European, Asian, and Indian. CONTACT: Tucson Festival Society, 425 W. Paseo Redondo, Suite #4, Tucson, AZ 85701, (602) 622-6911. 150,000

BILL WILLIAMS RENDEZVOUS DAYS *Memorial Day weekend (late May)*, Williams, Coconino Co., at the Kalbab National Forest in northern Arizona. "Historical recreation of the mountain men, specifically William S. Williams, the town's namesake." Parade, arts and crafts, pioneer food shows, Monte Carlo Night, carnival, Black-powder shoot, evening whooplas, best pioneer costume contest, roping, barn dance. FOODS SERVED: pioneer foods, pancake breakfast, barbecues. ADMISSION: varies. ACCOMMODATIONS: motels, campgrounds, RV parks. RESTAURANTS: fast foods, family, Mexican. CONTACT: Williams–Grand Canyon Chamber of Commerce, P.O. Box 235, Williams, AZ 86406, (602) 635-2041.

ARIZONA SUMMER ARTS FESTIVAL *June 1 through August 10*, Tucson, Pima Co., to celebrate the arts. More than sixty events including children's concerts, jazz, musical theatre and drama, classical music to modern art and other visual arts, performance art, lectures, workshops, film, video art, and opera. FOODS SERVED: "any and all." ADMISSION: $5.00–$8.00. ACCOMMODATIONS: motels and hotels, B&B's, campgrounds, RV parks. RESTAURANTS: fast foods, family, elegant, Mexican, Asian. CONTACT: University of Arizona, Faculty of Fine Arts, Office of the Dean, Tucson, AZ 85721, (602) 621-1302.

OLDTIME COUNTRY MUSIC & BLUEGRASS FESTIVAL *third weekend in June*, Payson, Gila Co., at the Rodeo Grounds. Payson calls itself the "Festival Capital of Arizona." Arts and crafts booths, two days of "good old-time country music." FOODS SERVED: several food booths available. ADMISSION: charge. ACCOMMODATIONS: motels, campgrounds. RESTAURANTS: fast foods, family. CONTACT: Payson Chamber of Commerce, Drawer A, Payson, AZ 85541, (602) 474-4515.

LOGGERS SAWDUST FESTIVAL *last weekend in July*, Payson, Gila Co., at the Rodeo Grounds. Logging events, the winners of which go on to the national Tournament of Kings. Contests include cross-cut sawing, chain sawing, ax cutting, pole climbing, log burling in water. Family events for spectators include pinecone toss for children, burrowing in sawdust pile for coins and the "Fire Fighting Contest" in which men smoke cigars and the cigars' fire is extinguished by water-filled balloons; arts and crafts. FOODS SERVED: several food booths. ADMISSION: charge. ACCOMMODATIONS: motels and campgrounds. RESTAURANTS: fast foods, family. CONTACT: Payson Chamber of Commerce, Drawer A, Payson, AZ 85541, (602) 474-4515.

OLD-TIME FIDDLERS CONTEST & FESTIVAL *third weekend in September,* Payson, Gila Co., at the Rodeo Grounds. Annual Arizona State Fiddlers Contest is two days of old-time fiddle music with jam sessions Saturday evening. FOODS SERVED: concessions. ADMISSION: charge. ACCOMMODATIONS: motels, campgrounds. RESTAURANTS: fast foods, family. CONTACT: Payson Chamber of Commerce, Drawer A, Payson, AZ 85541, (602) 474-4515.

CALL OF THE CANYON FESTIVAL OF THE ARTS *third weekend in September,* Sedona, Coconino Co., in the Verde Valley. Artists from all over the western states come to show and sell their works. FOODS SERVED: sidewalk vendors and local cafes. ADMISSION: free. ACCOMMODATIONS: motels and hotels, B&B's, RV parks. RESTAURANTS: fast foods, family, elegant. CONTACT: Sedona–Oak Creek Canyon Chamber of Commerce, Inc., P.O. Box 478, Sedona, AZ 86336, (602) 282-7888. 5,000

FALL FESTIVAL *last weekend in September,* Pinetop, Navajo Co. in the White Mountains, to celebrate the turning of leaves. Parades, "backstage theatre," 10k Run, arts and crafts shows, antique and car shows. FOODS SERVED: Indian, Asian, Mexican, burgers. ADMISSION: free. ACCOMMODATIONS: motels and hotels, campgrounds, RV parks. RESTAURANTS: fast foods, family, elegant, including Mexican, Asian, Italian. CONTACT: Pinetop–Lakeside Chamber of Commerce, P.O. Box 266, Pinetop, AZ 85935, (602) 367-4290. 15,000

LONDON BRIDGE DAYS *first two weeks in October,* Lake Havasu City, Mohave Co., to commemorate the dedication of London Bridge in Lake Havasu City. Adult and children's English-style costume contests, Fun Faire and carnival, wrist-wrestling competition, beard contest, grande parade, City of London Quit Rent Ceremony, triathlon, art shows, Senior Citizen Recognition Day, softball tournament, baking contest. Entertainment includes Blue Water Swingers Square Dancing, Honeybear Cloggers, Bill Miller Native American Folk Singer, London Bridge Christian Committee, various military bands. FOODS SERVED: Texas barbecue, pancake breakfast, many English specialties. ADMISSION: free. ACCOMMODATIONS: motels and hotels, campgrounds, RV parks. RESTAURANTS: fast foods, family, elegant. CONTACT: Lake Havasu Area Visitor and Convention Bureau, 1930 Mesquite Ave., Suite 3, Lake Havasu City, AZ 86403, (602) 453-3444. 5,000

REX ALLEN DAYS *first weekend in October,* Willcox, Cochise Co., in the Sulphur Springs Valley, honoring hometown hero, movie and recording star Rex Allen. Western parade, turtle derby, PRCA rodeo, stage show, golf tournament, arts and crafts, dances, western music. FOODS SERVED: chuckwagon barbecue. ADMISSION: charges vary by event. ACCOMMODATIONS: motels, campgrounds, RV park. RESTAURANTS: family, Mexican. CONTACT: Willcox Chamber of Commerce and Agriculture, 1500 N. Circle I Road, Willcox, AZ 85643, (602) 384-2272.

BILLY MOORE DAYS *third weekend in October,* Avondale, Maricopa Co., in the metro Phoenix area, honoring one of the original settlers of Avondale. Western theme parade, Miss Billy Moore Beauty Pageant, carnival. FOODS SERVED: barbecue, Mexican, American. ADMISSION: free. ACCOMMODATIONS: motels and hotels, campgrounds, RV parks. CONTACT: Avondale-Goodyear-Litchfield Park Chamber of Commerce, P.O. Box 327, Goodyear, AZ 85323, (602) 932-2260. 10,000

FOUR CORNER STATES BLUEGRASS FESTIVAL *second weekend in November,* Wickenburg, Maricopa Co., at the Rodeo Grounds. Three days of solid bluegrass music and band contests with contestants vying for more than $6,500 in prizes. Performers include Jethro Burns, U.S. Air Force Band, Shadow Mountain Band. FOODS SERVED: concessions available. ADMISSION: adults $6.00, seniors $5.00. ACCOMMODATIONS: motels and ho-tels, campgrounds, RV parks. RESTAU-RANTS: fast foods, family, elegant. CON-TACT: Wickenburg Chamber of Commerce, Drawer CC, Wickenburg, AZ 85358, (602) 684-7524. 20,000

COLORADO

ULLR FEST *third week in January,* Breckenridge, Summit Co., to recognize Ullr, the Norwegian god of winter. Breck-enridge becomes an independent kingdom since it's never been included in any U.S. land surveys. Broomball tournament, town skiing championships, Ullr Play, Nordic ski celebration, skiing along lan-tern–lit trails, ice sculpture, fireworks, bonfires, Grand Ullr Ball, wine tasting party, hockey game, Norwegian dancing. FOODS SERVED: Scandinavian. ADMISSION: free, some events $5.00–$10.00. ACCOM-MODATIONS: motels and hotels, B&B's. RESTAURANTS: family, elegant, continen-tal. CONTACT: Breckenridge Resort Cham-ber, P.O. Box 1909, Breckenridge, CO 80424, (800) 525-9189. 5,000

WINTERSKOL *third weekend in January,* Snowmass Village, Pitkin Co., near As-pen. Hot air balloon races over Snowmass ski area, Ankle Biters' Ski Race, chili shoot-out, Air Force Show, Queen of Hearts Ski and Tea Party, ice and snow sculpture judging, free telemark ski les-sons, children's free tethered hot air bal-loon rides, children's free movie during Winterskol Aprés-Ski Party, impromptu magic shows, torchlight descent of moun-tain on skis, Mad Hatter's Ball with "Doc-tor Sadistic and the Silverking Crybabies." FOODS SERVED: lots of chili. ADMISSION: $1.00 for Winterskol button. ACCOMMO-DATIONS: motels and hotels, B&B's. RES-TAURANTS: fast foods, family, elegant. CONTACT: Snowmass Resort Association, P.O. Box 5566, Snowmass Village, CO 81615, (303) 923-2000. 3,000

WHITE RIVER WINTER RENDEZ-VOUS *last weekend in January through first week in February,* Meeker, Rio Blanco Co. Craft show, snowmobile hill climbs, snowmobile drags and snocross races, black-powder shoots, archery contests, dog sledding, ice skating exhibitions, ice sculpting. FOODS SERVED: western, con-cessions. ADMISSION: free. ACCOMMODA-TIONS: motels and hotels, B&B's, camp-grounds, RV parks. RESTAURANTS: fast foods, family. CONTACT: White River Win-ter Rendezvous, P.O. Box 365, Meeker, CO 81641 or the Meeker Chamber of Commerce, P.O. Box 869, Meeker, CO 81641, (303) 878-5510. 5,000

WINTER FEST *first weekend in February,* Pagosa Springs, Archuleta Co., in the San Juan Mountains, "just minutes away from the Wolf Creek Ski Area . . . internation-ally famous for its powder snow and un-crowded slopes." Sled races, ice hockey, parade, water basketball, dog sled races, cross-country and downhill ski races, ice fishing competition, hot air balloons, snowmobile sprints, snow and ice sculp-ture competitions, square dance jubilee, melodrama. FOODS SERVED: Tex–Mex. ADMISSION: free, except $4.00 to melo-drama. ACCOMMODATIONS: motels and ho-tels, B&B's, campgrounds, RV park. RES-TAURANTS: family, elegant, French. CONTACT: Winter Fest Board, P.O. Box 382, Pagosa Springs, CO 81147, (303) 264-4141. 1,500

SNOWMASS/ASPEN BANANA SEASON *April 4–12,* Snowmass Village,

Pitkin Co., in recognition of the end of the ski season. "On-mountain" events include Banana Bonanza Hunt (finding prizes in plastic bananas hidden on the mountain), Banana Limbo Obstacle Race, Village Fruit Cup, kid's costume parade, Banana Boat Relay Race, Banana Olympic Games, Banana Beach Party, Banana Ball, Carmen Miranda Look-Alike Contest. FOODS SERVED: banana specialties. ADMISSION: Banana button $2.00 for discount admission to events. ACCOMMODATIONS: motels and hotels, B&B's. RESTAURANTS: fast foods, family, elegant. CONTACT: Snowmass Resort Association, P.O. Box 5566, Snowmass Village, CO 81615, (303) 923-2000. 3,000

SUNSHINE FESTIVAL *first full weekend in June,* Alamosa, Alamosa Co., in the San Luis Valley on the banks of the Rio Grande. "This is the first big community party after the long cold winter and everyone comes out and has a good time." More than 100 arts and crafts and food booths, free activities and games for children, dog show, indoor juried art show, live entertainment from ballet to flamenco, country music, fiddling, rock 'n' roll, barbershop quartets; horseshoe and softball tournaments, 3.6mi. Run. FOODS SERVED: "American, Japanese, Mexican food and Slovenian sausage." ADMISSION: adults $1.00, children free. ACCOMMODATIONS: motels and hotels, campgrounds, RV parks. RESTAURANTS: fast foods, family, Mexican, Chinese. CONTACT: Rio Grande Arts Center, Inc., P.O. Box 875, Alamosa, CO 81101, (303) 589-5772. 5,000

CENTRAL CITY ARTS FESTIVAL *June 7 through September 13,* Central City, Gilpin Co., to feature the works of Colorado artists. Juried comprehensive show and sale including painting, crafts, sculpture, photography. ADMISSION: free. ACCOMMODATIONS: motels and hotels, B&B, campgrounds, RV park. RESTAURANTS: family, elegant, Mexican, German. CONTACT: Kay Russell at (303) 582-5574 or City Hall, Central City, CO 80427, (303) 573-0247 or (303) 582-5251. 20,000

TELLURIDE BLUEGRASS AND COUNTRY MUSIC FESTIVAL *third Wednesday through third Sunday in June,* Telluride, San Miguel Co. Workshops, banjo, guitar, mandolin, and band contests, music all-day long Saturday and Sunday on an outdoor stage at the base of 13,000-foot peaks of the Rocky Mountains. Musicians who have appeared include Michael Martin Murphy, New Grass Revival, John Hartford, David Grisman Quartet, Leo Kotke, Chris Daniels, Nanci Griffith, and David Bromkey; crafts. FOODS SERVED: twenty international booths including Chinese, Mexican, ribs. ADMISSION: weekend $63.00, Friday only $23.00, Saturday or Sunday only $27.00. ACCOMMODATIONS: hotels, B&B's, condominiums, campgrounds, RV parks. RESTAURANTS: family, elegant, Italian. CONTACT: general information Telluride Chamber Resort Association, P.O. Box 653, Telluride, CO 81435, (303) 728-3041; for ticket and accommodations information and reservations, (303) 728-4431 instate or (800) 525-3455 from outside Colorado. 8,000

STRAWBERRY DAYS *third weekend in June,* Glenwood Springs, Garfield Co. Juried crafts fair, arts and crafts exhibition, parade, talent show, concert featuring big-name entertainers such as Martha Reeves and the Vandellas, Garfield the Cat Look-Alike Contest, other family events. FOODS SERVED: concessions and strawberries. ADMISSION: free to most events. ACCOMMODATIONS: motels and hotels, B&B's, campgrounds, RV parks. RESTAURANTS: fast foods, family, elegant, Hungarian, German, Swiss, Italian. CONTACT: Glenwood Springs Area Chamber of Commerce, 1102 Grand Ave., Glenwood Springs, CO 81601, (303) 945-6589. 10,000

ASPEN MUSIC FESTIVAL AND SCHOOL *last week in June through third week in August,* Aspen, Pitkin Co., in the Rocky Mountains. More than 130 events including concerts of symphonic, chamber, choral, opera, and jazz music daily for nine weeks. Each year composers of a specific country are featured and their work is intermingled with that of other greats. Benefit concerts, dinner dance featuring the Aspen Jazz Ensemble with special guests, a popular artist benefit concert which in the past has included such performers as Itzhak Perlman, John Denver, Glenn Frey, Dionne Warwick, and the late Danny Kaye. Guest conductors have included Jorge Mester, James DePriest, Lawrence Foster, Claudio Scimone, Murry Sidlin, Stanislaw Skrowaczewski, and Yoav Talmi. Guest artists have included The American Brass Quintet, American String Quartet, Jan De-Gaetani, Yefim Bronfman, Misha Dichter, Cho-Liang Lin, Mi Dori, Andreas Diaz, Lynn Harrell, and Gary Hoffman. Educational activities included major studies in strings, woodwinds, brass, percussion, piano, voice, conducting, and composition. Master classes and young artists concerts are offered daily and are open to the public. ADMISSION: $7.00–$30.00 per event. ACCOMMODATIONS: motels and hotels, B&B's, campgrounds, RV parks. RESTAURANTS: fast foods, family, elegant, international. CONTACT: Music Associates of Aspen, Box AA, Aspen, CO 81612, (303) 925-3254, or the Aspen Resort Association, 303 E. Main St., Aspen, CO 81612, (303) 925-1940. 50,000

ORO CITY REBIRTH OF A MINERS' CAMP *last weekend in June and first three weekends in July,* Leadville, Lake Co. An extensive festival of arts and crafts, yarn spinning, demonstrations of rug braiding, paper making, gunsmithing, instrument making, quilting, mining and panning, pottery, woodstove baking, goldsmithing, weaving, spinning, stained glass, and woodcarving; bluegrass, country and folk music, "saloon" entertainment, jam sessions every night. FOODS SERVED: "ethnic." ADMISSION: adults $3.50, seniors and children 12 and under $1.50. ACCOMMODATIONS: motels and hotels, B&B's, campgrounds, RV parks. RESTAURANTS: fast foods, family, elegant. CONTACT: Rick Christmas at Colorado Mountain College,

Timberline Campus, Leadville, CO 80461, (303) 486-2015. 7,500

BACH, BEETHOVEN OR BRECKENRIDGE: FESTIVAL OF MUSIC AT THE SUMMIT *July 3 through August 2,* Breckenridge, Summit Co., in the Central Rocky Mountains, to celebrate music in the mountains. Music workshops, recitals, chamber concerts, opening gala banquet with guest artists such as Robin Sutherland and Emil Miland of the San Francisco Symphony, Shari Anderson, Frank Speller, Grace Nash, and Luis Toro, Jr. FOODS SERVED: banquet dinner. ADMISSION: to recitals adults $3.50, senior citizens and children $2.50; concerts adults $7.50, senior citizens and children $5.00. ACCOMMODATIONS: motels and hotels, B&B's, campgrounds, RV parks. RESTAURANTS: fast foods, family, elegant, Asian, German, Mexican. CONTACT: Breckenridge Resort Chamber, P.O. Box 1909, Breckenridge, CO 80424, (303) 453-2913. 1,500

RANGE CALL CELEBRATION *four days around July 4th,* Meeker, Rio Blanco Co., in the White River Valley. Parade, antique car show, concert by "big-name entertainer" such as Reba McEntire, Charly McClain, Wayne Massey, The Younger Brothers, Dan Seals Show, dance, three rodeos, Meeker Massacre Pageant. FOODS SERVED: concessions. ADMISSION: package ticket price $12.00. ACCOMMODATIONS: motels and hotels, campgrounds, RV parks. RESTAURANTS: fast foods, family. CONTACT: Range Call, P.O. Box 253, Meeker, CO 81641, (303) 878-3138. 3,000

TELLURIDE JAZZ FESTIVAL *third weekend in July,* Telluride, San Miguel Co. Daytime "headliners" in Town Park and jazz all day and night featuring artists such as Art Blakey and the Jazz Messengers, Alex Degrani, Aquito D'Rivera, Etta James Band, McCoy Tyner, Spyro Gyra, Bonnie Raitt, Maynard Ferguson, High Voltage, and the Hot Tomatoes. FOODS

SERVED: concessions. ADMISSION: weekend $52.00, two days $48.00, one day $26.00. ACCOMMODATIONS: hotels, B&B's, campgrounds, RV parks, condominiums. RESTAURANTS: family, elegant, Italian. CONTACT: general information, Telluride Chamber Resort Association, P.O. Box 653, Telluride, CO 81435, (303) 728-3041; for ticket and accommodations information and reservations, (303) 728-4431 instate or (800) 525-3455 from outside Colorado. 5,000

SKI HI STAMPEDE *last full weekend in July,* Monte Vista, Rio Grande Co., in the San Luis Valley. Three days of the "oldest rodeo in the state of Colorado," parades, evening dances, rodeos, carnival for children, crafts booths. FOODS SERVED: barbecue, Mexican, American. ADMISSION: $4.00–$6.00. ACCOMMODATIONS: motels and hotels, campgrounds, RV parks. RESTAURANTS: fast foods, family, elegant, Mexican. CONTACT: Ski Hi Stampede, Inc., Box 152, Monte Vista, CO 81144 or the Chamber of Commerce, 1125 Park Ave., Monte Vista, CO 81144, (303) 852-2731. 15,000

TOP OF THE ROCKIES LEADVILLE MUSIC FESTIVAL *last week in July through first week in August,* Leadville, Lake Co., in conjunction with Loyola University of New Orleans, LA. "Hello, New Orleans" welcome performance, one-man musical variety show, Jazz Brunch New Orleans Style, sacred music concert, dinner show, Boom Days music, art songs, arias, choral concert, seminars, workshops. FOODS SERVED: dinner at dinner show. ADMISSION: $3.00 to performances, dinner show $25.00, Jazz Brunch $9.00. ACCOMMODATIONS: motels and hotels, B&B's, campgrounds, RV parks. RESTAURANTS: fast foods, family, elegant. CONTACT: Leadville-Lake Co. Chamber of Commerce, P.O. Box 861, Leadville, CO 80461, (303) 486-3900. 10,000

AMC SUMMITFEST *first weekend in August,* Dillon and Keystone, Summit Co., an exciting benefit for the AMC Cancer Research Center in Denver. Fireworks over Lake Dillon, rowing race, 10k Run, scenic lift rides, Lake Dillon Arts Guild Art and Music Festival, children's matinees and games, bingo, children's theatre by the Cut and Paste Players, tombola (fishbowl drawing), live music from chamber to country-western, AMC/Dillon Open Sailing Classic with 200 boats of all classes, firefighter olympics. FOODS SERVED: pancake breakfast, food fair, steak fry. ADMISSION: varies by event. ACCOMMODATIONS: motels and hotels, B&B's, campgrounds, RV parks, condominiums. RESTAURANTS: fast foods, family, elegant, continental, Mexican, Chinese. CONTACT: AMC Summitfest, 1600 Pierce St., Denver, CO 80214, (303) 233-6501. 10,000

BOOM DAYS CELEBRATION/INTERNATIONAL PACK BURRO RACES *second weekend in August,* Leadville, Lake Co., to celebrate Leadville's mining history. Women's and men's burro races, over 13,000-feet elevation course, cocktail waitress race, Rock Drilling Contest, Mucking Contest, bed race, softball, queen coronation, Raider Shenanigans, mining events, parade, children's events, dance, crafts fair, Leadville Rod and Gun Club show, music by local bands, burro-race guessing, street fair with arts and food booths. FOODS SERVED: pancake breakfasts, "various ethnic." ADMISSION: free, $1.00 for burro-race guessing. ACCOMMODATIONS: motels and hotels, B&B's, campgrounds, RV parks. RESTAURANTS: fast foods, family, elegant. CONTACT: Leadville-Lake Co. Chamber of Commerce, P.O. Box 861, Leadville, CO 80461, (303) 486-3900. 10,000

CENTRAL CITY JAZZ FESTIVAL *third weekend in August,* Central City, Gilpin Co., to honor traditional jazz and ragtime. At least fifteen jazz bands and pianists from the U.S., Canada, Europe, and South America play at different locations around the city. ADMISSION: $15.00 per day per person. ACCOMMODATIONS: motels and hotels, B&B, campgrounds, RV park. RESTAURANTS: family, elegant, Mexican, German. CONTACT: City Hall, Central City, CO 80427, (303) 573-0247 or 582-5251. 4,000

TELLURIDE FILM FESTIVAL *Labor Day weekend (early September),* Telluride, San Miguel Co. One of the world's best film festivals featuring national and international premieres, innovative and experimental film art, daily free seminars and discussions uniting masters and admirers of film. Stars featured each year are never announced prior to festival, although recent visitors have included Robin Williams and Jimmy Stewart; picnic seminars at top of chair lift. ADMISSION: general $150.00, opera house $250.00, patron $750.00, individual screening tickets available at door. ACCOMMODATIONS: hotels, B&B's, campgrounds, RV parks, condominiums. RESTAURANTS: family, elegant, Italian. CONTACT: general information, Telluride Chamber Resort Association, P.O. Box 653, Telluride, CO 81435, (303) 728-3041; for ticket information and reservations, National Film Preserve, Box B-1156, Hanover, NH 03755, (603) 643-1255. Tickets go on sale in May. 4,000

OKTOBERFEST *second weekend in September,* Glenwood Springs, Garfield Co. Two days of Bavarian music, food, and dancing, arts fair, outdoor polka dances. FOODS SERVED: German. ADMISSION: free. ACCOMMODATIONS: motels and hotels, B&B's, campgrounds. RESTAURANTS: fast foods, family, elegant, Hungarian, German, Swiss, Italian. CONTACT: Glenwood Springs Area Chamber of Commerce, 1102 Grand Ave., Glenwood Springs, CO 81601, (303) 945-6589. 5,000

BRECKENRIDGE FESTIVAL OF FILM *third weekend in September,* Breckenridge, Summit Co., in the Rocky Mountains. Celebrities, foreign films, premieres, children's programs, gala parties, documentaries, outdoor film forum. Stars who have appeared include Rod Steiger, Elliott Gould, Jeffrey Lyons, Donald Sutherland, Sydney Pollack, Sam Waterston, Jonathan Demme, and Malcolm McDowell. ADMISSION: general admission $5.00, movie and season passes available. ACCOMMODATIONS: motels and hotels, B&B's, campgrounds, RV parks. RESTAURANTS: fast foods, family, elegant. CONTACT: Breckenridge Festival of Film, P.O. Box 1639, Breckenridge, CO 80424, (303) 453-6200. 5,000

NEW MEXICO

GATHERING OF NATIONS POW-WOW *third Friday and Saturday in April,* University of New Mexico Arena, Albuquerque, Bernalillo Co. One thousand Indian dancers compete for $28,000 in prize money, Miss Indian World Contest, 5k and 10k runs, 1mi. Walk, 200 Indian dancers an Miss Indian World march in Old Town Easter Parade. FOODS SERVED: Indian specialties. ADMISSION: $4.00 per day, $7.00 both days, parade free. ACCOMMODATIONS: motels and hotels, campgrounds, RV parks. RESTAURANTS: fast foods, family, elegant, international. CON-TACT: Albuquerque Convention and Visitors Bureau, P.O. Box 26866, Albuquerque, NM, (800) 321-6979.

MAYFAIR *Memorial Day weekend (late May),* Cloudcroft, Otero Co., at Zenith Park on Highway 82. Juried arts and crafts fair, hay rides, horseshoe tournament, square dancing, mountain men demonstration. FOODS SERVED: Mexican, American. ADMISSION: free. ACCOMMODATIONS: motels and hotels, campgrounds, RV parks. RESTAURANTS: fast foods, family, elegant. CONTACT: Cloudcraft Chamber of

Commerce, P.O. Box 125, Cloudcroft, NM 88317, (505) 682-2733. 5,000

TAOS SPRING ARTS CELEBRATION

Memorial Day (late May) and first three weekends in June, Taos, Taos Co., to celebrate the arts. Artists' studio tours, Native American and Hispanic traditional and contemporary music and dance, hands-on workshops, lectures, performance poetry, performance arts, and live entertainment which in the past has included Dennis Hopper, Cloris Leachman, Peter Fonda, and Ruth Warrick. FOODS SERVED: Native American, Hispanic. ADMISSION: varies by event. ACCOMMODATIONS: motels and hotels, B&B's, campgrounds, RV parks. RESTAURANTS: fast foods, family, elegant, continental. CONTACT: Rita Sutcliffe, Director, Taos Spring Arts Celebration, Box 1691, Taos, NM 87571, (505) 758-0516. 6,000

TAOS SCHOOL OF MUSIC SUMMER CHAMBER MUSIC FESTIVAL

last week in June through first week in August, Taos, Taos Co. Chamber music concerts and seminars in the inspiring setting of Taos; artists have included the American String Quartet and pianist Robert McDonald. ADMISSION: free to some events, to $6.00 for others. ACCOMMODATIONS: motels and hotels, B&B's, campgrounds, RV parks. RESTAURANTS: fast foods, family, elegant, continental. CONTACT: Chilton Anderson, Box 1879, Taos, NM 87571, (505) 776-2388. 1,600

PIÑATA *last weekend in June,* Tucumcari, Quay Co. Fun Run, swim races, softball and golf tournaments, Piñata Queen's Pageant, Prince Tocom and Princess Kari Pageant, gospel sing-a-long, chili cook-off, parade, rodeo, street dance, local musical performances. FOODS SERVED: "three cultures—Spanish, Anglo, and Indian." ADMISSION: free. ACCOMMODATIONS: motels and hotels, campgrounds, RV parks. RESTAURANTS: fast foods, family, elegant, Eurasian. CONTACT: Tucumcari–Quay Co. Chamber of Commerce, Drawer E, Tucumcari, NM 88401, (505) 461-1694.

SOUTHEASTERN NEW MEXICO FOURTH OF JULY CELEBRATION

July 4th, Lovington, Lea Co., at Chaparral Park, to celebrate Independence Day. "World's Greatest Lizard Race (must be seen to be believed)," large fireworks display, games, musical entertainment. FOODS SERVED: booths offering barbecue, Mexican, fast foods. ADMISSION: free. ACCOMMODATIONS: motels and hotels, RV parks. RESTAURANTS: fast foods, family, Mexican. CONTACT: Lovington Chamber of Commerce, P.O. Box 1347, Lovington, NM 88260, (505) 396-5311. 20,000

RUIDOSO ART FESTIVAL *last full weekend in July,* Ruidoso, Lincoln Co., in the Ruidoso Valley. More than 110 artists display their works outdoors under large tents in this juried show of original art, with continuous entertainment by local talent. FOODS SERVED: variety of food booths including Mescalero Apache Indian fry bread. ADMISSION: adults $2.00, children $1.00. ACCOMMODATIONS: motels and hotels, B&B's, campgrounds, RV parks. RESTAURANTS: fast foods, family, elegant, French, Chinese, Mexican. CONTACT: Ruidoso Valley Chamber of Commerce, P.O. Box 698, Ruidoso, NM 88345, (505) 257-7395. 8,000

INTER-TRIBAL INDIAN CEREMONIAL *second weekend in August,* near Gallup, McKinley Co., at Red Rock State Park, "The Gateway to Indian Country . . . where the sun shines on many cultures," to celebrate Indian culture. American Indian ceremonial dances featuring more than twelve tribes, more than "$10,000,000.00 worth of Indian fine art on display and for sale," Indian craft demonstrations, Indian professional rodeos, Indian sports and games, storytellers, singers, musicians, and dancers who perform the Basket Dance, Navajo Yeibeichai, Buffalo Dance, Rain, Mountain Spirits, Corn, and War dances, and the Hoop Dance. Participants include members of more than fifty tribes from throughout the U.S. FOODS SERVED: Indian foods and "typical fair concessions." ADMISSION: adults

$2.00–$9.00, children $1.00–$5.00. ACCOMMODATIONS: nearby motels and hotels, campgrounds, RV parks. RESTAURANTS: nearby fast foods, family. CONTACT: Inter-Tribal Indian Ceremonial Association, P.O. Box One, Church Rock, NM 87311, (505) 863-3896. 30,000

MUSIC FROM ANGEL FIRE FESTIVAL last three weeks in August through first week in September, at Angel Fire, Taos, Red River, Eagle Nest, Raton, and Mora, NM and Las Vegas, NV featuring "chamber music and jazz at its highest level!" Concerts and performances by internationally renowned artists including Ida Kavafian, James Walker, Walter Trammpler and Andre-Michel Schub and jazz group "Free Flight," John W. Giovando, general director; festival-benefit auction and dinner at Angel Fire resort. ADMISSION: charge. ACCOMMODATIONS: motels and hotels, campgrounds, RV parks, resorts. RESTAURANTS: fast foods, family, elegant, Mexican-Spanish. CONTACT: Music From Angel Fire, P.O. Box 502, Angel Fire, NM 87710, (505) 984-8548 or the Angel Fire Chamber of Commerce, Box 547, Angel Fire, NM 87710, (505) 377-6353.

FIESTA DE SANTA FE Labor Day weekend through second weekend in September, Santa Fe, Santa Fe Co., in the Plaza de Santa Fe, to celebrate and remember the peaceful resettlement in Nuevo Mejico by the Spanish Colonists. Pregon de la Fiesta and General Don Diego de Vargas Mass with burning of Zozobra (Old Man Gloom), Entrada (reenactment of resettlement), Mariachi Mass and Mass of Thanksgiving, Procession of the Cross of the Martyrs, carnival rides, fiesta show and sale, Gran Charreada (Mexican rodeo), La Marcha de la Reina parade, Plaza entertainment such as mariachis from New Mexico, Arizona, and Mexico, Navajo band, steel bands, Indian dancers, Fiesta Melodrama by Santa Fe Community Theatre, arts and crafts market, Baile de la Gente (people's ball or street dance), Desfile de los Niños (children's pet parade), Pontifical Fiesta Mass and Mass of Thanksgiving, mariachi concert. FOODS SERVED: Navajo tacos, Mexican, American. ADMISSION: free, charges for some events. ACCOMMODATIONS: motels and hotels, B&B's, campgrounds, RV parks. RESTAURANTS: fast foods, family, elegant, Mexican, continental. CONTACT: Santa Fe Fiesta Council, P.O. Box 4516, Santa Fe, NM 87501, (505) 988-7575. 100,000

TAOS ARTS FESTIVAL last week in September through first week in October, Taos, Taos Co., to celebrate the arts in this unique southwestern center for artists and writers. Major art shows, lectures, arts and crafts fairs, photography and jewelry shows, major Indian ceremonial at the Taos Indian Pueblo, theatrical presentations. FOODS SERVED: "Indian, Hispanic, and Anglo." ADMISSION: free. ACCOMMODATIONS: motels and hotels, B&B's, campgrounds, RV parks. RESTAURANTS: fast foods, family, elegant, northern New Mexican, French, Swiss. CONTACT: Taos Arts Festival, P.O. Box 2915, Taos, NM 87571, (505) 732-8267. 10,000

THE WHOLE ENCHILADA FIESTA first weekend in October, Las Cruces, Dona Ana Co., to celebrate "the food, music, cultural heritage of the area. Chile (peppers) are major crop and Mexican-style food, particularly enchiladas, is a principal attraction of the area." Watch the cooking and sample the "World's Largest Enchilada," gala parade of floats and marching bands, Fun Run, Fiesta Mexicana, Las Cruces Farmers and crafts market, Whole Enchilada Run includes 3mi. Run for Your Life and 10k Run, World Championship New Mexico Chili Cook-off, creative enchilada recipe contest, Los Vaqueros, Teatro de Las Cruces, western dance, bicycle races, Grocery Cart Race, live entertainment including mariachis, country-western music, square dancing, and street dancing. FOODS SERVED: enchiladas!, gorditas, fajitas, tomales, chile, "continuous enchilada supper," concessions, beer and wine gardens. ADMISSION:

free. ACCOMMODATIONS: motels and hotels, campgrounds, RV parks. RESTAURANTS: fast foods, family, elegant, Mexican, Chinese. CONTACT: Las Cruces Chamber of Commerce, P.O. Drawer 519, Las Cruces, NM 88005, (505) 523-1968.

ALBUQUERQUE INTERNATIONAL BALLOON FIESTA *first full weekend in October and eight following days,* Albuquerque, Bernalillo Co., the "largest ballooning event in the world." Air show, parade, U.S. Air Force Thunderbirds, sunrise prayer service, high school band performances, U.S. Navy Leapfrogs parachute team, mass ascension of balloons daily, balloon flying events, Key Grab Contest, picnic, awards banquet featuring more than 500 colorful, giant hot air balloons launching from a mile-high site, gas balloon races, sky divers, educational exhibits, photo contests. Truly "one of the world's most colorful spectacles." FOODS SERVED: international concessions. ADMIS-SION: adults $1.00. ACCOMMODATIONS: motels and hotels, campgrounds, RV parks. RESTAURANTS: fast foods, family, elegant, Mexican. CONTACT: International Balloon Fiesta, 4804 Hawkins, N.E., Albuquerque, NM 87109, (505) 344-3501. 500,000

SOUTHEASTERN NEW MEXICO ARTS AND CRAFTS FESTIVAL *first weekend in November,* Lovington, Lea Co., at the County Fairgrounds, to celebrate the arts. Art show, sales, and displays featuring artists from New Mexico, Texas, Colorado, California, and Washington. FOODS SERVED: Mexican, concessions. ADMISSION: free. ACCOMMODATIONS: motels and hotels, RV parks. RESTAURANTS: fast foods, family, Mexican. CONTACT: Lovington Chamber of Commerce, P.O. Box 1347, Lovington, NM 88260, (505) 396-5311. 10,000

TEXAS

LOVELADY LOVE FEST *weekend closest to February 14,* Lovelady, Houston Co., to celebrate Valentine's Day. Bunny rabbit catching contest, Calf Scramble, greased-pig contest, chili-BBQ Cook-off, Baby Beauty Contest, arts and crafts, games, domino tournament. FOODS SERVED: "all kinds." ADMISSION: free. ACCOMMODATIONS: motels and hotels. RESTAURANTS: fast food, family. CONTACT: Houston Co. Chamber of Commerce, P.O. Box 307, Crockett, TX 75835, (409) 544-2359.

SWEETWATER "WORLD'S LARGEST RATTLESNAKE ROUNDUP" *second weekend in March,* Sweetwater, Nolan Co., as the "rounding up of rattlesnakes to rid the countryside of the varmint." Rattlesnakes caught and turned in at the roundup, snake-handling demonstrations, snake exhibits, sports celebrities such as Dallas Cowboys "Too Tall" Jones and Danny White. FOODS SERVED: fried rattlesnake meat. ADMISSION: free. ACCOMMODATIONS: motels and hotels, campgrounds, RV parks. RESTAURANTS: fast foods, family. CONTACT: Sweetwater Chamber of Commerce, P.O. Box 1148, Sweetwater, TX 79556, (915) 235-5488. 30,000

DERRICK DAYS *last weekend in March through first weekend in April,* Corsicana, Navarro Co., in Texas' Golden Circle, to celebrate Corsicana's "oil heritage" which claims the "first oil field in Texas." Juried art show, Mayor's Cup Regatta, Derrick Days Derby, Derrick Days Revue, chili cook-off, Oil-Town Minithon Fun Run, Oil and Energy Museum, book bazaar, children's activities, Roughneck Rodeo, Corsicana Spill Canoe Race, Junior Olympics,

Armadillo Race, miniature golf tournament, Old Homebodies Home Tour, antique car exhibition, melodrama of oil heritage, music in the park. FOODS SERVED: chili, food booths. ADMISSION: most events free, charges for revue and melodrama. ACCOMMODATIONS: motels and hotels, B&B's, campgrounds. RESTAURANTS: fast foods, family, Mexican, Chinese. CONTACT: City of Corsicana Annual Event, Inc., P.O. Box 426, Corsicana, TX 75110, (214) 874-4731. 10,000

TYLER COUNTY DOGWOOD FESTIVAL *last weekend in March and first weekend in April,* Woodville, Tyler Co., "celebrating the beauty of springtime in East Texas." The March weekend is called "Western Weekend" and includes a Western trail-ride, Playday events, Trailride Dances, Western Trail-ride Parade featuring more than 1,800 riders with wagons, buggies, and oxen, beard contest, Sweetheart Contest, Wild West Rodeo, Western Dance. The first weekend in April, known as "Dogwood Queen's Weekend" includes an arts and crafts show, marathon and 10k races, antique and classic car show, Dogwood Queen's Parade, queen's coronation and historical pageant, and the Dogwood Dance and Queen's Ball, fireworks. FOODS SERVED: concessions. ADMISSION: free. ACCOMMODATIONS: motels and hotels, B&B, campground nearby. RESTAURANTS: family. CONTACT: Tyler Co. Chamber of Commerce, 507 N. Pine, Woodville, TX 75979, (409) 283-2632. 15,000

PRAIRIE DOG CHILI COOK-OFF AND WORLD CHAMPIONSHIP OF PICKLED QUAIL EGG EATING *first weekend in April,* Grand Prairie, Tarrant Co. in the Dallas/Fort Worth area at Traders Village, to salute the "official state dish of Texas chili." This tongue-in-cheek celebration is "the most fun you can have with your clothes on" and includes chili cooking, sampling, and showmanship at elaborate cooksite booths, World Championship Pickled Quail Egg Eating, costumes, skits with audience participation,

country-western dance, free contests for public participation including the Cuzin Homer Page Invitational Eat-and-Run Stewed-Prune Pit-Spitting Contest and many more. FOODS SERVED: chili with jalapeño pepper chasers. ADMISSION: free, parking $1.25 per vehicle. ACCOMMODATIONS: motels and hotels, RV park on grounds. RESTAURANTS: fast foods, family. CONTACT: Doug Beich, Traders Village, 2602 Mayfield Rd., Grand Prairie, TX 75051, (214) 647-2331. 80,000

RIOFEST *second weekend in April,* Harlingen, Cameron Co., at Fair Park, in the Rio Grande Valley, to celebrate the arts and culture of the Rio Grande Valley and Mexico. Art and crafts exhibits, sporting events, children's activities, horse show, rock bands, folk singers, Cajun and gospel music. FOODS SERVED: Mexican, Scottish, American. ADMISSION: $1.00. ACCOMMODATIONS: motels and hotels, campgrounds, RV parks. RESTAURANTS: fast foods, family, Mexican. CONTACT: RioFest Office, P.O. Box 1105, Harlingen, TX 78551, (512) 425-2705. 30,000

HUMBLE GOOD OIL DAYS *fourth Saturday in April,* Humble, Harris Co., on Main Street, to celebrate good oil days. Arts and crafts, dancing, eating, contests for young and old, parades, square dancing, country-western bands featuring local talent. FOODS SERVED: "down-home country cookin' and Texas barbecue." ADMISSION: free. ACCOMMODATIONS: motels and hotels, campground. RESTAURANTS: fast foods, family, elegant, French, Italian, Mexican. CONTACT: Humble Downtown Business Association, 626 Ferguson St., Humble, TX 77338, (713) 446-6184. 5,000

LUBBOCK ARTS FESTIVAL *fourth weekend in April,* Lubbock, Lubbock Co., in the South Plains area of Texas, to celebrate "all art forms." Visual art exhibits and sales, art demonstrations, children's crafts, exhibits by local cultural organizations, Children's Theatre production, preview gala, live entertainment by local choral groups and orchestras, instrumental and vocal soloists, Theatre Mask Ensemble, and big–name entertainers such as Burl Ives, Carol Lawrence, Ink Spots, Preservation Hall Jazz Band. FOODS SERVED: Spanish, Italian, Chinese, Indian, Greek, German, French. ADMISSION: free. ACCOMMODATIONS: motels and hotels, campgrounds, RV parks. RESTAURANTS: fast foods, family, elegant, international. CONTACT: Lubbock Cultural Affairs Council, P.O. Box 561, Lubbock, TX 79408 or the Lubbock Chamber of Commerce and Board of City Development, P.O. Box 561, Lubbock, TX 79408, (806) 763-4666. 85,000

STRAWBERRY FESTIVAL *fourth weekend in April*, Pasadena, Harris Co., at the Pasadena Convention Center, to celebrate and honor local strawberry growers and history and to promote the observance of San Jacinto Day. Arts and crafts, strawberry eating, growing, and cooking contests, beauty contests, auction, gumbo cook-off, elephant and camel rides, magic show, San Jacinto dog show, parade, costume contest, air show with skydivers, celebrity dunking booth, children's petting zoo, mud volleyball, turkey shoot, street rod car show, polo tournament, carnival, helicopter rides, costume ball, fireworks. FOODS SERVED: Italian, Tex-Mex, lots of strawberries, American. ADMISSION: free. ACCOMMODATIONS: motels and hotels, RV parks. RESTAURANTS: fast foods, family, elegant, international. CONTACT: San Jacinto Day Foundation, P.O. Box 4710, Pasadena, TX 77502, (713) 472-1211. 40,000

NECHES RIVER FESTIVAL *last week in April through first weekend in May*, Beaumont, Jefferson Co. Boat races and other water sports and demonstrations, air show at the municipal airport, Queen's Ball, coronation pageant. FOODS SERVED: concessions. ADMISSION: varies. ACCOMMODATIONS: motels and hotels, RV parks. RESTAURANTS: fast foods, family, elegant, international. CONTACT: Neches River Festival Committee at (409) 892-5124 or

the Beaumont Chamber of Commerce, P.O. Box 3150, Beaumont, TX 77704, (409) 838-6581. 100,000

TEXAS STATE FESTIVAL OF ETHNIC CULTURES AND ARTS AND CRAFTS SHOW *last weekend in April*, Ballinger, Runnels Co., in Central-west Texas, to honor the cultures of early Runnels County settlers. Arts and crafts, River Raft Race, pinto bean cook-off, parade, trap shoot, bass tournament, Fun Run, tennis tournaments, fiddlers contest, local entertainers such as Jerry Clower, Mary Jo Pierce, Mrs. America. FOODS SERVED: English, German, Czech, Italian, Indian, soul food, Mexican, French, Irish. ADMISSION: free. ACCOMMODATIONS: motels and hotels, campgrounds, RV parks. RESTAURANTS: fast foods, family, elegant. CONTACT: Ballinger Chamber of Commerce, P.O. Box 577, Ballinger, TX 76821, (915) 365-2333. 8,000

WILDFLOWER TRAILS OF TEXAS *last weekend in April*, Hughes Springs, Avinger, and Linden, Cass Co., to celebrate the blooming of wildflowers in this triangle of cities known as Triangle In The Pines of Texas. Events in Hughes Springs include Miss Wildflower Pageant, treasure hunt, carnival, art exhibition, children's art contest, country cottage featuring home-baked goods, crafts and food, Dan Barth Old-Time Medicine Show, historical displays, Western Day, Outhouse Dash, parade, ugly truck contest, and the Mason-Dixon Concert, cake walk, fish fry, street dance, gospel music celebration, and all-breed dog show. Avinger boasts a trail ride, fish fry, hickory-smoke barbecue, flea market and swap meet, antique car display, parade, break dance contest, games, old-fashioned shootout, and bluegrass, country-western, and other bands. Linden's celebration includes junior wildflower trails pageant, treasure hunt, D.D.'s Silver Dollar Saloon, street dances, Western Day, food fair, 4mi. Race, chili cook-off, Western Melodrama, egg toss, arts and crafts fair, fiddlers contest, mechanical armadillo races, cake walk, carnival, games, and a fish fry. Entertainers have included Rex Allen Jr. and Mason Dixon. FOODS SERVED: chili, fish fry, barbecue, sausage-on-a-stick, French waffles, funnel cakes, concessions. ADMISSION: free. ACCOMMODATIONS: motels and hotels, campgrounds, RV parks. RESTAURANTS: fast foods, family. CONTACT: Barbara Wakefield, Wildflower Trails, c/o Hughes Springs Chamber of Commerce, Box 218, Hughes Springs, TX 95656, (214) 639-2351. 50,000

SCARBOROUGH FAIRE *all weekends from late April through early June*, Waxahachie, Ellis Co., to celebrate "Old English Renaissance days." Authentic jousting, artists and craftspeople, plays and shows for children, live entertainment, puppet shows, Rogue, Oaf, and Fool. FOODS SERVED: Old English. ADMISSION: adults $9.00, children $4.00. ACCOMMODATIONS: motels and hotels, RV parks. RESTAURANTS: fast foods, family. CONTACT: Richard Holeyfield at (214) 937-6130 or the Waxahachie Chamber of Commerce, P.O. Box 187, Waxahachie, TX 75165, (214) 937-2390. 100,000

CINCO DE MAYO FESTIVAL *first weekend in May*, Grand Prairie, Tarrant Co. at Traders Village, to celebrate Cinco de Mayo, Mexican's Independence Day. Folklorico dancers, mariachi bands, and Latino bands provide continuous entertainment all afternoon both days. FOODS SERVED: Latin American. ADMISSION: free, parking $1.25. ACCOMMODATIONS: RV parks. RESTAURANTS: fast foods, family. CONTACT: Doug Beich at (214) 647-2331 or the Grand Prairie Chamber of Commerce, 900 Conover Dr., Grand Prairie, TX 75051, (214) 264-1558.

ENNIS POLKA FESTIVAL *first full weekend in May*, Ennis, Ellis Co., to celebrate local residents' Czechoslovakian heritage in downtown Ennis and at four Czech Halls. National Polka Festival featuring Texas' "finest polka bands" and "out-of-state polka bands" playing polkas

and waltzes, parade including colorful Czech costumes, folk dancing, gymnastics, street dancing, Beseda Dancers. FOODS SERVED: downtown and at all four halls, Czech foods and pastries including kolaches and klobase. ADMISSION: outdoor festivities free, $3.00–$5.00 to halls. ACCOMMODATIONS: motels and hotels, campgrounds, RV parks. RESTAURANTS: fast foods, family. CONTACT: Ennis Chamber of Commerce, P.O. Box 1177, Ennis, TX 75119, (214) 875-2625. 12,000

FORT BEND COUNTY CZECH FEST *first full weekend in May*, Rosenberg, Fort Bend Co., at the County Fairgrounds, to celebrate the Czechoslovakian heritage of many residents at "Texas' largest Czech festival." Arts and crafts including domestic and Czech imports, Czech costumes, Fun Run, children's events and carnival, polka and country-western music, Bohemian Garden, Czechoslovakian, German, and Polish singers, choirs and dancers, skits, jugglers and mimes. FOODS SERVED: loads of Czech delicacies, Mexican, and "walk-around food" including kolaches, sausages, corn on-the-cob, and potato pancakes. ADMISSION: adults $3.00, children under 12 $1.00. ACCOMMODATIONS: motels and hotels, RV park. RESTAURANTS: fast foods, family, elegant. CONTACT: Czech Fest, 4120 Avenue H, Rosenberg, TX 77471, (713) 342-5464.

KALEIDOSCOPE *Mothers' Day weekend (early May)*, Beaumont, Jefferson Co., on the grounds of the Beaumont Arts Museum. Art show featuring seventy-four juried artists, kids' Kaleidoscope activity tents with participatory activities with art to take home, Clothesline Art Contest for high school students, Art Alive on-site artists' demonstrations, computer graphics art contest, marching band and drill team, and Arts-on-Parade Walkathon. FOODS SERVED: "variety." ADMISSION: adults $2.50, senior citizens $2.00, children $1.00. ACCOMMODATIONS: motels and hotels, RV parks. RESTAURANTS: fast foods, family, elegant, international. CONTACT: Beaumont Art Museum, 1111 9th

St., Beaumont, TX 77704, (409) 832-3432 or (409) 832-8143. 20,000

KERRVILLE FOLK FESTIVAL *Memorial Day weekend (late May)*, and eighteen days following, 9 miles south of Kerrville, Kerr Co., at the Outdoor Theatre of Quiet Valley Ranch, to honor and celebrate the work of more than 107 original songwriters, and featuring more than 140 artists. Eleven six-hour evening concerts, five two-hour sundown concerts, three Folk Mass celebrations, three "New Folk" concerts of emerging songwriters, eight two-hour Ballad Trees for unknown songwriters, Lecture Series on the "History of American Popular Music," Anniversary Ball, seventy crafts booths. This festival is known as "America's leading songwriters festival" and is known for presenting and preserving one-of-a-kind original performers. Participating musicians have included Allen Damron, Carolyn Hestor, Steven Fromholz, Odetta, Peter Yarrow, Riders in the Sky, Gary P. Nunn, Jerry Jeff Walker, Ian Tyson, Bob Gibson, David Amram, Marcia Ball, Peter Rowan, and Tom Rush. FOODS SERVED: concessions. ADMISSION: from $8.00–$12.00 per day, packages of three days $21.00, five days $30.00, eight days $50.00, 11 days $60.00, and 18 days $100.00. ACCOMMODATIONS: motels and hotels, campgrounds, RV parks, camping free at site with minimum of three-day ticket. RESTAURANTS: fast foods, family, Italian, Mexican. CONTACT: Rod Kennedy Presents, P.O. Box 1466, Kerrville, TX 78029, (512) 257-3600. 30,000

TEXAS STATE ARTS AND CRAFTS FAIR *Memorial Day weekend and the following weekend (late May and early June)*, Kerrville, Kerr Co., in the Texas Hill country, to celebrate Texas arts and crafts, food, and music. More than 235 "carefully selected artists and crafters," educational programs, live entertainment which has included Lightcrust Dough Boys, Dallas Black Dance Theatre, the Poverty Playboys Bluegrass, jazz, country-western, vintage rock 'n' roll, historic-

costume show, and a children's circus. FOODS SERVED: wide range at thirty-five food booths. ADMISSION: adults $5.00, children $3.00, group rates available. ACCOMMODATIONS: motels and hotels, B&B's, campgrounds, RV parks. RESTAURANTS: fast foods, family, elegant, Mideastern, Chinese. CONTACT: Texas Arts and Crafts Foundation, P.O. Box 1527, Kerrville, TX 78029-1527, (512) 896-5711 or the Kerrville Area Chamber of Commerce, P.O. Box 790, Kerrville, TX 78029, (512) 896-1155. 37,500

STRANGE FAMILY BLUEGRASS FESTIVAL *Memorial Day weekend (late May) and Labor Day weekend (early September)*, Texarkana, Bowie Co., in the Liberty–Eylau community, to celebrate the joys of bluegrass music. Arts and crafts exhibits, bluegrass jamming, fourteen "booked bands," open stage and camping (". . . when bluegrass music lovers and performers get together"), music from noon to midnight, Wednesdays are Fiddlers Nights. FOODS SERVED: fast foods, concessions. ADMISSION: from $3.00–$7.00, five-day pass $20.00. ACCOMMODATIONS: motels and hotels, campgrounds, RV parks. RESTAURANTS: (nearby) fast foods, family, elegant. CONTACT: Patsy Holder, 111 Brookfield, Texarkana, TX 75501, (214) 832-1464 or the Texarkana Chamber of Commerce, P.O. Box 1468, Texarkana, TX 75504, (214) 792-7191. 20,000

LULING WATERMELON THUMP *last weekend in June*, Luling, Caldwell Co., in South-central Texas, to celebrate the watermelon harvest. Arts and crafts, watermelon eating contests for all ages, Champion Melon judging, Champion Melon Auction, watermelon seed-spitting contests by age groups, team seed-spitting contests, Championship Seed Spit-off, carnival, kiddie rides, concessions, flea market, open rodeo, street dance, 10,000m Marathon, golf, softball, and bowling tournaments, parade, Car Rallye, old-time fiddlers, local dance bands. FOODS SERVED: watermelon, American,

Mexican-American. ADMISSION: free, charge for street dances. ACCOMMODATIONS: motels and hotels, campgrounds and RV parks nearby. RESTAURANTS: fast foods, family, Mexican. CONTACT: Luling Watermelon Thump Association, P.O. Box 710, Luling, TX 78648, (512) 875-3214. 33,000

SAINTS ROOST CELEBRATION *July 4th weekend,* Clarendon Donley Co., in the Texas Greenbelt. Craft fair, art show, fiddlers' contest, Old Settlers Reunion, turtle race, parade. FOODS SERVED: barbecue. ADMISSION: free to some events, charges for others. ACCOMMODATIONS: motels and hotels, campgrounds, RV parks. RESTAURANTS: fast foods, family, elegant. CONTACT: Clarendon Chamber of Commerce, P.O. Box 730, Clarendon, TX 79226, (806) 874-2421. 4,000

BLACK-EYED PEA JAMBOREE *third weekend in July,* Athens, Henderson Co., at the Fairgrounds, to celebrate the black-eyed pea. Arts and crafts show, black-eyed pea cook-off, black-eyed pea taste-in, pie eating contests, pea poppin' and pea shellin' contests, terrapin races, rodeo, beauty pageant, parade, 10k Jaunt, 5k Run, 1mi. Fun Run, bicycle tour, carnival, gospel concert. FOODS SERVED: black-eyed pea concoctions, concessions. ADMISSION: free, charges for some events. ACCOMMODATIONS: motels and hotels, campgrounds, RV parks. RESTAURANTS: fast foods, family. CONTACT: Athens Chamber of Commerce, P.O. Box 2600, Athens, TX 75751, (214) 675-5181. 40,000

AUSTIN AQUA FESTIVAL *first nine days in August,* Austin, Travis Co., at Auditorium Shores. "Pre-festival events" include the Governor's Cup Sailing Regatta, night auto cross, a youth basketball tournament, Jr. Open Tennis Tournament, jet ski and volleyball tournaments, Disabled Feats and Record-Breaking Madness, and an arts and crafts extravaganza. The actual festival includes Texas Watercolor Society Exhibition, pet parade, Sheriff's Rodeo, Lone Star Truck and Tractor Pull, Capital Art Society Show, horseshoe pitching, bicycle race, judo meet, Hill Country Road Rally, beauty pageants, fencing tournament, Quarter Midget Race, Great River Raft Race, state wheelchair basketball tournament, swim meet, ice hockey tournament, horse show, Renaissance Market, motorcycle races, barefoot water ski competition, skeet shoot, Aerofest, children's art show, teen essay contest, shuffleboard tournament, nightlighted water parade and fireworks display, gymnastics, BMX races, small fry fishing derby, 5k Run, Mustang Car Show, International Folk Dance Workshop, softball and basketball tournaments, trap shoot, River City Pops concerts, and more than 100 bands and entertainers which have included the Miami Sound Machine, The Jets, Will Sexton and the Kill, Marcia Ball, La Mafia, Beto Y Los Fairlanes, Three Dog Night, Gary P. Nunn, Randy Travis, The Sardines, Peoples Choice, Texas Fever, Extreme Heat, Boys Don't Cry, and Ruben and Alfonso Ramos. "Post-festival events" include a Volunteer Appreciation Party, novice ski tournament, and the Texas Water Ski Championships. FOODS SERVED: concessions. ADMISSION: many events free, charges for others. ACCOMMODATIONS: motels and hotels. RESTAURANTS: fast foods, family, elegant, international. CONTACT: Austin Aqua Festival, P.O. Box 1967, Austin, TX 78767, (512) 472-5664. 250,000

TEXAS FOLKLIFE FESTIVAL *first weekend in August,* San Antonio, Bexar Co., at the University of Texas Institute of Texan Cultures, downtown, to celebrate the "ethnic diversity and pioneer heritage of Texas." Nearly 6,000 participants from thirty ethnic groups and nationalities present their cultures and traditions through crafts, music, dance, and food. The program for this festival is a true guide to the festival which includes a schedule of all performances, a menu of all foods available from every country and culture represented and which ones offer recipes, a listing of all crafts and craftspeople, all demonstrations and participatory events for guests from crafts to cooking, games and special events. Texas Lace Day includes exhibits and demonstrations of lace making, crafts and skills shown include adobe brick making, basketmaking, antique tools, beekeeping, blacksmithing, bobbin lace, bocce, bootmaking, chair caning, children's folk games, corn shucking, fortune telling, goose plucking, gourds, horsehair rope making, horseshoe pitching and tobacco spitting, kite making, lye-soap making, net tying, Native American arts, piñatas, Polish needlework, quilting, roof thatching, snake skinning and tanning, and steel pan tuning, and whittling. Continuous entertainment involving ten stages includes performances by all thirty ethnic groups ranging from Highlander bagpipes and the Nacogdoches Jazz Band to mariachis, Ballet Folklorico de San Antonio, Ballet Artes de Mexico, Lebanese Folk Dancers, Bavarian Village Band, fiddlers, Indian dancers, cloggers, storytellers, blues, ventriloquists, Cajun dancers, harps, steel bands. FOODS SERVED: vast array of ethnic specialties, some with recipes. ADMISSION: adults $5.00, children 6–12 $1.00, children under 6 free. ACCOMMODATIONS: motels and hotels. RESTAURANTS: fast foods, family, elegant, international. CONTACT: Texas Folklife Festival, The University of Texas Institute of Texan Cultures at San Antonio, P.O. Box 1226, San Antonio, TX 78294, (512) 226-7651. 100,000

SCHULENBURG FESTIVAL *first weekend in August,* Schulenburg, Fayette Co., at Wolters Park, to celebrate homecoming. Arts and crafts show, cow-chip throwing contest, egg toss, musical and theatrical productions, Fun Run, chili cook-off, ladies' softball tournament, live entertainers such as Eddy Raven and B. J. Thomas. FOODS SERVED: Czech/German, Mexican, American such as sausage, hamburgers, barbecued chicken. ADMISSION: free, $5.00 for big-name entertainment. ACCOMMODATIONS: motels and hotels, campgrounds, RV parks. RESTAURANTS: fast

foods, family. CONTACT: Schulenburg Chamber of Commerce, P.O. Box 65, Schulenburg, TX 78956, (409) 743-3023. 30,000

XIT RODEO AND REUNION *first full weekend in August,* near Dalhart, Dallam–Hartley counties, at the XIT Ranch which in the 1880s was "the largest range in the world under fence" including three million acres (XIT apparently stands for "Ten in Texas" referring to the ten counties the ranch covered within Texas.), to honor its cowhands. Antique car show, parade, rodeos, Empty Saddle Run, dances, entertainment which has included stars such as Lacy J. Dalton and Mo Bandy. FOODS SERVED: barbecue. ADMISSION: free, rodeo $5.00, dances $10.00. ACCOMMODATIONS: motels and hotels, campground, RV parks. RESTAURANTS: fast foods, family. CONTACT: Ron Hanbury, President, XIT Rodeo and Reunion Association, c/o the Dalhart Area Chamber of Commerce, P.O. Box 967, Dalhart, TX 79022, (806) 249-5646. 22,000

ST. LOUIS DAY *Sunday closest to August 25,* Castroville, Medina Co., at Koenig Park, to celebrate the "birthdate of Patron Saint of St. Louis Parish (who) was also Louis IX, King of France" in Castroville, known as "The Little Alsace of Texas." Arts and crafts, Alsatian Dancers of Texas, auction, kiddie land, gunslingers, choral groups. FOODS SERVED: Alsatian barbecue dinner with sausage, beef brisket, concessions. ADMISSION: free, Alsatian meal $4.00. ACCOMMODATIONS: motels and hotels, campground, RV park. RESTAURANTS: fast foods, family, elegant, Alsatian. CONTACT: St. Louis Rectory, Box 500, Castroville, TX 78009, (512) 538-2267 or the Castroville Chamber of Commerce, P.O. Box 572, Castroville, TX 78009, (512) 538-3142. 10,000

WESTFEST *Labor Day weekend (early September),* West, McLennan Co., to celebrate "Czech tradition." Arts and crafts, Kolache 5000, 3mi. foot race, Parade of

Authentic Costumes, Ukranian Dancers of Dallas, Sokol Gymnastics Exhibition, Polish, German, Italian, and Czech folk dancers, El Folklorico Juveniles of Waco, polka and other dance bands from throughout the Southwest, petting zoo. FOODS SERVED: Czech, German, Mexican, American including kolaches, cabbage rolls, sausage rolls, funnel cakes, tamales, potato pancakes, pretzels, barbecue, hamburgers, and concessions. ADMISSION: adults $3.00, children 6–12 $1.00. ACCOMMODATIONS: motels and hotels, campgrounds, RV park outside grounds. RESTAURANTS: family. CONTACT: Nita Gerik, P.O. Box 326, West, TX 76691, (817) 826-5452 or Westfest, P.O. Box 65, West, TX 76691, (817) 826-5058. 40,000

NATIONAL CHAMPIONSHIP INDIAN POWWOW *weekend after Labor Day (early September)*, Grand Prairie, Tarrant Co., at Traders Village, to celebrate Native American culture. More than twenty-five Indian tribes participate in championship dance competitions in full regalia, vying in more than twelve different dance categories, Indian arts and crafts show, homemade teepee village. FOODS SERVED: Indian. ADMISSION: free, parking $1.25 per vehicle. ACCOMMODATIONS: motels and hotels, RV park on grounds. RESTAURANTS: fast foods, family. CONTACT: Doug Beich, Traders Village, 2602 Mayfield Rd., Grand Prairie, TX 75051, (214) 647-2331. 85,000

KOLACHE FESTIVAL *second Saturday in September*, Caldwell, Burleson Co. on the Town Square, in central Texas, to celebrate the Czech heritage of many local residents and the Czech wedding pastry kolache. Kolache state bake contest and show, arts and crafts show and demonstrations including stenciling, basket weaving, egg decorating, quilting, woodcraft, carving, sculpting, tatting; antiques including Czechoslovakian lead crystal and antique Czech Easter eggs; culinary arts demonstrations of kolache baking, pasta making, farmer's cheese, butter churning, and sausage stuffing; antique automobile

show and classic motorcars, Czech flag ceremony, singing of the Czech national anthem, local museums of Czech history; live entertainment including the Beseda, Czech dancers, The Sokol, Lee Roy Matocha Polka Band, Wendish and Slovak Music, Czech Choir, Czech dulcimers, accordian players, strolling musicians, and the Burleson County Opry Members and Band. FOODS SERVED: kolache and many other Czechoslovakian specialties, in the Czech Gardens and the Kolache Kafe. ADMISSION: free. ACCOMMODATIONS: motels, campgrounds. RESTAURANTS: fast foods, family. CONTACT: Kolache Festival, c/o Caldwell Chamber of Commerce, P.O. Box 126, Caldwell, TX 77836, (409) 567-3218 or (409) 567-7979.

OAK CLIFF URBAN PIONEER FESTIVAL AND HOMES TOUR *third weekend in September*, Oak Cliff, Dallas Co., at Kidd Springs Park, to celebrate urban pioneering. Arts and crafts, live entertainment including the Sox Off Blues Band playing blues, country, and rock, "fiddlers and pickers, cloggers and singers, shuckers and jivers." Homes Tour "spotlights historic structures in various stages of rebirth." FOODS SERVED: "tasty cooking." ADMISSION: free. ACCOMMODATIONS: motels and hotels. RESTAURANTS: fast foods, family, elegant, international. CONTACT: Ross Ramsey, President, Old Oak Cliff Conservation League at (214) 720-6929 or the Dallas Chamber of Commerce, 1507 Pacific Ave., Dallas, TX 75201-3481, (214) 954-1111.

CITY FEST–HIGHLAND GAMES *third weekend in September*, Plano, Collin Co., on the campus of Plano Senior High School in the Dallas–Fort Worth area. Ukranian and Hispanic folkloric dancers, Highland bagpipers, North Texas Celtic Society musical groups, ugliest dog contest, crowning of King and Queen of City Fest, fiddlers contest and hoedown. FOODS SERVED: "smorgasbord of ethnic foods." ADMISSION: free. ACCOMMODATIONS: motels and hotels, campgrounds, RV parks. RESTAURANTS: fast foods, family, elegant, international. CONTACT: Plano Cultural Arts Center, 811 N. Central Expressway, #1076, Plano, TX 75075, (214) 423-7809. 15,000

TEXAS INTERNATIONAL WINE CLASSIC *fourth weekend in September,* Lubbock, Lubbock Co., at the Lubbock Plaza Hotel, as a salute to the wine industry and grape growers. Grand tasting of wines from more than fifty wineries throughout the U.S., seminars, gourmet lunches featuring wines, gourmet dinner featuring seven wines and speaker from featured winery, jazz Friday night, symphony orchestra performances Saturday night. FOODS SERVED: gourmet lunch and dinner. ADMISSION: wine tasting $20.00, lunches $15.00, dinner $50.00, all events $95.00. ACCOMMODATIONS: motels and hotels, campgrounds, RV parks. RESTAURANTS: fast foods, family, elegant, international. CONTACT: Lubbock Chamber of Commerce, P.O. Box 561, Lubbock, TX 79408, (806) 763-4666. 1,200

TEXAS RICE FESTIVAL *first Wednesday through Saturday in October,* Winnie, Chambers Co., at Winnie–Stowell Park, to celebrate local agriculture and the rice harvest. Arts and crafts, rice cooking contest, rice eating contest, parades, street dances, carnival, horse show, farm equipment display, continuous entertainment on stage. FOODS SERVED: rice concoctions, concessions. ADMISSION: adults $1.00, students $.50. ACCOMMODATIONS: motels and hotels. RESTAURANTS: fast foods, family. CONTACT: Winnie–Stowell Area Chamber of Commerce, P.O. Box 147, Winnie, TX 77665, (409) 296-2231. 50,000

SHRIMPOREE *first weekend in October,* Aransas Pass, San Patricio Co., at the Roosevelt Stadium Shrimporee Grounds, to celebrate the local seafood industry. Arts and crafts, shrimp eating contest, Fun Run, Outhouse Race, bicycle decorating contest, beauty pageant, men's sexy legs contest, children's area featur-

ing clowns, face painting, games, magician, balloons, folk singing, sea shell crafts, photo boards, hopscotch, and basketball; parade, Texas Riviera Cloggers, country-western music on stage during afternoons and evenings, gospel music. FOODS SERVED: shrimp on a stick, fried shrimp and oysters, shrimp creole, crab cake sandwiches, Mexican, snowballs, baked potatoes, fried mushrooms, corn on the cob, red beans, cornbread, and more. ADMISSION: free. ACCOMMODATIONS: motels and hotels, campgrounds, RV parks. RESTAURANTS: fast foods, family, seafood. CONTACT: Aransas Pass Chamber of Commerce, 452 W. Cleveland Blvd., Aransas Pass, TX 78336, (512) 758-2750. 40,000

SEAFAIR *second weekend in October,* Rockport, Aransas Co. Arts and crafts exhibits, crab races, sailing regatta, gumbo cook-off, Anything That Floats But a Boat Race, melodrama, Miss Seafair Pageant, local bands and cloggers, karate demonstrations, belly and Polynesian dancers. FOODS SERVED: seafood specialties, gumbo. ADMISSION: free. ACCOMMODATIONS: motels and hotels, campgrounds, RV parks. RESTAURANTS: fast foods, family, elegant. CONTACT: Rockport Seafair Inc., 1014 Wharf, Rockport, TX 78382, (512) 729-3312 or the Rockport–Fulton Area Chamber of Commerce, P.O. Box 1055, Rockport, TX 78382, (512) 729-6445. 50,000

EAST TEXAS YAMBOREE *third weekend in Ocober,* Gilmer, Upshur Co., in East Texas, to salute the sweet potato or yam. Art show, hobby and craft show, yam and corn contest, sweet potato pie judging, Tater Trot, bicycle tour, carnival on the square, pageant, parades, fiddlers contest, livstock show and sale, tennis tournament, performances at bandstands of gospel, bluegrass, country-western, and a barn dance at which Joe Stampley and Con Hunley have performed. FOODS SERVED: sweet potatoes in everything, other concessions. ADMISSION: most events free, charges for others. ACCOM-

MODATIONS: motel, B&B, campground, RV park. RESTAURANTS: fast foods, family, Mexican. CONTACT: East Texas Yamboree Association, Box 854, Gilmer, TX 75644 or the Upshur Co. Chamber of Commerce, P.O. Box 854, Gilmer, TX 75644, (214) 843-2413. 50,000

WESTERN DAYS CELEBRATION *third weekend in October,* Yorktown, DeWitt Co., at the City Park. Arts and crafts; chili, bean, and barbecue cook-offs, Little Miss and Mister Contest, fiddlers contest, Western Parade, children's parade, western bands. FOODS SERVED: Polish, Spanish, Cajun, Italian, Chinese, Mexican, gumbo, chili, barbecue. ADMISSION: free. ACCOMMODATIONS: motels and hotels, campground, RV park. RESTAURANTS: fast foods, family, Mexican. CONTACT: Yorktown Chamber of Commerce, P.O. Box 488, Yorktown, TX 78164, (512) 564-2661. 7,000

OLD FIDDLER'S FESTIVAL *last weekend in October,* Sinton, San Patricio Co., in South Texas. Arts and crafts, fiddling contest, carnival with games and rides, teen and children's areas, parade, Miss Sinton Contest, continuous entertainment in biergarten, local bands and entertainers such as Frenchie Burke and James and Michael Younger. FOODS SERVED: "all kinds." ADMISSION: $2.00 per person, children under 6 free. ACCOMMODATIONS: motels and hotels, RV parks. RESTAURANTS: fast foods, family, elegant, Mexican, seafood. CONTACT: Old Fiddler's Festival, c/o Sinton Chamber of Commerce, P.O. Box 217, Sinton, TX 78387, (512) 364-2307. 25,000

CZHILISPIEL *fourth full weekend in October,* Flatonia, Fayette Co. Arts and crafts, chili cook-off, barbecue cook-off, "World's Largest Biergarten," parade, street dances, variety of live entertainment including German songs and waltzes, The Velvets of Flatonia, the Lee Roy Matocha Band, The Jimmy Brosch Band, country and rock 'n' roll music. FOODS SERVED: chili and barbecue, food booths. ADMISSION: free. ACCOMMODATIONS: motels and hotels, RV park nearby. RESTAURANTS: fast foods, family. CONTACT: Flatonia Chamber of Commerce, P.O. Box 651, Flatonia, TX 78941, (512) 865-3920. 10,000

PEANUT FESTIVAL *October during football homecoming,* Grapeland, Houston Co., at Community Park, to celebrate the peanut harvest. Arts and crafts, carnival, local musical entertainers. FOODS SERVED: peanut specialties, "many different kinds." ADMISSION: free. ACCOMMODATIONS: campgrounds, RV parks. RESTAURANTS: fast foods, family. CONTACT: Houston Co. Chamber of Commerce, P.O. Box 307, Crockett, TX 75835, (409) 544-2359.

SYMPHONY OF TREES *first weekend in December,* Beaumont, Jefferson Co., at the Beaumont Civic Center, to celebrate Christmas. Arts and crafts exhibits, ice skating, Christmas trees exhibit, children's activities, entertainment by the Beaumont Symphony Orchestra, and local dance groups, choirs, and bands. ADMISSION: $2.50. ACCOMMODATIONS: motels and hotels, RV parks. RESTAURANTS: fast foods, family, elegant. CONTACT: Julie Randolph at (409) 866-3115 or the Beaumont Chamber of Commerce, P.O. Box 3150, Beaumont, TX 77704, (409) 838-6581. 15,000

UTAH

UNITED STATES FILM FESTIVAL *mid-January,* Park City, Summit Co., in the Salt Lake City–Wasatch Mountain Area, sponsored by Robert Redford's Sundance Institute. More than thirty-five independently produced American films are shown, screenings of Canadian and other foreign films. Judges have included Randa Haines, director of "Children of a Lesser God"; Paul Bartel, director of "Eating Raoul" and "Death Race 2000"; Los Angeles Times film critic Sheila Benson, and L.M. "Kit" Carson, screen writer of "Paris, Texas" and "Texas Chainsaw Massacre 2." ADMISSION: varies by event. ACCOMMODATIONS: motels and hotels, B&B's, campgrounds, RV parks. RESTAURANTS: fast foods, family, elegant, international. CONTACT: Sundance Institute, c/o Park City Chamber of Commerce–Convention and Visitors Bureau, P.O. Box 1630, Park City, UT 84060, (801) 649-6100, (800) 453-1360, or (801) 322-FILM.

UTAH SHAKESPEAREAN FESTIVAL *July 16 to September 5,* Cedar City, Iron Co., on the campus of Southern Utah State College, to celebrate the works of William Shakespeare. Performances of three Shakespearean plays in repertory on an outdoor stage, complimentary Greenshow of festive dancing, singing, storytelling, mime and specialty acts, Renaissance Feaste of "excellent food and riotous food humor," Costume Cavalcade including sixty costumes originally designed for Utah Shakespearean Festival for productions from the Dark Ages through the reign of James I, A Royal Tea with Chamber Consort musicians performing on authentic Renaissance instruments, fruit drinks, teas, and crumpets; backstage tours of the costume shop, makeup room and scene shop; literary seminars, production seminars, educational services including a study guide which provides background materials, "Words you May Not Know" and "Who's Who," synopses, and descriptions of characters in the current year's productions. FOODS SERVED: English with 16th century Elizabethan dinners and treats, teas. ADMISSION: from $10.00–$14.00, group services available. ACCOMMODATIONS: motels and hotels, B&B's, campgrounds, RV parks. RESTAURANTS: fast foods, family, elegant, Mexican, German, Chinese. CONTACT: Utah Shakespearean Festival, Cedar City, UT 84720, (801) 586-7880. 51,000

DAYS OF '47 PIONEER CELEBRATION *third weekend through fourth week in July,* Salt Lake City, Salt Lake Co., to celebrate the arrival of the Mormon pioneers in the Salt Lake Valley. Statewide fairs, festivals, parades, pageants, rodeos, "third largest parade in the United States," Horse Parade, nightly professional rodeo, children's parade, fireworks, theatrical presentations such as "Here is Brother Brigham" and "Promised Valley" musical presentations. The Vocal Majority Barbershop Chorus, Mitch Miller, and the Beach Boys. FOODS SERVED: "all kinds of foods." ADMISSION: varies by event, some free. ACCOMMODATIONS: motels and hotels, B&B's, campgrounds, RV parks. RESTAURANTS: fast foods, family, elegant. CONTACT: Utah Travel Council, Department of Community and Economic Development, Council Hall, Capitol Hill, Salt Lake City, UT 84114, (801) 533-5681 or the Salt Lake Area Chamber of Commerce, 175 E. 400 S., Salt Lake City, UT 84111, (801) 364-3631. 200,000

FESTIVAL OF THE AMERICAN WEST *last weekend in July through first weekend in August,* Logan, Cache Co., on the campus of Utah State University, to celebrate the lifestyle of settlers of the west. Artists and craftspeople demonstrate traditional life skills and crafts, American Dutch-oven cook-off, Historical Pageant, quilt show, medicine show, American Folk Ballet, folk music, square dancing, clogging, Indian chants and dances. FOODS SERVED: traditional foods prepared over open fires such as Dutch oven potatoes, crepes, Mormon jonny cakes, Navajo tacos, Indian fry bread, buffalo stew, buffalo burgers, lots more. ADMISSION: charges vary by event, some events free. ACCOMMODATIONS: motels and hotels, campgrounds. RESTAURANTS: fast foods, family, elegant. CONTACT: Festival of the American West, Utah State University, Logan, UT 84322-0125, (801) 750-1143. 42,000

MAIN STREET U.S.A. SUMMER-FEST *first week in August,* Bountiful, Davis Co., at Main and Center streets, to celebrate the visual and performing arts. More than sixty-five artists and craftspeople exhibit fine art, handmade dolls, weaving, ceramics, photography, and works of other disciplines, Children's Theatre, Scottish bagpipe band, John Phillip Sousa Brass Band, cloggers, folk and ethnic music, excerpts from Broadway musicals. FOODS SERVED: Maori, Filipino, Mexican, American. ADMISSION: free. ACCOMMODATIONS: motel, campgrounds, RV parks. RESTAURANTS: fast foods, family, Asian, Mexican, others in Salt Lake City. CONTACT: Bountiful–Davis Art Center, 2175 S. Main St., Bountiful, UT 84010, (801) 292-0367 or the Bountiful Area Chamber of Commerce, P.O. Box 99, Bountiful, UT 84010, (801) 295-6944. 3,500

PARK CITY ART FESTIVAL *first weekend in August,* Park City, Summit Co., in the Salt Lake City–Wasatch Mountain area. More than 200 artists from throughout the U.S. show their works in this juried art show on historic Main Street, Utah entertainers perform on two stages such as the Utah Opera, Salt Lake Chamber Ensemble, and shows such as "Kismet" have been performed. FOODS SERVED: food booths by Park City-area restaurants. ADMISSION: $1.00 per per-

son. ACCOMMODATIONS: motels and hotels, B&B's, campgrounds, RV parks. RESTAURANTS: fast foods, family, elegant, international. CONTACT: Kimball Art Center, P.O. Box 1478, Park City, UT 84060, (801) 649-8882 or the Park City Chamber of Commerce–Convention and Visitors Bureau, P.O. Box 1630, Park City, UT 84060, (801) 649-6100 or (800) 453-1360. 100,000

SPRINGVILLE WORLD FOLKFEST *second weekend through third weekend in August,* Springville, Utah Co. An international festival honoring countries such as Greece, Japan, Bulgaria, Lithuania, Italy and China featuring cultural programs of those countries such as dancing, artists, singing, concession stands and food booths. FOODS SERVED: Chinese, Japanese, Greek, American. ADMISSION: adults $4.00, senior citizens and children under 12 $3.00, family pass $12.00. ACCOMMODATIONS: motels and hotels, campgrounds, RV parks. RESTAURANTS: fast foods, family, Chinese, Mexican. CONTACT: Springville Arts Commission, 50 S. Main, Springville, UT 84663, (801) 489-3263 or the Springville Chamber of Commerce, P.O. Box 189, Springville, UT 85663, (801) 489-4681. 40,000

SWISS DAYS *Labor Day weekend (early September),* Midway, Wasatch Co., to celebrate Swiss heritage of local residents in "The Alps of Utah." Swiss folk plays, Swiss entertainment and music, arts and crafts booths. FOODS SERVED: Swiss and Bavarian, such as knockwurst and sauerkraut. ADMISSION: free. ACCOMMODATIONS: motels and hotels, B&B, campground, RV park. RESTAURANTS: fast foods, family, elegant. CONTACT: Wasatch Chamber of Commerce, P.O. Box 427, Heber City, UT 84032, (801) 654-3666. 30,000

PEACH DAYS *weekend following Labor Day (early September),* Brigham City, Box Elder Co., to celebrate the peach harvest. Art show, Peach Queen Scholarship Pageant, 11.1mi. Road Race, street festival including arts and crafts, window displays, car show, Golden Spike Bicycle Classic, fruit display, carnival, two parades, softball, tennis, and bowling tournaments, flea market, concerts in the park, art festival, model airplane demonstrations, Home Enterprise Fair, library used-book fair, square dancing, street dance, bluegrass, bagpipers, and drummers. FOODS SERVED: peach-baked goods, concessions. ADMISSION: free. ACCOMMODATIONS: motels and hotels, campgrounds, RV parks. RESTAURANTS: fast foods, family. CONTACT: Greater Brigham City Chamber of Commerce, P.O. Box 458, Brigham City, UT 84302, (801) 723-3931. 40,000

GLOSSARY

The "definitions" of many words and phrases below are not found in dictionaries. They are oral descriptions provided the author by the sources of material on festivals, and thereby are deemed to be the regional, popular interpretations or applications of the words.

Acadian Sometimes shortened to Cajun. Pertains to descendants of Nova Scotia expatriots who settled in Louisiana.

atlatl An archeological Ice Age tool originally made of bone and now made of wood that is used to extend one's leverage in throwing a spear.

ATV All Terrain Vehicle

bale bucking Throwing of hay bales.

blue crabs Crabs that have just molted and whose shells have not yet hardened; characteristic of the East Coast of the United States.

brats shortened form of bratwurst, a German-style sausage.

bridies Meat pies that might contain sausage or kidneys.

Brunswick stew A stew that might include pork, beef, or chicken or any combination thereof, plus tomatoes, okra, corn, hot peppers, Tabasco sauce, catsup, bread cubes, or potatoes, and a few dozen other things.

buck dancing Individual square dance to lively country music with lots of free expression.

burgoo A soupy stew that might include shanks of pork, veal, and beef, breast of lamb, potatoes, onions, carrots, green peppers, okra, cabbage, corn, red pepper, Tabasco, and other seasonings.

cafe con leche Coffee with milk.

Cajun Acadian or a term referring to the cuisine originating in Louisiana featuring local seafood and spices, and combining French, southern, and islands cooking practices.

cannoli Italian pastry tube filled with a cheese cake-like mixture and sometimes chocolate chips.

capoiera A combination of dance and martial art native to African slaves in Brazil.

ceilidh Scottish, Welsh, or Irish party.

chalo nitka Big bass in the Miccasukie Indian language.

Chautauqua Lectures or talks derived from early 20th century lecture circuit which originated in Chautauqua, New York.

cheese grits The white meal of corn kernels mixed with cheese.

chorizo A Mexican sausage.

clam fritter Minced clams dipped in batter and deep fried.

clogging A country dance during which participants wear shoes similar to tap shoes and stomp their feet to country or mountain music. Often bold plaids and crinoline skirts are worn by women and cowboy hats (and other clothes) are worn by men.

conch Small shellfish or mollusk with a large, often colorful shell.

contra dancing Line dancing of European origin, originally called "contre danse" in French. Contra dancing is believed by many people to be the forerunner of square dancing.

corridos Traditional Mexican ballads.

crab cakes A fried patty of crab chunks from the back fin of blue crabs, mayonnaise, and seasonings.

crab fluff Minced crab dipped in butter and deep fried until it fluffs.

criterium A team bicycle race consisting of repeated laps around a fixed course in a city.

dagoes Italian meat loaf sliced and served on Italian bread and covered with tomato sauce and hot peppers.

elephant ears Fried dough the shape of an elephant's ear with sugar sprinkled on top.

fais-do-do A party to which parents bring their children. The term comes from French "faire dormir" which translates "to make sleep," but means take yourself off to bed, which is what parents would say to children as the party and evening wear on.

fjord horse A docile Norwegian horse of exceptional strength.

flintknapping The native American art of making arrowheads, spear points or stone tools from flint or other hard materials such as animal bone, horns, and antlers.

fried pie Fruit or other filling is dipped into batter and then fried in hot oil.

funnel cake A fried cake made from pancake batter which is poured into a funnel while you hold your finger over the hole at the small end. When you remove your finger, you swirl the batter in circles into a skillet of hot oil, and sprinkle the top with powdered sugar.

ghost bread "Probably isn't there."

golumbki Cabbage leaf stuffed with ground beef and rice.

gumbo Soup thickened with okra which also might include local fish, or shellfish, chicken.

haggis A traditionally Scottish dish consisting of the heart, liver, and lungs of a sheep or a calf, minced with suet, onions, oatmeal, and seasonings, and boiled in the stomach of the animal.

halau Hawaiian school.

hawktawk Discussion of habits and lifestyle of a hawk with one present.

hjemkomst A Viking ship, now used as a term for "homecoming" in Minnesota.

Ho'olaule'a Street parties in Hawaii.

hoppin' john A mixture of cowpeas, black-eyed peas, or canned peas with rice, fried bacon, and bacon grease.

hush puppies 1) A side dish made with corn meal, chopped onion, and sugar, which is dropped by the spoonful into hot oil and fried. 2) shoes.

Hutterite food German-American foods resembling Amish foods and might include cabbage rolls and noodles, home-smoked hams, bacon, and sauerkraut.

kielbasa Spicy sausage.

kolache Czechoslovakian-Moravian wedding pastry filled with fruit, cheese, cabbage, or poppy seeds.

krewe An association or club of men found in the Deep South.

kringla A Norwegian cake shaped somewhat like a pretzel.

krumkake   Egg-based thin waffle often rolled in the shape of a cone or cylinder, often filled with whipped cream or ice cream.

kuchen   German coffee cake.

landlubber   A person who prefers not to venture out onto the open seas.

lefse   Norwegian flat flour dough bread.

Lowcountry cooking   Cuisine of the marshy area around Charleston, South Carolina, at sea level, which features fried chicken, red rice, deviled crab, and a general combination of Cajun and soul food.

lutefisk   A Norwegian delicacy of dried and then soaked cod fish which is baked and served with butter or cream sauce, also referred to as a "stinky old fish."

maque-chou   Corn off the cob mixed with cream or mushroom sauce and green-bell peppers.

Montana Ranch food   Features outdoor cooking of beef, beans, wild game, home-baked breads and desserts.

Mormon Jonny cakes   Flapjacks or pancakes.

moussaka   Eggplant casserole.

mudbug   Crawfish.

musky   A fighting fish more formally known as the muskellunge whose minimum keepable size is 32".

Navajo taco   Ingredients of a taco such as hamburger meat, beans, lettuce, tomatoes and cheese are placed on top of Indian fry bread.

pan con lechon   Pork sandwich.

pastichio   Greek casserole resembling lasagna including noodles, cheese and beef.

Philly-style cheese steaks   A "sub" sandwich with "Steak-ums" including thinly sliced steak covered with melted mozzarella cheese, sauteed green onions, mushrooms, and lettuce.

pierogis   Filled dumpling.

pig pickin'   A gathering at which guests file by a barbecued or pit roasted pig and pick off the meat.

P.R.C.A.   Professional Rodeo Cowboys Association

quahog   Clam-like mollusk of the Northeastern U.S.

sandbakkel   A dough heavy with butter and sugar with a little flour, molded into a small pie-shaped tin and baked. While they look as though they should be filled, they are usually served empty.

Seminole fry bread   Made from dough which might combine flour and pumpkin or flour and corn meal fried in hot oil.

shake-up   A drink made of lemon or orange juice, ice, water, and sugar in a cup upon which is placed a glass upside down and then shaken.

shoofly pie   A pie which includes a crumb mixture of flour, cinnamon, and sometimes cloves, plus a liquid mixture based on molasses, all of which attracts a lot of flies.

snoball   Crushed ice formed into a ball shape and flavored with fruit juice or syrup poured over it.

soft-shell crabs   Blue crabs in soft-shell stage.

sorghum   A grass used for grain or syrup.

spotza   Pennsylvania Dutch term stemming from maple syrup drops on the snow, and now applied to mixing hot syrup with ice, creating a soft caramel.

stone crabs   Similar to Dungeness crabs with hard shells and whitish meat in both body and claws.

swamp cabbage   "Hearts of palm" from Florida's Sabal Palm trees.

switchel   A drink made of molasses, brown sugar, vinegar, and water, which is best served cold or with ice.

Syttenda Mai   Norwegian Independence Day

tabouli salad   A Mideastern salad made of bulgar wheat, coriander, onions, garlic, mint leaves, tomatoes, lemon juice, and other variables.

tamburitzan   Slovakian dance group.

tombola   Basque village fair.

varpa   Swedish stone throwing game in which participants throw flat stones at other flat stones.

woosterbrodjes   "Pigs in a blanket" or hot dogs in flour dough.

W.R.A.   Western Rodeo Association

yaki soba   Japanese stir-fry vegetables.

INDEX

NOTE: *FESTIVAL U.S.A.*'s index excludes those categories of activities that are simply too enormous to list, such as arts and crafts and some of the foods served at festivals.

Arts and crafts are sold or demonstrated at almost all festivals in the United States, and vary from fine arts to cottage crafts. Their origins are as varied as the many countries and cultures represented in this book.

Foods are served at most festivals and vary according to the local harvest or national origins of festival organizers. The foods and nationalities listed here are just those that are the main attraction or focus of a festival.

Occasionally events, particular foods, and nationalities are mentioned more than once on a page, so be sure to read each festival listing and page thoroughly.

A

Acadian, 106
Aerobatics, 3
Agricultural exhibits, 27
Airplanes
  model, 134
  remote control, 108, 111
Air shows, 3, 26, 105, 110, 130, 144, 168, 174, 215, 217
Alligators, 107
  eating contests, 107
Antiques, 10, 16, 20, 28, 37, 41, 43, 47, 54, 61, 65, 76, 83, 85, 97, 120, 126, 127, 130, 131, 138, 139, 146, 147, 148, 156, 159, 161, 193, 207
Apples and apple products, 6, 22, 41, 45, 56, 58, 60, 69, 72, 79, 112, 148, 153, 154, 164, 201
  blossoms, 2
Apricots, 174
Archery, 7, 55, 60, 137, 157
Asparagus, 134
Austrian, 140
Automobiles. *See* Cars

B

Bagpipes and bagpipe competitions, 18
Balloon races, 5
Barnum, Phineas Taylor, 3
Baseball, 187

Basketball tournaments, 7, 17, 128, 149, 199, 220
Basque, 191, 192
Bavarian, 134
Beauty pageants, 5, 7, 20, 44, 52, 55, 56, 57, 65, 67, 69, 72, 76, 78, 86, 87, 88, 90, 91, 100, 104, 105, 111, 113, 119, 120, 121, 133, 135, 142, 149, 151, 157, 172, 174, 177, 179, 184, 189, 196, 207, 212, 213, 217, 220, 223
Bed races, 6, 7, 117, 121, 122, 123, 124, 131, 135, 136, 137, 138, 160, 178, 189, 197, 198, 199, 211
Beef, 131
Biathalon, 120
Bicycle races, 5, 6, 7, 9, 10, 11, 15, 16, 37, 46, 55, 62, 66, 75, 87, 94, 103, 106, 112, 121, 127, 131, 132, 139, 140, 141, 146, 149, 162, 193, 194, 201, 205, 214, 220, 227
  tours, 64, 139, 153, 177, 220, 223
Bingo, 7, 118, 130, 134, 135, 136, 142, 159, 163, 176, 187
Blackberries, 196
Black-eyed peas, 220
Black heritage, 71, 106, 163
Black walnuts, 78
Blessing of the Fleet, 9, 106, 167, 168, 172, 181
Blessing of the Grapes, 181
Blessing of the Hounds, 79
Blueberries, 84, 136, 151
Blue crab. *See* Seafood

233

Boats
  antique, 150
  canal, 41
  displays and shows, 5, 20, 21, 89, 108
  model, 150
  parades, 16, 88, 106, 114, 118, 130,
    135, 137, 142, 145, 167, 172, 220
  races, 5, 8, 9, 10, 26, 46, 76, 77, 89,
    112, 120, 128, 130, 141, 147, 150,
    177, 193, 194, 199, 200, 211, 217
  regattas, 15, 41, 45, 75, 98, 141, 142,
    200, 215, 220, 223
  rides, 5, 25, 36, 104, 123, 128, 135,
    141, 150
  steamboats, 118, 125
  tugboats, 135
  yachts, 10, 46
Body building, 75, 141, 168
Boomerang Meet, 16
Bowling and bowling tournaments, 44, 75,
    87, 123, 149, 219, 227
Boxing, 21
Bratwurst, 152
Brussels sprouts, 182
Buckwheat, 78

C

Cajun, 106
Calf Fry, 158
Canoe races, 7, 10, 16, 46, 63, 76, 78,
    111, 128, 136, 138, 157, 184, 200,
    215
  tours, 19, 103
Carnivals, 3, 5, 6, 7, 11, 20, 28, 29, 45,
    46, 51, 52, 65, 75, 78, 90, 91, 95,
    100, 106, 110, 113, 117, 118, 119,
    120, 121, 122, 124, 128, 129, 133,
    134, 135, 136, 137, 140, 141, 142,
    145, 152, 156, 160, 163, 164, 167,
    169, 172, 173, 174, 178, 187, 191,
    193, 194, 198, 199, 200, 201, 206,
    211, 217, 218, 219, 220, 223, 224,
    227
Carrots, 169
Cars
  antique, 10, 15, 22, 25, 26, 27, 28, 51,
    52, 53, 54, 60, 75, 78, 79, 84, 86, 87,
    89, 94, 95, 100, 101, 108, 109, 119,
    120, 125, 126, 128, 130, 132, 135,
    137, 141, 145, 151, 153, 154, 155,
    157, 159, 160, 162, 174, 180, 194,
    198, 210, 216, 217, 221, 222
  British, 47, 123
  classic, 3, 9, 22, 52, 123, 137, 146, 154,
    198, 216, 222
  custom, 125, 132, 160
  model, 26
  racing, 46, 111, 132, 155, 194
  shows, 3, 20, 22, 23, 24, 28, 29, 47,
    52, 53, 59, 63, 67, 78, 120, 121, 141,
    151, 154, 164, 173, 193, 207, 227
  stock, 28
  street rods, 22, 28, 52, 133, 134, 142,
    217
Catfish, 95, 108, 114
  eating contests, 108
  also see Seafood
Celtic, 18, 37, 175, *also see* Scottish
Checkers, 62, 154
Cheese, 156, 159, 182, 193
Cherries, 136
Cherry blossoms, 35, 171, 184, 189
Chess tournaments, 88, 133, 141, 146,
    154
Chicken, 35, 44, 111, 147
Children's activities and events, 3, 7, 9,
    10, 11, 13, 19, 21, 23, 26, 30, 35, 41,
    44, 47, 51, 54, 56, 58, 59, 62, 64, 69,
    71, 76, 86, 88, 89, 91, 100, 106, 109,
    111, 118, 119, 120, 123, 124, 129,
    130, 138, 140, 141, 150, 156, 159,
    160, 161, 163, 178, 186, 188, 190,
    198, 206, 211, 215, 216, 223
Circus, 3, 16, 87, 99, 201
Clans, Scottish, 37, 58
Coal, 74, 77
Coffee, 139, 186
Collards, 101
Cooking
  contests, 41, 51, 63, 71, 77, 78, 79, 94,
    104, 108, 136, 145, 150, 151, 152,
    182, 192, 199, 201, 207, 214, 217,
    222, 223
  demonstrations, 3, 184
Cook-offs
  barbecue, 51, 70
  beef, 183
  black-eyed peas, 220
  catfish, 63
  chili, 54, 62, 69, 100, 155, 158, 160,
    167, 172, 178, 183, 189, 201, 208,
    213, 214, 215, 216, 217, 221, 224

chowder, 197
duck gumbo, 90
Dutch oven, 226
fish, 170
garlic, 177
gumbo, 217, 223
huckleberries, 188
pinto bean, 217
pork, 72, 103
slugs, 170
sweet onion, 103
wild game, 170
Corn, 86, 152, 153. *Also see* Sweet corn
Costumes, 23, 83, 125, 139, 145, 147,
    148, 167, 182, 206, 216, 219
colonial, 26
Czech, 147, 155, 218, 222
Dutch, 162
German, 89, 141, 142, 163
Greek, 5
international, 23
Italian, 4
Mexican, 163
Norwegian, 168
Polish, 164
Scandinavian, 140, 175, 196, 198
Swedish, 147
Swiss, 154
Costume contests, 69, 217
Cotton, 109, 110, 205
Country Music. *See* Music,
    country/western
Covered bridges, 6, 124, 126
Cow chip throwing, 87, 88, 147, 156, 221
Crabs and clams, 40, 57
Cranberries, 11
Czech, 128, 147, 155, 158, 222, 224

D

Dancing, 12, 14
Appalachian, 58
ballet, 44, 46, 95, 96, 97, 98, 105, 109,
    112, 114, 120, 121, 195, 226
Basque, 191, 192
belly, 5, 99, 126, 174, 223
Buck, 67, 68, 69
Caddo Indian, 89
Cajun, 221
Cherokee, 60
Choctaw, 110

clogging, 19, 23, 37, 46, 52, 55, 57, 58,
    59, 60, 61, 62, 63, 67, 69, 72, 73, 76,
    89, 91, 95, 96, 104, 112, 125, 126,
    130, 131, 143, 145, 148, 164, 172,
    176, 180, 195, 197, 206, 221
Contra, 20
Crow Indian, 190
Czech, 158, 222
Dutch, 126, 162
Estonian, 180
folk, 5, 51, 71, 123, 155, 156, 190
German, 16, 85, 114, 146, 156, 200,
    212, 222
Greek, 5, 11, 83, 198, 200
Highland, 58, 150, 175
Hula, 184, 185, 186
Iriquois, 18
Irish, 13, 19, 27, 126, 146, 147, 163,
    175
Italian, 76, 77, 125, 162, 163, 200, 221
Japanese, 16, 63, 92, 195
jazz, 5
Latin, 36
Macedonian, 11
Mexican, 170, 177, 179, 206, 218, 220,
    222
Native American, Indian, 18, 40, 42, 57,
    73, 96, 117, 119, 139, 146, 149, 159,
    160, 172, 179, 200, 205, 212, 221,
    222, 226
Native American, Indian, ceremonial,
    42, 196, 213
Norwegian, 128, 168, 190, 208
Polish, 4
Polka, 4, 5, 17, 128, 164
Portuguese, 10, 24
Scandinavian, 175, 190, 196, 197, 198
Spanish, 177
square dancing, 7, 20, 23, 38, 52, 54,
    58, 59, 60, 61, 62, 63, 67, 71, 72, 75,
    76, 78, 79, 87, 88, 89, 103, 104, 118,
    121, 124, 126, 131, 134, 145, 146,
    149, 157, 160, 164, 172, 197, 199,
    207, 208, 212, 214, 216, 227
theatre, 14, 16, 64
Dandelions, 75
Danish, 27, 137, 180
Dart tournaments, 154
Dates, 169
Dog shows, 5, 120, 209, 217
Dogwood trees, 3, 37, 55, 62, 63, 187,
    216

Doll shows, 21, 47, 190
Dumplings, 67
Dutch, 162

E

Eggs, 71
  quail, 216
Enchiladas, 215
Engines,
  antique, 124
  gas, 19, 22, 39, 94
  steam, 19, 39, 94

F

Fall foliage, 8, 11, 20, 21, 28, 43, 47, 60,
  61, 72, 113, 124, 133, 138, 164, 207
Farm equipment, vintage, 20
Farmers' markets, 16, 20, 46, 72, 91,
  120, 123, 124, 148, 164
Fashion shows, 3, 24, 35, 43, 46, 52, 66,
  94, 102, 121, 123, 124, 133, 138,
  148, 149, 152, 175, 179, 190, 205
Films, 5, 9, 10, 21, 25, 29, 64, 106, 107,
  110, 114, 148, 162, 169, 170, 180,
  186, 212, 225
Firemen's musters, 7
Fireworks, 4, 5, 7, 8, 9, 11, 13, 14, 15,
  17, 21, 36, 37, 38, 41, 45, 46, 51, 56,
  66, 70, 75, 84, 87, 91, 94, 95, 98, 99,
  105, 109, 118, 119, 120, 123, 125,
  127, 129, 130, 134, 136, 140, 141,
  142, 151, 152, 162, 164, 174, 179,
  187, 194, 198, 199, 201, 205, 208,
  211, 213, 216, 217, 225
Fishing contests and derbies, 7, 16, 41,
  55, 57, 62, 88, 92, 100, 109, 111,
  134, 137, 141, 161, 163, 178, 217
Flea markets, 7, 10, 17, 19, 21, 26, 28,
  35, 39, 45, 47, 51, 52, 53, 54, 55, 58,
  67, 94, 109, 110, 117, 118, 120, 121,
  122, 123, 124, 129, 134, 135, 138,
  139, 141, 145, 146, 147, 148, 150,
  153, 159, 164, 167, 176, 197, 198,
  201, 217, 219, 227
Flowers and flower shows, 3, 46, 62, 76,
  104, 111, 120, 132, 134, 136, 141,
  168, 169, 176, 190
  Azaleas, 64, 110, 155

Chrysanthemums, 5, 61, 153
Confederate Daisies, 104
Daffodils, 9
Easter Lilies, 176
Marigolds, 104, 120
Narcissus, 184
Orchids, 90, 170, 182
Petunias, 118
Rhododendrons, 57, 67, 193, 197
Roses, 96, 111, 179
Tulips, 13, 126
Wildflowers, 4
Yellow Daisies, 104
Folklife, 17, 19, 22, 27, 36, 39, 40, 43, 47,
  61, 69, 70, 71, 97, 100, 103, 122,
  127, 145, 198, 210, 220
Folk music. *See* Music, folk
Football
  Little League, 79
  Pro, 152
French, 6, 162
Frisbees, 36, 87, 141, 148, 158
Frogs and frog jumping, 7, 37, 61, 84,
  107, 144, 173
Frog eating contests, 107

G

Garden tours, 3, 90, 111
Garlic, 176, 177
Gem and mineral shows, 47, 169, 170
German, 16, 41, 52, 71, 73, 85, 89, 114,
  121, 125, 138, 143, 146, 148, 149,
  162
Goebelfest, 16
Golden oldies, 18
Golf
  miniature, 42, 216
  tournaments, 7, 9, 10, 28, 43, 44, 46,
    53, 55, 56, 57, 58, 59, 62, 63, 65, 87,
    91, 92, 102, 103, 107, 111, 112, 128,
    131, 132, 134, 136, 142, 149, 158,
    168, 172, 173, 174, 187, 193, 207,
    213, 219
Go-karts, 4
Gourds, 154
Greased pole climb, 18, 84, 88, 121, 176
Greek, 5, 11, 83, 198
Gyro, 5

H

Hang gliders, 26, 167
Herring, 167
Hiking meet, 21
Historic tours, 9, 28, 38, 77, 83, 90, 110,
    114, 122, 125, 126, 133, 135, 136,
    187, 206, 216, 222
Hobos, 129
Hockey, 149
Honey, 78, 121, 153
Horse races, 37
Horse shows, 7, 47, 52, 53, 54, 58, 59,
    62, 117, 139, 142, 151, 189, 216,
    220, 223
Horseshoes and horseshoe tournaments,
    7, 20, 55, 58, 61, 67, 69, 77, 78, 87,
    101, 130, 133, 135, 147, 148, 157,
    158, 171, 172, 174, 190, 205, 209,
    212, 220, 221
Hot air balloons, 6, 20, 24, 26, 37, 68, 77,
    78, 84, 91, 95, 100, 105, 110, 111,
    114, 118, 119, 121, 123, 125, 129,
    131, 141, 149, 153, 160, 161, 167,
    173, 174, 197, 208, 215
Huckleberries, 188

I

Ice sculpture, 11, 149, 160, 208
Ice skating, 149
Indian. *See* Native American
Irish, 13, 19, 27, 102, 126, 131, 146, 163
Italian, 4, 14, 17, 23, 38, 39, 68, 76, 77,
    125, 156, 162, 181

J

Jai Alai, 3
Japanese, 144, 195
Jazz. *See* Music, jazz

K

Karate, 7, 8, 47, 86, 87, 163, 175, 223
Kayak races, 63
Kielbasa, 10
Kilt races, 65

Kite flying, 10, 35, 42, 43, 62, 76, 93,
    124, 137, 172, 197, 220
Kolache, 147, 155, 222

L

Latin American, 36
Laurel, 24
Lewis, Sinclair, 141
Lights, Christmas, 21, 73, 74, 108, 114
Lobster. *See* Seafood
Log races, 3
Logging shows, 199, 206
Lotus blossoms, 39
Low country cooking, 112, 113
Lumberjack contests, 7, 24, 54, 74, 119,
    137, 157, 161, 176, 177, 189, 199,
    200, 206
Lutefisk, 139, 197. *Also see* Seafood

M

Macadamia nuts, 185
Magdalena, Santa Maria, 4
Magic, 3, 10, 21, 44, 72, 75, 91, 111, 117,
    118, 125, 131, 132, 141, 158, 163,
    172, 174, 176, 177, 180, 217, 223
Maple and maple products, 22, 29
Marine exhibits, 7
Marketplace, Greek, 5
Marksmanship, 69
McDonald, Ronald, 7, 173
Mennonite, 26
Mexican, 163, 173, 214, 218
Military exhibits, 29, 47, 53, 105, 128,
    150, 153
Military reenactments, 10, 28, 47, 52, 61,
    77, 94, 117, 120, 121, 142, 150
Milk, 117
Mimes, 4, 8, 12, 13, 14, 20, 60, 61, 73,
    91, 96, 97, 105, 114, 124, 126, 127,
    129, 132, 138, 139, 141, 151, 158,
    172, 173, 189, 218
Moonshine, 149, 150
Motorcycle
    races, 51
    shows, 28
Mountain climbing, 75
Moussaka, 5

Mudbug, 105
Mules, 62
Mullet, 99
Mushrooms, 143
Music
  Afro-American, 163, 195
  Appalachian, 58
  Bach choir, 64
  Bach, Johann Sebastian, music of, 14,
    22, 23, 30, 93, 176, 194, 210
  bagpipes, 57, 58, 175, 176, 195, 200,
    221, 222, 226, 227
  banjo and banjo contests, 7, 23, 26, 27,
    39, 43, 67, 68, 75, 76, 78, 97, 119,
    123, 133, 146
  barbershop quartets, 7, 21, 24, 55, 85
  Bavarian, 57, 71, 76, 212, 221
  beach, 43, 44, 45, 47, 56, 59, 111
  Beethoven, Ludwig von, music of, 210
  Beiderbeck, Bix, music of, 129
  Big Band, 24, 25, 42, 60, 91, 98, 118,
    123, 131, 154, 161, 163, 174, 195
  bluegrass, 7, 8, 17, 19, 22, 26, 29, 38,
    39, 41, 45, 47, 51, 52, 53, 54, 56, 58,
    59, 61, 62, 63, 66, 67, 68, 72, 73, 75,
    76, 78, 84, 85, 86, 89, 91, 94, 95,
    102, 104, 106, 110, 117, 120, 122,
    123, 124, 127, 132, 133, 134, 136,
    137, 142, 157, 158, 160, 161, 172,
    174, 176, 182, 183, 189, 195, 198,
    199, 206, 207, 209, 210, 217, 219,
    223, 227
  blues, 75, 85, 105, 106, 128, 136, 161,
    182, 198, 206, 221, 222
  brass, 64
  Cajun, 105, 106, 107, 108, 198, 216,
    221
  Celtic, 18
  Cherokee gospel, 60
  classical, 7, 8, 9, 25, 29, 44, 46, 51, 57,
    58, 59, 62, 64, 68, 69, 98, 112, 140,
    176, 179, 189, 194, 201, 206, 209,
    210, 211, 213, 214, 223, 224, 226
  country/western, 6, 7, 11, 16, 19, 21,
    22, 23, 24, 25, 26, 27, 28, 29, 40, 42,
    44, 47, 53, 54, 59, 60, 61, 64, 65, 66,
    67, 68, 70, 71, 72, 73, 76, 78, 85, 86,
    87, 88, 89, 91, 93, 94, 95, 97, 98, 99,
    101, 103, 104, 105, 108, 109, 112,
    113, 114, 118, 119, 120, 121, 123,
    124, 125, 127, 128, 130, 131, 132,
    133, 135, 136, 140, 142, 145, 146,

    150, 154, 156, 157, 160, 162, 169,
    171, 174, 176, 178, 180, 181, 183,
    188, 191, 193, 194, 198, 201, 206,
    207, 209, 214, 216, 217, 218, 219,
    223, 224
  Croatian, 132
  Cuban, 91
  Czech, 147
  Danish, 137
  Delius, Frederick, music of, 93
  Dixieland jazz, 16, 19, 42, 45, 64, 86,
    91, 123, 124, 128, 136, 164, 171,
    172, 173, 174, 179, 189, 191
  Dulcimer, 27, 87, 97, 130, 133
  Dutch, 13, 126
  ethnic, 8, 9, 15
  fiddles and fiddle contests, 17, 23, 24,
    25, 27, 38, 39, 43, 45, 56, 61, 67, 68,
    75, 76, 78, 88, 97, 108, 123, 127,
    130, 132, 133, 143, 145, 146, 154,
    157, 158, 162, 168, 172, 174, 175,
    182, 187, 189, 190, 194, 198, 200,
    201, 206, 207, 209, 217, 219, 220,
    221, 222, 223, 224
  folk, 4, 8, 11, 12, 13, 19, 23, 25, 26,
    44, 47, 57, 58, 60, 61, 67, 76, 136,
    140, 155, 156, 161, 164, 176, 179,
    183, 188, 190, 206, 210, 219
  Franco-American, 8
  German, 7, 26, 40, 41, 73, 85, 89, 111,
    114, 120, 122, 123, 125, 134, 135,
    146, 190, 193, 212, 224
  gospel, 17, 21, 24, 39, 47, 51, 53, 54,
    58, 59, 60, 64, 67, 68, 73, 76, 78, 87,
    88, 95, 97, 103, 106, 108, 130, 137,
    188, 206, 213, 217, 220, 223
  Greek, 5, 11, 83
  Handy, W. C., music of, 85
  Hawaiian, 184, 185, 186
  Irish, 7, 13, 27, 102, 163
  Italian, 4, 15, 23, 39, 76, 77, 91, 125,
    162, 181
  Japanese, 184
  jazz, 7, 8, 10, 11, 14, 17, 21, 25, 28,
    29, 30, 42, 44, 59, 60, 61, 63, 68, 72,
    73, 76, 85, 86, 95, 98, 99, 102, 103,
    109, 110, 113, 117, 118, 119, 123,
    127, 128, 129, 135, 136, 137, 140,
    143, 144, 151, 152, 156, 183, 188,
    193, 194, 195, 196, 197, 199, 200,
    206, 209, 210, 211, 214, 216, 219,
    223

Latin, 8, 36, 91, 94, 100, 101, 138, 179,
    195, 218, 220
Lithuanian, 132
lumberjack, 142
Mariachi, 132, 138, 163, 170, 179, 199,
    205, 214, 218, 221
military, 20, 29, 41, 42, 69, 77, 86, 88,
    101, 102, 104, 107, 129, 136, 151,
    161, 168, 172, 180, 194, 208
Miller, Glenn, music of, 127
minstrel, 21
mountain, 47, 56, 60, 61, 68
Mozart, Wolfgang Amadeus, music of,
    30, 36
Native American, Indian, 179, 198, 205,
    213
Norwegian, 129, 140
opera, 4, 15, 46, 57, 62, 129, 175, 181,
    209
Ozark, 89
piano competition, 40
Polish, 4, 11, 19, 22, 38, 132
polka, 17, 24, 118, 119, 121, 128, 130,
    136, 138, 140, 147, 148, 154, 158,
    160, 164, 190, 218, 222
Portuguese, 10, 28
ragtime, 42, 143, 144, 180, 194, 206
reggae, 8, 17, 36, 59, 183
rhythm and blues, 17, 59, 68, 119, 172,
    179
rock, 7, 8, 26, 59, 62, 63, 65, 68, 73,
    88, 97, 99, 101, 105, 110, 114, 118,
    119, 121, 130, 131, 135, 140, 154,
    156, 161, 173, 174, 180, 199, 209,
    216, 219, 222
Rodgers, Jimmie, music of, 109
Russian folk, 63
Scandinavian, 175
Scottish fiddling, 37
Scottish Highland, 65, 134, 150
Sligo, 27
steel band, 21, 113, 117, 119, 200, 214,
    221
swing, 64
Tamburitzans, 24
top 40, 44, 86
vesper, 26
whistling, 5, 130, 179, 192
Musky, 161. *Also see* Seafood

N

Native Americans, 40, 60, 149, 159, 171,
    190, 213
Nature walks, 19
Norwegian, 129, 168, 190, 197, 208

O

Onions, 103, 199
Oranges, 91
Oysters, 5, 20, 60, 110
    shucking contests, 5, 20. *Also see* Sea-
    food

P

Paddlesurfing, 46
Parachuting, 3, 75
Parades, 3, 5, 6, 7, 8, 11, 13, 14, 15, 17,
    20, 21, 22, 23, 24, 28, 35, 37, 38, 42,
    43, 44, 45, 46, 47, 51, 52, 53, 54, 56,
    58, 59, 60, 62, 63, 65, 66, 69, 70, 74,
    75, 78, 79, 83, 87, 91, 93, 94, 95, 96,
    98, 100, 104, 105, 106, 108, 109,
    111, 117, 118, 119, 120, 121, 122,
    123, 124, 125, 127, 128, 129, 130,
    137, 133, 134, 135, 136, 138, 139,
    140, 141, 143, 144, 146, 147, 148,
    149, 150, 151, 152, 153, 154, 156,
    157, 158, 159, 160, 163, 164, 168,
    169, 170, 171, 173, 174, 176, 177,
    178, 179, 180, 182, 183, 185, 188,
    188, 189, 190, 191, 192, 193, 194,
    196, 197, 198, 199, 200, 201, 205,
    206, 207, 208, 209, 210, 211, 212,
    213, 214, 215, 216, 217, 218, 219,
    220, 221, 223, 224, 227
    boat. *See* Boats, parades
    hobo, 108
    torchlight, 129, 138, 141, 160, 161,
        187, 197, 220
Peaches, 226
Peanuts, 47, 87, 224
Pear blossoms, 193
Peppers, 163
Pet shows, 12, 59, 77, 78, 89, 194
Petting zoos, 19, 20, 21, 22, 28, 29, 47,
    61, 77, 118, 131, 217

Photography, 9, 12, 20, 30, 56, 60, 61, 94, 95, 111, 118, 148, 154, 157, 158, 167, 193, 209, 214, 215, 226
Pickles, 59
Pie eating contests, 19, 20, 22, 66, 119, 121, 136, 138, 182, 220
Poetry and poetry reading, 25, 77, 113, 126, 160, 175, 190, 213
Polish, 22, 38, 164
Popcorn, 124
Pork, 72, 102, 121
Portuguese, 24
Potatoes, 51, 152
Potato blossoms, 7
Poultry, 44
Pulaski, General Casimir, 22
Pumpkins, 121, 138, 154, 182
Puppets, 10, 11, 12, 16, 20, 21, 25, 26, 43, 46, 47, 59, 60, 62, 64, 76, 87, 88, 90, 91, 97, 104, 111, 113, 114, 123, 124, 126, 131, 132, 141, 152, 173, 176, 180

R

Racquetball and racquetball tournaments, 84, 87, 123
Rafting and raft races, 5, 6, 7, 45, 46, 88, 95, 110, 118, 123, 140, 141, 189, 220
Railroad memorabilia, 77
Railroads. *See* Trains
Railroads, model. *See* Trains, model
Rattlesnakes, 155, 215
Recipe contests, 10, 87, 113, 134, 170, 177
Religious processions, 4, 5
Rice, 223
Riverboat rides, 16, 17
Road races, 6. *Also see* Running marathons, races
Rodeos, 63, 87, 92, 95, 102, 127, 131, 132, 139, 142, 146, 147, 149, 153, 157, 159, 173, 177, 178, 183, 190, 191, 199, 200, 201, 205, 206, 207, 210, 211, 213, 214, 215, 219, 220, 221, 225, 226
Rugby and rugby tournaments, 37, 128, 131, 150
Running marathons, 6, 29, 35, 41, 57, 144, 168, 171, 189, 193, 216, 219
races, 5, 6, 7, 8, 10, 16, 17, 21, 22, 28, 29, 37, 43, 45, 46, 47, 51, 52, 53, 56, 58, 59, 60, 62, 63, 64, 66, 69, 70, 71, 72, 73, 75, 77, 78, 79, 83, 88, 89, 90, 91, 92, 95, 96, 99, 102, 103, 104, 107, 108, 109, 111, 112, 118, 119, 120, 121, 122, 123, 127, 129, 131, 132, 133, 134, 135, 136, 137, 138, 140, 141, 145, 146, 147, 148, 151, 153, 154, 157, 159, 162, 164, 170, 172, 177, 178, 179, 184, 185, 187, 188, 189, 190, 193, 194, 196, 197, 198, 199, 200, 205, 207, 209, 212, 213, 214, 215, 216, 217, 218, 220, 221, 223
Rutabagas, 163

S

Sailboarding, 93, 193
Sailing races, 46
Salmon, 177, 196. *Also see* Seafood
Sandcastles, 46, 136
Sand sculpture, 86, 96
Sauerkraut, 17, 155
Sausage, 158, 159
Scandinavian, 129, 140, 175, 196, 198
Scottish, 58, 90, 150. *Also see* Celtic
Seafood, 3, 4, 5, 7, 8, 9, 10, 11, 20, 21, 22, 40, 41, 45, 46, 47, 51, 55, 57, 60, 63, 86, 91, 95, 97, 98, 99, 100, 101, 106, 108, 110, 112, 114, 134, 150, 161, 162, 167, 168, 169, 170, 172, 177, 193, 196, 201, 223
Shakespeare, William, 85, 177, 192, 193, 225
Shrimp. *See* Seafood
Singing
a cappella, 27
barbershop, 7, 21, 24, 55, 124, 125, 131, 179, 189, 206, 209
black choir, 71
choral, 25
Christmas, 74
Czech, 218, 222
Danish, 137
folk, 103, 105, 124, 134, 138, 139, 146, 164, 216
German, 144, 218, 224
gospel, 88, 94, 101, 104, 105, 112, 123, 125, 145, 146, 157, 179, 198, 216
Irish, 175

Italian, 77
Japanese, 144
madrigal, 25, 132
Native American, Indian, 149
Polish, 218
Scandinavian, 175, 196
Scottish, 175
sea chanties, 3
shape-note, 56
Also see Music
Skiing and ski races, 6, 13, 37, 133, 139,
      148, 149, 160, 168, 170, 187, 208,
      209
Sky diving, 5, 19, 20, 84, 113, 128, 150,
      160, 162, 193, 197, 215, 217
Sled dog races, 6, 160, 167, 168, 208
Slugs, 170, 193
Snowmobile races, 138, 187, 208
Snow sculpture, 138, 148, 187, 208
Softball and softball tournaments, 6, 7, 8,
      38, 55, 58, 63, 67, 84, 89, 96, 102,
      111, 119, 123, 131, 132, 133, 138,
      139, 142, 146, 147, 149, 160, 163,
      189, 194, 201, 207, 209, 211, 213,
      219, 220, 221, 227
Soccer, 24, 63, 190, 199
Songwriting, 8
Sorghum, 53, 54, 158
Soup-off, 149
Soybeans, 86, 145
Speckled perch, 95
speedskating, 138
Square dancing. *See* Dancing
Stickball, 109
Storytelling, 8, 11, 18, 20, 26, 54, 55, 56,
      60, 63, 71, 72, 74, 76, 86, 97, 103,
      107, 113, 117, 129, 130, 138, 140,
      143, 146, 151, 160, 164, 176, 180,
      200, 206, 213, 221
Strawberries, 14, 15, 65, 75, 93, 135,
      150, 156, 173, 194, 199, 209, 217
Street fairs, 7, 24, 56
Surfing, 96, 98, 184
Sushi eating contests, 92
Swedish, 118, 147
Sweet corn, 98, 119, 120, 121, 163
Sweet potatoes, 51, 105, 113, 223
Swim meets, 7, 93, 141, 179, 213, 220
Swiss, 154, 226

T

Tall ships, 36, 37, 46
Tea party reenactment, 37
Teddy bear contests, 15
Tennis and tennis tournaments, 6, 9, 28,
      41, 44, 46, 55, 58, 62, 65, 75, 84, 87,
      88, 100, 103, 107, 111, 115, 118,
      119, 121, 123, 128, 131, 133, 141,
      157, 173, 194, 205, 207, 220, 227
Theatre, 5, 11, 13, 14, 19, 20, 23, 30, 37,
      43, 65, 90, 97, 104, 111, 113, 121,
      139, 142, 151, 153, 156, 157, 167,
      172, 188, 201, 214, 216, 217
Tobacco, 54, 73
      spitting contests, 39, 54, 59, 87, 88,
      151, 157, 171, 221
Tomatoes, 8
Toys, antique, 26
Trains, 77, 108, 119, 123
      model and toy, 21, 28, 47, 111, 119,
      123, 170, 171
Tree sitting contests, 21
Triathalon, 24, 46, 64, 141, 149, 151, 160,
      198, 201, 207
Trout, 134, 201. *Also see* Seafood
Truck and tractor pulls, 117, 120, 128,
      142, 169, 220
Turkeys, 124
      turkey calling contests, 74, 78

V

Vaudeville, 20
Videos, 24, 105, 106, 107
Volleyball and volleyball tournaments, 6,
      46, 103, 133, 136, 149, 158, 160,
      197, 199, 205, 220

W

Wagon rides, horse-drawn, 20
Walleye, 161. *Also see* Seafood
Walnuts, 78
Watermelon, 88, 121, 219
Water skiing, 26, 36, 56, 118, 119, 130,
      135, 136, 139, 140, 141, 142, 151,
      160, 199, 220
Whales, 170
Wheat, 132

Wine and wine tasting, 3, 5, 15, 20, 38, 42, 45, 68, 75, 76, 77, 88, 99, 137, 164, 173, 175, 177, 178, 180, 181, 182, 193, 196, 197, 208, 223
   wine making contests, 68, 77
Windsurfing, 42, 46, 95, 96, 136, 188
Woodsmen's events, 18, 27. *Also see* Lumberjack contests

Woolly worms, 61
Wrestling, 8
Wrist and arm wrestling, 62, 78, 167, 207

Y

Yacht races, 10, 46. *Also see* Boats, racing